198870

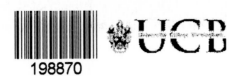

KU-360-770

AN INTRODUCTION TO

HACCP

BY QAMRUL A. KHANSON

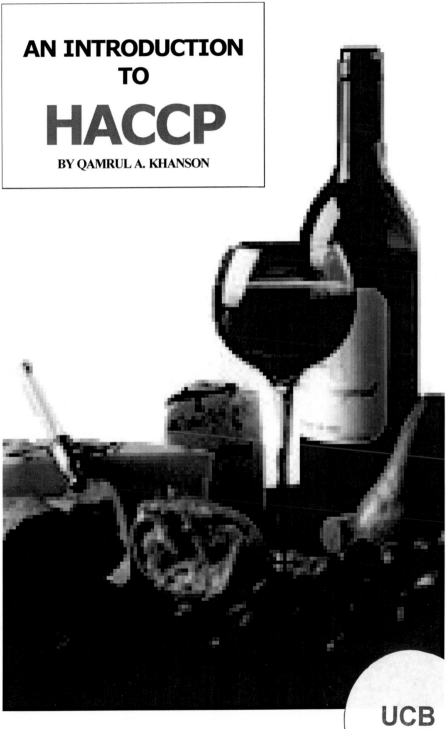

UCB
198870

Copyright © 2010 by Qamrul A. Khan (Khanson)

All rights reserved. No part of this book may be reproduced, stored, or transmitted by any means whether auditory, graphic, mechanical, or electronic without written permission of the author, except in the case of brief excerpts used in critical articles and reviews.

Unauthorized reproduction of any part of this work is illegal and is punishable by law.

Book: An Introduction to HACCP
ISBN 978 – 0 – 9739024 – 4 - 0

PREFACE

The book **"An Introduction to HACCP"** has been written to provide general guidance and information regarding the food safety issues being faced by the food industry in the western world and catching speedy momentum in the developing world. The book brings you the two-decade experience of the author with the food safety issues, its evolution, and transformation on to a concept, which is now a necessity to safe food consumption and safeguarding human health.

The traditional food practices, nature, and extent of information utilised, safety, education initiatives, and scope of food regulation guide the decision-making with relation to the quality and food safety. The food supply of Canada and the United States is among the worlds safest and most wholesome, however, significant food safety problems can cause human illness, long-term squeal, death and severe economic losses that threaten the competitiveness of Canadian and U.S. Agriculture. This book introduces Hazard Analysis Critical Control Point (HACCP) from the basic overview to overall acceptance by the food industry. Then taken down to each of the most prevalent food products with their criticality where the danger lies for food spoilage and human illness.

The discussion starts with the concept of food safety covering bakery, beverage, dairy, and meat, seafood with respect to existing concerns with relation to food manufacturing and catering businesses. To enable the food operators and consumers understand the safety matters in food business, valuing the different segments of food industry, the need for a food safety system, the benefit measurement its legal implications have been discussed in Chapter: 02. The critics label HACCP system as a costly expense with no significant benefit in real economic terms. An attempt to counter that labelling has been made in Chapter: 03 where different elements of HACCP costs have been discussed to justify the utmost importance of the food safety system. Further, down the line, text on the evolution of HACCP provides an opportunity to upheld reasons and importance of HACCP safety system in the food industry. The identification of risks, its characterization, communication, and responsibilities shared by the manufacturers, regulatory agencies and consumers are discussed.

Since the book has been written in Canada, a special attention was granted to elaborate The Canadian Food Safety System with affiliated discussion on United States Food Safety System although copyright constraints did not allow detailed elaborations. Though both systems have a long history of collaboration, a detailed study by visiting their respective food safety official sites would enhance the knowledge.

Chapter: 05 have been exclusively allocated to the basis of HACCP system on which the whole system has been based. The seven principles of HACCP applications have been convoluted so that its application in practical situations becomes easier. The current state of food safety situation in North America and need of the future is the most needed piece of investigative literature to keep the continual momentum of food safety drive in the industry. Whole book has been devoted for that purpose.

HACCP as a scientifically sound standard with international uniformity and acceptance has given hope to consumers. Recent advances by Codex Alimentarius and its acceptance by Canada, USA, UK, Japan, and few other trading partners of Canada have been discussed in Chapter: 09.

Chapter: 10 is a section of the book categorically devoted for food operators to develop their HACCP system for different segments of the food industry any where in the world. Effective management of GMPs, SSOPs, QAP, state of art technology available with adequately trained staff can make a positive difference in the confidence of any country's manufactured foods. HACCP audits and documentations have been discussed in Chapter: 11 & 12 but its coverage will provide information for any food operator who would find it compatible for international applications and different regional needs.

By reading each chapter of this book, a food operator, technologist, coordinator and manager would be in a position to independently manage a HACCP system based on legal, scientific and consumers demand. This book is intended to provide a detailed discussion of diverse subjects with relation to food safety related to bakery, beverage, dairy, fish, and meat industries. It is well suited for under-graduate, post-graduate university students who are in dairy or food technology fields needing education in food safety and the HACCP system. This book will equally serve the food processing courses, industry sponsored courses and in plant HACCP training courses for the staff.

The author expresses profound gratitude to Canadian Food Inspection Agency, Agri-Canada, Environment Canada, United States Food Safety Inspection System (US-FSIS), and United States Department of Agriculture (USDA) for providing assistance in up to date technical information and continual support. The references provided at the end of this book would guide you to reach the knowledge areas, which not necessarily contributed to this book due to copyright constraints.

I express deep appreciation of some authors; Dr. Douglas Powell, Katherine Ralston, Victoria Salin, Sheila A. Martin and Donald W. Anderson and many other renowned scientists whose work has been referenced with gratitude and who gave permission to reproduce and take excerpts to add value to this book. I appreciate the guidance of my family physician Dr Nadeem Ashraf Khan and Cardiologist Dr El Zhawi in keeping my health under control during the writing of this book.

Qamrul A. Khanson   **June 01 - 2010**
The Author

List of Contents

Qamrul A. Khanson

Chapter: 01
FOOD SAFETY CONCEPT

Overview:

Food safety is dependent on microbiological control, toxicological prevention, Physical and Chemical hazards elimination, Good Hygiene Standard (GHS), Adequate Sanitation, Trained Food Personnel (TFP), Standard Operating Procedures (SOPs) Good Manufacturing Practices (GMPs), Good Laboratory Practices (GLPs) Innovative Food Technologies (IFTs), Compliance to Regulations (CTR), Conformance for Performance (CFP), Consumers satisfaction by documenting and enforcing all Do's according to the seven principles of HACCP. The food safety concept is designed to assist food manufacturers in incorporating food safety assurance technologies into the product development, manufacturing, and packaging process. The use of detective, quantitative, microbial, chemical and physical risk assessment as tools for assessing, characterizing risk and emphasis on the development of prerequisite programs form the foundation for the Hazard Analysis Critical Control Points (HACCP) concept. HACCP is unique to its sole purpose of food safety.

Consumer's choice of food and beverage preferences is the first step towards one's own health protection. The manufacturers of food have an obligation to produce food, which is free from biological, chemical, physical, and environmental hazards. Law to highlight and label allergens present in food so that consumers could make their preference to consumption mandates the manufacturers of food. They are required to use food processing, production, packaging, and storage parameters, which are legal, scientifically proven, and free from risks to human health. The regulatory agencies like CFIA (Canada) and FSIS (USA) are in their home jurisdictions to enforce respective government's food safety regulations. Therefore, food safety is a tripartite axis between manufacturers, regulatory agencies, and consumers in serving the greater interest of North American healthy society.

HACCP (Hazard Analysis Critical Control Point) is a system to help food industry guarantee the safety of cultivated and manufactured food products by controlling breeding, harvesting, food ingredients, food raw materials, food processing, packaging materials, and food storage. People should understand the importance and benefits of HACCP safety system in the food business and they should strive to achieve these safeties by implementing HACCP.

HACCP has gained international recognition as being one of the most efficient ways to ensure the safety of food products. The first key to the success of a HACCP system is through demonstrated leadership and commitment of management.

Each year in Canada, over $82 billion in domestic retail and food service sales are generated by the Agri-food industry. The Agri-food sector is one of the most important in Canada's economy. It is the second-largest manufacturing sector, the source of one in seven Canadian jobs, and is valued at approximately $130 billion. Therefore, its security and safety are the first priority of Canadian people and the government of Canada. In USA, Food Processing industry is worth $500 billion-67.

Traditionally, industry and regulators have depended on spot-checks of manufacturing conditions and random sampling of final products to ensure safe food. This approach however, tends to be reactive, rather than preventive, and can be less efficient than the hazard analysis critical control system. HACCP helps food processors lower their overall cost up to a significant level by reducing and subsequently eliminating product recalls and product wastages, while increasing profits by proper decision-making and proper ingredients resourcing system. By reducing cost, an increase in profit is impacted by product reputation, customer satisfaction, customer confidence, openings in export market and attaining a compatible edge in the competitive market. HACCP can improve the safety of the foods being produced as well as company's productivity, marketing capabilities, and most importantly- profitability while managing risk.

Government of Canada has provided and allocated resources to help food manufacturers implement food safety programs in there manufacturing units. In Canada, many federally registered food-processing facilities can get continual assistance from Agriculture & Agri-Food Canada (AAFC) inspectors, who are trained professionals in HACCP system implementation on generic models.

A number of quality registrar companies within Canada and across the border in the United States also exist to assist food companies in implementing HACCP. These registrar companies provide materials, tools, and training and help to implement the Food Safety HACCP system.

The educational institutions like The Guelph Food Technology Centre (GFTC), in partnership with the University of Guelph (U of G), are providing training and technical assistance with the implementation of HACCP. GFTC approaches HACCP from a business perspective, helping the clients in the food industry to develop a program that leads to cost savings on the production floor-109.

When we discuss the HACCP principles, we will understand that those principles form the success note in the food safety. One of those principles stipulates identification of Critical Control Points (CCPs). Only trained people in hygiene, microbiology, chemistry, and the processing technology could easily identify questionable hazards and CCPs in the food manufacturing plants. A proper controlling of the CCPs is a key to the success of whole system.

Let us review the example of an advisory from a government agency in the United States of America (USA). On May 25, 1999, Food Safety and Inspection Services (FSIS) announced several steps to help the meat industry control bacterium *Listeria monocytogenes* in ready-to-eat (RTE) meat products. FSIS advised large and small meat plants to reassess their HACCP plan to ensure that their plans were adequately addressing the *Listeria sp.,* hazard in RTE meat products. FSIS also provided guidance to the meat industry recommending environmental and finished-product testing, for the evaluation of *Listeria monocytogenes*. This announcement did not state that a CCP had to be in every HACCP plan relating to a fully cooked product for the detection of *L. monocytogenes*. Many quality professionals interpreted and emphasised that the proper controlling of the CCPs is between cooking and packaging. This should pave the way for the reassessment of *Listeria monocytogenes* plans-141. The meat processors should have identified questionable hazards specifically during the cooking and packaging process. That is where the main hazard exists and to prescribe proper Critical Control Limits (CCLs) to prevent hazard.

A paceful continual assessment either by internal auditing or by first party, second party, or the third party will create the way for the identification of missing links and subsequent corrective actions. Corrective actions are taken to eliminate recurrence. A corrective action in this case would be taken after self-assessment or if need be, the services of a third party auditor could be materialised. FSIS had shown concern that some companies have not reassessed their HACCP plans following the food borne illness outbreaks and recalls of meat products earlier in the year. As it is presented in most introductory HACCP training courses, HACCP plan reassessment is always expected to occur when there is new information regarding food product related outbreaks or new regulatory recommendations.

FSIS recommended food-manufacturing plants to reassess the potential for *L. monocytogenes* contamination of raw meat materials that they procure. Plants must validate their cooking process and ensure it is effective in destroying *L. monocytogenes*. FSIS also advised that environmental sampling (floors, walls, drains, etc.) and testing for *L. monocytogenes* would validate the effectiveness of a plant's Standard Operating Procedures (SOPs). In this case, if establishments have records to show that *L. monocytogenes* is reasonably likely to occur as a hazard in finished product due to raw materials, processing failures, packaging materials and environmental contamination, they are encouraged and directed to lift their procedures for preventing *L. monocytogenes* contamination from their SOPs and convert them into a CCP.

Another example of a proper critical control point could be taken from Canadian Turkey producers in Alberta. The On Farm Food Safety Program (OFFSP) in Alberta provides growers of turkey with the most current information on animal husbandry and bio-security that will assist in controlling *Salmonella sp.* and other pathogens on-farm; minimizing the risk of animal disease transmission to commercial flocks. Thus ensuring those turkeys grown in Canada meet or surpass the standards of international competitors; and, that the turkeys marketed are free of residues that may adversely affect food safety and the consuming public. This program is based on Hazard Analysis Critical Control Point or HACCP. This comprehensive bio-security and quality assurance program consists of two sections: Good Management Practices (GMPs) and Critical Control Points (CCPs) in the Production of Turkeys.

We are referring to their second section dealing specifically with Critical Control Points (CCPs) in the production of turkeys. CCPs are those points in the production cycle of turkey where the lack of grower control may potentially result in a human health risk. When contamination occurs in turkey birds on farm level then it is not possible to process the contaminating hazard out of the turkey meat during evisceration, processing, cooking and packing stages; thus initial contamination at farm level should be eliminated through proper farm management.

Based on this preventive sensitivity, the following three management practices have been classified as CCPs at this time: Cleaning of Turkey Barns; Rodent-Pest Control; and, Administration of Medications and Vaccines. In all three instances, the lack of proper management increases the risk of chemical contamination, which cannot be removed through processing or cooking stages. Thus, the importance of an audit, corrective action, and verification for these three practices is highly significant in this example-158.

Most food and beverage manufacturers in Canada will need to consult with the Canadian Food Inspection Agency (CFIA), as the CFIA is responsible for administering and enforcing the following Acts: Canada Agricultural Products Act; dairy, eggs, fresh fruits, vegetables, honey, livestock, poultry, maple products, and processed products regulations. Consumer Packaging and Labelling Act which is applicable to food, Fertilizers Act and Fish Inspection Act. Food and Drugs Act; as it relates to food Meat Inspection Act, Plant Breeders' Rights Act and Seeds Act.

In the following text, the author has identified important food safety issues related to different food sectors, which are helpful to prepare a comprehensive Food Safety Program through HACCP.

A.Critical Control & Bakery:

Canadian bakery industry includes two distinct segments classed as "Wholesale bakers" and "Retail bakers". Retail bakers produce and sell on the premises and cater to the demand for fresh baked goods such as bread, rolls, and pastries, made from "scratch" or from frozen dough supplied by wholesale bakers. Wholesale bakers are part of the manufacturing sector of the economy and, for statistical purposes, are referred to under Standard Industrial Classification (SIC) 1072 as Bread and Bakery Products' Manufacturers.

A key characteristic of this industry is the perishable nature of many of its mainstream products, which cannot be kept for a very long period under ambient as well as under refrigerated temperatures. The concept of long life bakery products rarely exists. For this reason, distribution costs and the management of product on the retail shelf is an integral part of the bakery business; it also imparts a relatively higher cost structure to bakers than other food processors. The government has had the bright idea to offer a solution by introducing programs that would help food processors to develop modern food safety standards, quality assurance training, and hire food safety experts.

Ontario government in 1999 designed a program called Healthy Futures for Ontario Agriculture (HFOA) to promote safe water, safe food, and develop new markets. Critical control points in bakery industry are steps at which control can be applied and is essential to prevent or eliminate a food safety hazard or reduce it to an acceptable level in the bakery production. If the controls applied are not adequate and products are contaminated, food may go out to the consumer creating health hazard to the population. That is why these steps are critical to bakery food safety.

Water crisis involving _E. coli_ in Walkerton is an example of what can happen when standards are lacking or not fully implemented. Bakery processing plants, restaurants, and other food operations are not restricted to critical control from water. The recent warnings (in a few cases closings) issued to restaurants, bakeries are a reminder that standards need to be improved, and that "business as usual" is not acceptable by the regulatory authorities in Canada.

The ingredients control for any food manufacturing is the starting point to accomplish a control. The main ingredients of the bakery food are grains and cereals. Cereals are unique in bakery food because of their bulk usage and good keeping qualities. They remain an important food for the majority of humans. The grains and cereals used in the bakery are wheat (_Triticum aestivum_ L), barley (_Hordeum vulgare_ L), oat (_Avena sativa_ L), corn (_Zeamays indentata_) (_Zea saccharata_) (_Zeamays everta_), Sorghum (_Sorghum sp._) buckwheat (_Fagopyrum esculentum_ Moench), Millet (_Pennisetum glaucum_), Rice (_Oryza stiva_ L.), Basmati rice, pre-boiled rice, rye (_Secale cereale_ L.), sago (_Metroxylon sagu_), and Tapioca (_Manibot utilissima_) etc. The only safety concern from the grains and cereals is that the products should be free from disease, remain dry and free from fungal infections. The pure, clean, and healthy grains and cereals free from impurities are most suitable for safer bakery production.

Flour is another major ingredient in the bakery, which is prepared from grains and cereals. Any edible substance from grains and cereals is called flour. Wheat flour is extremely important to the bakery industry due to gluten (protein fraction of flour), which enables wheat flour mixtures to be leavened for the manufacture of baked produce. The flours used in the bakery are Wheat flour, Baker's flour, barley flour, Gram flour (Indian Besan), Continental flour, Corn flour, Gluten, Malt flour, Rice flour, Rye flour, Soya flour, unbleached flour, wholemeal flour and white flour etc. Different ingredients bring the possibility of diverse risks prompting a preventive measure commensurate to the nature of risk.

Many examples of critical control points in bakery industry should be studied and understood before starting the bakery business. As a supplement to Good Manufacturing Process (GMP) and quality control system, bakery industry in Belgium started implementing a product safety system based on Hazard Analysis Critical Control Points (HACCP) - Systematic Risk Identification Analysis (SRIA) that is applied to all critical processes in the bakery manufacturing and packaging[-12].

Temperature control during dough making plays an important role in the final quality of baked products. Controlling the dough-temperature optimizes dough development with all related connections like the safety and final quality of baked goods. For this reason, a technique has been developed with process-controlled module for direct production of CO_2-snow, which is used to cool the dough directly during the mixing operation. At the same time, the CO_2-gas will be separated and removed from the mixing vessel. The communication of this CO2-injector with a temperature - sensor, like an infrared-sensor, enables the bakers to reach the wanted dough-temperature exactly. This is a critical control point for a baker's dough making system necessary to safeguard the dough from extra microbial activity prior to baking or other proceedings -117.

Critical point for Metal detection is crucial for the bread making companies. A piece of equipment that detects metal in food is a substantial remedy. In the process of detection, the wrapped loaf is passed through a metal detector at the end of the production process. However, prevention of metal falling during the recombination, processing, and packing remains the first priority.

Sieving of basic bakery ingredients is a very well known critical point. Bagged ingredients, such as flour, are passed through a fine sieve to remove any material that may have got into the raw ingredient, such as metal, wood, stones, etc. Even if a manual sieving is done, chances of foreign materials like hairs from personnel, rubber-pencil-coins etc., kept in workers pocket may fall in to the flour; sieve may contain threads etc., which may fall during the sieving process. Thus, proper personnel protective uniform and proper equipments of operation are necessary to eliminate such divergence. The criticality of the process is to eliminate the foreign body.

Hippocrates, the father of medicine, first recorded allergens in food. It is important for consumers to identify their allergens so that one can eat safely with the minimum of dietary reactions. A little intelligent detective work can be done to identify the food allergens by the consumer and doctors could help identify the process by skin-pick test. Food manufactures and regulatory agencies will make sure that all allergens are definitely labelled so that consumers could make a choice. Allergen control in bakery products have been monitored by manufacturers and CFIA in Canada. A proper labelling is required to indicate the presence of any allergen to safeguard sensitive consumers.

In the United States, retail bakeries are covered by the statute of The Perishable Agricultural Commodities Act (PACA). Such units must obtain a license. This statute requires food processors buying fresh or frozen in quantities of a ton or more on any given day, to get a license from the U.S. Department of Agriculture (USDA).

In the United States and Canada, major customers demand that bakery suppliers implement GMP's and HACCP programs. Further, if bakery suppliers intend to export, then HACCP becomes a prerequisite. By implementing a food safety and food quality program, manufacturers can eliminate costs that result from poor quality and unsafe food products. Poor quality in a bakery is an easy affair to detect, for example, it can be spotted by visual aids whenever a defective product is looked upon, from the wastage a defective nature of the products can be identified with in the processing section and visibly spoilt product returns can be investigated for the cause of spoilage.

The critical points in bakery manufacturing should be controlled to enhance shelf life and safety to human consumption. Bakery products like breads and rolls when stored at ambient temperatures undergo a progressive deterioration of quality commonly known as staling. The fresh bakery products (without any preservatives) at both wholesale and retail levels are highly subjected to deterioration, limiting their shelf life to only several days at ambient temperature. It has been observed that the higher the moisture content of the product in its fresh state, the more pronounced are the changes resulting from staling. Products such as breads, yeast-raised sweet goods, and cakes stale much more markedly than do cookies and crackers, which have much lower initial moisture contents. Controlling water activity of this product should be critically analysed. Modified atmosphere packaging (MAP) has become increasingly popular as a method to extend the mold-free shelf life of bakery products. The gases most commonly used in MAP of bakery products are N_2 and CO_2. Samples packed with MAP alone are less moist in the beginning period of storage, but with better microbiological quality. Development of many baked products involves maximizing the moisture content to produce the best possible eating qualities while minimizing Aw (water activity). Lowering the Aw increases product stability in terms of susceptibility to microbial growth. The ethanol vapour can help to maintain the moisture of the pastries and suppress mold growth though its usage may be restricted due to religious and cultural diversity in Canadian society.

Many baked products, such as pies and fillings, have water activities above 0.85 and relatively neutral pH conditions that are even conducive to the growth of pathogens such as *Staphylococcus aureus*. Incidence of mycelial growth in baked products is more

26

than other pathogens commonly found in non-baked products. The critical factor in bakery products comes from meat, dairy, and vegetable toppings particularly if these toppings are not pasteurized and contaminated. It should be critically looked upon and controlled. Most cakes and pastries are highly energized bakery foods. A typical cake could contain principally flour, milk fat, vegetable fat, eggs, and sugar, which are good nutrients providing constituents for human consumption and at the same time provide a good media to lactose fermenters from Enterobacteriaceae, which are usually pathogenic. With the presence of such nutrients, it also provides a good media for the bacteria from *Streptococcaceae*, *Lactobacillaceae,* and *Pseudomonadaceae*, which are mostly spoilage organisms. The cakes, which need extra care, are Angel cakes, Carrot cake, Chocolate cake, Christmas cake, Cream pastries, and Sponge cakes etc.

Pastries are manufactured from ingredients principally flour, milk, butterfat, ghee, eggs, honey, sesame seeds, cinnamon and other sweet spices and nuts which are added to append the value. The preventive measures necessitate the added ingredients and their types, which are required to safeguard the pastry products from spoilage and from harbouring pathogenic microorganisms. The products, which are most common in this category, are Choux pastry, File pastry, Hot water pastry, Citify pastry, and Puff pastry etc.

Desserts and Puddings are the most vulnerable bakery products to pathogens and need scientific preventive measures to safeguard their wholesomeness. The dessert may be a simple fruit dessert, milk pudding, rice pudding, hearty steamed fruit pudding, treacle tart, and custard. What makes these bakery products highly perishable is their moisture content in the presence of carbohydrates and added sugar. The critical control points during their processing, postproduction packing and storage conditions are detrimental to their safe consumption. The products under this category are Cereal dessert, Fruit dessert, Apple and Rhubarb crumble, Milk Pudding, Pavlova and Meringue, Lemon Meringue pie, Mango mousse, Indian Kheer and Christmas pudding.

Pasta and noodles are also part of bakery foods and they are part of grain and cereal products and closely related with Canadian gourmet. Agnolotti is semicircular stuffed pasta, which is an important delicacy in bakery foods. Anelini, bucatini, cannelloni, ditalini, farfalle, farfallini, and Gnocchetti Saridi are the best-known examples of pasta available in food stores of Canada. Similarly, noodles are made by mixing flours with water, salt, alkaline salt, until homogeneous dough of crumbly consistency is produced. Once the dough sheet has been rolled out to the desired thickness, it is cut into noodle strands by passing it to cutting rollers. The same goes true with Pakistani Sewain delicacy, which is passed through minute metal sieve to get thinner strands. Fresh Raw noodles may be sold fresh and require refrigeration for 3-4 days at 39.20 °F (4 °C). Dried noodles are also raw noodles, which are sun dried or dried in ovens. They keep for at least a year under dry conditions. Dry noodles have negligible water activity and risks are minimal.

Confectionary is the sweetest segment of the long list of bakery food products. The sugar content in confectionaries could range from 10% in butterscotch to 95% in Fondant. The beauty of old time confectionary manufacturer was the usage of honey as a sweetening agent rather than modern day crystal clear sugar. Confectionary is thus an energy-dense food providing resistance to microbial spoilage due to high sugar and less water activity. Sugar acts as a preservative and shelf life of confectionary products is normally longer than chilled pudding and custard. Their critical safety factors are of minor importance as the processing and sugar content are self-preserving. However, a proper packaging and dry to chilled storage conditions as per the nature of the confectionary provides safety to the product and the consumers alike. The best examples of confectionary are Butterscotch, Caramel, Chocolate, Coconut ice, Fondant, Fruit paste, Fudge, Arabic Halawa, Pakistani Halwa, Indian Halwa, Health bar, Honey comb, Jellied confectionary, Marshmallow, Marzipan, Nougat, Pasteli, Pastille, Toffee, Turkish delight and Bangladeshi Rasogulla etc.

Steps should be taken to reduce the favourable conditions, which allow mold and bacterial growth in bakery products during transitional period to consumption. FDA approved mold inhibitors can be added to breads and other products to lengthen their shelf life and safety to health. However, such additions are never considered replacement of adequate processing techniques.

Post baking steps are the critical stages of bakery contamination. Baked products emerge from the oven, essentially sterile from a microbial point of view. To keep bakery products in sterile condition may not be possible but GMPs and good hygiene will definitely make the significant difference. Most contamination is not a result of inadequate heating of the product, but due to post-handling contamination from airborne contaminants, packaging equipments, packaging materials, and direct human contact by production personnel. Fillings made with cream and eggs can pose severe risk, but problems tend to come in post-baking handling of the bakery products. The food handling personnel should give the particular importance to hand washing and sanitizing practices. Insect and rodent infestations can compromise baking areas as well. That is where the pre-requisites of HACCP become indispensable.

Fermentation of sugar containing ingredients may cause problems in filled bakery products. The water activity of bakery products is considerably low; growth of microorganisms other than mold is not a major problem if preventive measures are adequately taken. Mold is an aerobic microorganism, and can be effectively controlled by carbon dioxide together with low residual oxygen levels (less than 1%), extending shelf life by many valuable days. MAP is especially suitable for rye bread, sweet bakery products, various pies, and pre-baked bread.

Bakers yeast is adversely affected due to abnormal refrigeration and freezing temperatures. Use of preservatives like Glucono Delta Lactone (GDL) is often the leavening agent of choice for refrigerated or frozen dough products. Acidulant sometimes help prevent bacterial problems in special dough products. Such Acidulant as GDL can help in the prevention of black spotting or grey discoloration in dough during refrigerated storage. GDL is also a helpful ingredient in preventing undesirable microbial growth in bakery fillings. Salmonellosis and staphylococcal food poisoning outbreaks can occur when filled bakery products are subjected to elevated temperatures and manual handling. For the bakery product safety controlling temperature, water activity, and pH are the real critical factors. In this role, GDL can be used to lower the pH and thus retard the growth of acido-phobic bacteria in bakery fillings and icings. When used in combination with sugar and salt to control water activity, GDL is extremely useful in adding safe commercial shelf life to filled bakery products. Therefore, the preservation with in the jurisdiction of local food preservative's law is a critical factor for the safety of bakery products.

In the case of breads, muffins, cakes, doughnuts and brownies, whey protein ingredients can help maintain crumb softness by reducing moisture migration and starch retrogradation. Wheat contains the proteins gliadin, and glutenin which, when mixed with water, form the elastic gluten which make it possible for dough to stretch and rise and bakers yeast ferments the sugars releasing carbon dioxide. Wheat flour, salt, yeast, water and optional ingredients are used to produce breads of different kinds where critical points are involved right from the spot on ingredients and follow on to the manufacturing process. Crusty breads are eaten preferably the same day; other breads could be stored at room temperature for immediate consumption. For longer storage, it can be frozen for a maximum of three months period depending on one likes and the variety of bread.

The normal bread like white bread, Scottish bap, whole grain bread, bread crumbs, Bagel, chapatti, crumpet, fruit bread, Lavash, Mixed grain bread, Pita bread, Arabic khubs and rye bread are all low fat food and remain less vulnerable to lipolytic bacterial spoilage resulting in rancid odour. Some foods, which are substitute of bread like Croissant, Damper, Danish pastry, Doughnut, Asian Paratha, Indian Puri and Indian Samosa, are high fat bakery products, which may require special care in preparation and storage due to their critical fat content, which would require proper preventive measures. Such products usually attract fungi and bacteria, which act on fat.

Packaging material is the last chain in factory process of manufacturing which is critical to final product safety. Baked products, whether designed to have a shelf life of two weeks or longer weeks, have probably achieved these goals largely due to packaging technology. Some of the latest technology includes adding gases to control the atmosphere within the package. As explained earlier, modified-atmosphere packaging (MAP) has given products like bagels or brownies sometimes weeks of added shelf life. However, issues with faulty seals, package integrity, leakers, and the amount of residual oxygen in the package play a role in the life and safety of a baked product. In concluding remarks, food product designers need to be conscious of temperature, Aw and pH conditions where growth can occur, as well as the conditions in which toxins are produced. Food companies face a challenge in determining acceptable MAP-defect levels, since defects might lead to a mouldy product or, more seriously, transfer of a food-borne illness to a consumer-135.

B. Critical Controls & Beverages:
When we discuss the issues related to Canadian beverage industry, we include alcoholic beverages, Fruit and nut liqueurs, Soft drinks, Coffee, Tea, Herbal tea, Fruit juices, Vegetable juices, Fruit drinks, soda water, tonic water and Mineral water. Since we are concerned with the critical control from raw material to processing and finally to consumption of beverages, we shall discuss the common points relating to the general beverage system. The adult human body is almost 60% water and beverages play an important role to maintain the level of water in the human body. All beverages contain at least 80% of water and the best beverage is pure water itself with no impurities.

The most harmful beverage to human health is an alcoholic beverage, which is one of the major health problems in modern times. It could be a one-third factor in all hospital admissions in North America. The best service to health conscious people is to eliminate alcoholic beverages from their diet. If some one makes a choice then the amount shall be with in the healthy limits provided by health directors. The examples of alcoholic beverages where CCPs are important factor include Advocaat, Beer, Brandy, Cider, Clear spirits, Coffee liqueurs, Crème liqueurs, Fortified wines, Herbal liqueurs, Rum, Whisky, Champagne and ginger wines etc. The critical points in their preparations start right from the raw materials and maintaining its safety during pasteurization, fermentation, maturity packing etc. It is more important to take alcoholic beverages in healthy amounts, as its keeping quality and disease risks from contaminants are minimal. The major risk remains from its volumetric consumption not from the way it is manufactured. Homemade wines in poor countries often are adulterated with cheap hydrocarbon liquids resulting in health hazard. Such incidents could be controlled through punitive and regulatory jurisdictions. Non-microbial contaminants require attention with critical angles to safeguard alcoholic beverages for human consumption.

The non-alcoholic beverages are healthy in choice, manufacturers and regulators have equal responsibilities to safeguard beverages through GMPs and regulatory parameters. Tea and coffee are the most popular beverages consumed world over since the cessation of hostilities in 1945. Tea, coffee, and cola are known stimulants to the central nervous system. It is agreed by most experts that a 300 mg intake of caffeine on a daily basis remains safe for human health. The indication of caffeine on labels is a requirement so that consumers could make their own choice.

The fruit juice, fruit juice drinks, fruit juice cordials and fruit flavoured belly wash drinks are available in Canadian market for the non-alcoholic consumers. The fruit juices are labelled to indicate a juice content of 100%, which means, it is not adulterated with un-natural juice ingredients. However, most of the fruit juices are prepared from natural concentrates like FCOJ but it may contain additives to safeguard shelf life according to one's state regulations. The critical safety matter is the amount of additives and its conformity with the regulation. Many countries specify the Vitamin C content in citrus and other fruit juices; the addition of Vitamin C is helpful in enhancing the shelf life and the nutritional value. Thus, the quantity and its addition is a pre-researched critical control factor otherwise, safety of juice remains doubtful. The fruit juice drinks are with added sugar and water, and may contain certain degree of juice content, which qualify such products for the given name. The fruit juice drinks could contain additives as per the recommended and permissible regulatory dosages. The fruit nectars are the fruit juice drinks with at least 30% of juice content. They may contain additives and sweetening agents like sucrose etc. Certain fruits like guava, mango etc., are converted in to fruit nectars because 100% juice content is not considered suitable for drinking purpose. Fruit juice cordials also fall in the same category where juice content is specified with added ingredients like sugar, water, and additives. Fruit flavoured drinks are without juice content and are composed of fruit flavours, sugar, water and additives like permitted food colours, cloudifers and stabilizers etc. In all categories of juices and drinks, the resourcing of raw materials, prepared compounds, fruit emulsions, sweetening agents, additives, formulations, processing, packing and storage temperatures play a definite role in their shelf life and consumer's safety.

Mineral water is a clear colourless beverage with little minerals of not significant nutritional values. Like all beverages, pasteurization of mineral water to make it pathogen free is an important factor. Some mineral waters coming from mountain rocks water reservoir may contain certain therapeutic values and it is consumed where natural water resources are doubtful. It is also mixed with fruit juices in domestic consumption due to its guaranteed processing and final regulatory parameters in the water bottling factories.

The wider spectrum of Canadian and U.S. population quenches their thirst by drinking orange juices, vegetable juices, or sparkling apple cider. It is rare to hear the cases of juice borne food poisoning. It seems majority of juices are safe for human consumption in North America. Thanks to cooler temperatures in northern portions of North America. However, the safety of juices in our market could not be ignored merely because of cooler atmospheric temperatures, acidic nature of beverages or even added preservatives. People have sporadically suffered from juice borne poisoning even though acidic nature of most of the juices and drinks retard the growth of pathogenic bacteria. However, juices by nature of their acidic quality remain a suitable medium for fungal growth.

Such was the 1996 case of a 16-month-old child in Colorado who died of heart damage and kidney failure after drinking contaminated apple juice. In another 1996 case involving contaminated apple juice, 3 1/2-year-old Amanda Berman of Chicago was hospitalized for 24 days. In both cases, the apple juice was Unpasteurized and the culprit was bacterium _E. coli_ O157:H7, the same microbe that claimed the lives of four children during a 1993 outbreak from undercooked hamburger. In this case, a proper heat treatment and subsequent cooling were ignored. In Unpasteurized juices, the chances of contaminants are from the surface of fruits, un-sanitized fruit juicer and crusher, contaminated utensils, prolonged storage, temperature of storage and unhygienic practices by vendors. The fresh healthy fruits containing juices in their tissues are the most reliable and safe to drink but added inadequate processing steps without a heat treatment often results in contamination. Food poisoning outbreaks have been traced to fresh juices that were not pasteurized or otherwise processed to eliminate harmful bacteria, the US-Food and Drug Administration proposed measures to reduce the risk of illness from disease-causing microbes in unpasteurized fruit and vegetable juices.

A 1997 study by US-FDA's Center for Food Safety and Applied Nutrition (CFSAN) found that while contamination of juice products most likely occurs during the growing and harvesting of the raw product, it may occur at any point between the orchard and the table. Therefore, US-FDA's proposed regulations will require juice processors to implement a Hazard Analysis and Critical Control Point (HACCP) plan that addresses all points of production. In addition to a number of U.S. food companies already using individually tailored HACCP systems in there manufacturing processes, systems are also in place in Canada and in other countries. In addition to HACCP, a warning is now required on Unpasteurized juices. The warning label must be visible on the information panel or on the principal display panel of the container's label and must read: "WARNING: This product has not been pasteurized and, therefore, may contain harmful bacteria that can cause serious illness in children, the elderly, and persons with weakened immune systems". For apple juice or apple cider, the warning statement was required beginning Sept. 8, 1998. For all other unpasteurized juices, the effective date had been Nov. 5, 1998-40.

The new labelling was only intended to be an interim measure because a 3-year phase-in period for processors to implement their HACCP programs had been proposed. Those individual firms requesting additional time were allowed until July 8, 1999, to comply with the warning label final rule.

US-FDA urges high-risk individuals-children, the elderly, and those with weakened immune systems - to drink only pasteurized juices. And while manufacturers were asked before the date in the regulation to voluntarily place warning statements on the labels of juices that haven't been pasteurized, the agency advises people to be aware that a product without a warning label at this time might still be Unpasteurized.

New challenges arising from the growing size of the food industry and the diversity of products and processes have prompted US-FDA to consider requiring HACCP regulations as a standard throughout much of the remaining U.S. food supply. The Center for Food Safety and Applied Nutrition (CFSAN) found in its preliminary study that unpasteurized juices accounted for 76 percent of contamination cases reported between 1993 and 1996. In addition, the study concluded that illnesses associated with unpasteurized juices tended to be more severe than those associated with pasteurized products were. Therefore, FDA believes that pasteurization, or a comparable process that would eliminate or reduce the level of harmful pathogens that can cause food-borne illness, appears to offer an effective way to control the significant hazards that have become a problem with juice.

In 1996, 69 people in Canada and the western U.S. became ill and one child died after consuming apple juice contaminated with _E. coli_ O157:H7. Unpasteurized orange juice caused a 1999 _Salmonella muenchen_ outbreak that sickened 423 people in 20 states and 3 provinces and caused one death. In 2000, unpasteurized orange juice was the culprit again, causing 88 _Salmonella enteritidis_ infections in six Western states. The number of juice-related illnesses annually is 16,000 to 48,000, according to US-FDA estimates. Action taken in response to the rule will prevent an estimated 6,000 of these illnesses.

Juice safety has been called into question in recent years due to an increase in the number of food borne illness outbreaks associated with juice. To protect consumers from pathogens in juices, the US-FDA announced a rule on January 18, 2001, requiring juice processors to use Hazard Analysis and Critical Control Point (HACCP) programs for juice processing. This rule went into effect on January 2002 for large companies. Small companies had until January 21, 2003, to comply and very small companies must implement HACCP programs by January 20, 2004.

The HACCP system for the juice processors will be required to include an analysis of potential hazards, determination of points in the manufacturing process where hazards can occur, developing appropriate control measures for the hazards, and implementing corrective actions for problems that occur. The elimination of recurrence will form the backbone of HACCP. The HACCP requirement to juice processors is not new in North America; meat, poultry, and seafood processors are already using HACCP systems.

Processors in United States must use control methods that achieve a 5-log, or 100,000 fold, reduction in the numbers of the most resistant microbes in their finished products versus levels in the untreated juice. The control methods processors can use include pasteurization, alternative technologies, such as UV irradiation technology, or a combination of the two. Citrus processors have the additional option of reducing pathogens by 5-logs on the surface of the fruit, in conjunction with testing the procedure to ensure that it is effective.

This new rule does not apply to retail establishments, such as juice bars, who sell juice to consumers directly. In addition, those who make shelf-stable juices or concentrates using a single thermal processing step do not need to meet the microbial hazard requirements of the juice HACCP regulation.

In Canada, Unpasteurized juices are very common and popular to consumers because of its freshness and psychological perceptions. To ensure that proper preparation methods are met, the CFIA has developed *The Code of Practice for the Production and Distribution of Unpasteurized Apple and Other Fruit Juice/Cider in Canada*. The Code outlines steps for producers, processors, distributors and retailers, which they can take to reduce possible contamination. The CFIA has increased processing plant inspections, juice sampling, and laboratory analysis. As well, Health Canada has introduced a policy encouraging producers to label unpasteurized drinks so consumers can take decisions that are more informed.

The CFIA advises people in the high-risk group to drink only those juices and ciders that are pasteurized, which includes any shelf stable product and most of the refrigerated products in the grocery stores. Unpasteurized juices and ciders are commonly found at roadside stands, farmers markets, and apple orchards.

Back in 1998, CFIA prepared a generic model to produce Aseptic Fruit Juices. It was designed to provide an example of how the Canadian Food Inspection Agency (CFIA) and its Food Safety Enhancement Program (FSEP) can be used to establish an effective Hazard Analysis Critical Control Point (HACCP) plan. This model has an unusual feature in that it was found to have a CCP only to screen the incoming ingredients and materials. Throughout the hazard analysis and CCP determination, prerequisite programs or the deployment of Good Manufacturing Practices (GMPs) was found to eliminate the necessity of a CCP. Though GMPs are not the replacement of CCPs they should be considered preventive measures in support of eliminating the risk from CCPs. The committee identified and analyzed the biological, chemical, and physical hazards. Particular attention was paid to biological hazards originating from yeasts and moulds as that could result in poisoning and spoilage, if not properly controlled. Because of the low pH of the apple juice, the bacterial hazards were not considered critical from a safety perspective. Some process steps were thought to be quality control points rather than critical control points. The chemical and physical hazards are controlled by prerequisite programs, and by strict ingredient and material specifications.

Only fungi (yeasts and moulds) and two main groups of bacteria, called "lactic acid bacteria" and "acetic acid bacteria," will grow in apple cider. Yeasts produce ethanol (ethyl alcohol) and carbon dioxide as by-products of growth and are probably the most important spoilage microbes present in cider. Lactic acid and acetic acid bacteria produce organic acids as a by-product of growth. At high enough concentrations, these acids will cause off-flavours.

Viruses, like the hepatitis A virus, and pathogenic protozoa, such as _Cryptosporidium parvum_, can only grow inside a host animal. Steve Ingham (2000) in his review of Basics of Microbiology for Apple Processors states that these microbes may survive in cider, but they will not grow. Pathogenic Microbes that may jeopardize Cider safety are _E. coli_ O157:H7, _Salmonella sp_, _Cryptosporidium parvum,_ and a potent toxin Patulin. Critical control points for these should be identified and prevented[199].

Pasteurized juices are encouraged for consumers as they are treated with heat to either kill all pathogenic organisms or reduce up to a level that will not cause illness to humans provided they are stored as per the manufacturer's recommendation. The endurance of pasteurized and refrigerated juices in the market shelves will depend on the quality assured from the manufacturing factory and subsequent handling during the transition from producer to consumer. In the quality assured pasteurized juices from the manufacturer, the spoilage organisms are reduced to such an extent that a threat to the shelf life of juices is minimised.

Table: 1(1) shows that there has been an increase in food borne illness linked to fresh produce including juice and cider products. A variety of pathogenic organisms such as _Escherichia coli_ O157:H7, _Salmonella sp._ and _Cryptosporidium sp._ have been known to cause human illness related to the consumption of juice/cider. _E. coli_ O157:H7 is the most frequently isolated of these strains, which are referred to as Enterohaemorrhagic _E. coli_. The table presents a history of reported unpasteurized juice/cider outbreaks since 1990.

Aseptic processing and packing of juices provide a better solution if the juice safety and long perseverance are the priorities. The chemical and physical hazards are controlled by prerequisite programs, and by strict ingredient and material specifications. It is of priority to have a CCP to screen the incoming ingredients and materials. The hazards identified with aseptic juice product can be adequately avoided by diligent adherence to ingredient, raw material specifications, and prerequisite programs throughout the establishment.

With aseptic fruit juices and drinks, good manufacturing practices (GMPs) with only one CCP will ensure a safe and wholesome product.

Table: 1(1)-Reported Food borne outbreaks linked to Unpasteurized juice/cider since 1990 -30

Year	Product	Pathogen	Location	Cases
1991	Apple cider	E. coli O157:H7	Massachusetts	23
1993	Apple cider	Cryptosporidium parvum	Maine	160
1995	Orange juice	Salmonella sp.	Florida	63
1996	Apple cider	E. coli O157:H7	Connecticut	10
1996 (1)	Apple cider	E. coli O157:H7	USA and Can.	66
1996	Apple cider	E. coli O157:H7	Washington	2
1996	Apple cider	Cryptosporidium parvum	New York	31
1998 (2)	Apple cider	E. coli O157:H7	Ontario	14
1999	Orange juice	Salmonella typhimurium	Australia	400

| 1999 | Orange juice | *Salmonella muenchen* | Arizona, Western USA and Canada | 200 |
| 1999 | Apple cider | *E. coli* O157:H7 | Oklahoma | 7 |

(1) Unpasteurized juice from California was involved. 14 of the 66 people affected were from British Columbia. One child died in the USA.

(2) Local health officials identified one batch of non-commercial, custom-pressed apple cider as the most likely source.

The package integrity of aseptic fruit juices and drinks is another critical control point where attention should be paid. A pinhole seal defect will render the packed juice unsuitable for long perseverance and spoilage could be noticed within a week of ambient storage.

C. Critical Control & Dairy:

The dairy industry may be defined as production of milk, milk powders, cream, butter, buttermilk and cheese. It may include many other products where milk based ingredients are playing a detrimental and significant role in the final quality and safety. Each of these poses operators and legislators with particular problems. In North America, cow's milk is the main raw material for the dairy industry. However, goat milk, sheep milk, and reindeer milk may find an important place through therapeutic and nurturing channels. Water buffalos have been farmed for whiter and richer dairy milk in India, Pakistan, Thailand, and Egypt. While some of the Arab countries have put a task to procure fresh camel milk for drinking and therapeutic benefits. It is very early to designate camel milk as a commercial dairy beverage but efforts in Mauritania, Saudi Arabia, and United Arab Emirates are moving ahead with untiring expedition.

Milk by its source and nature carries the risk of disease if the milking animal is suffering from diseases or kept under unhygienic conditions. Such milk may contain *Streptococcus pyogenes*, *Streptococcus equisimilis, and Streptococcus agalactiae* from the mastitis-infested cows. *Streptococcus faecalis* may get in from the faecal material of cows and humans. *Mycobacterium tuberculosis* is the cause of tuberculosis in human and cattle. *Mycobacterium paratuberculosis Staphylococcus aureus* and *Listeria sp*. could get in from diseased milk animals. *E. coli* is found in milk if contaminated by exterior of milk animals, *Salmonella sp.*, *Shigella sp.*, *Enterobacter sp.*, *Proteus sp.*, and many other bacteria could be found in milk if cowboys or milk cow handlers suffering from the disease come in contact of milk animals. *Streptococcus lactis*, *Streptococcus cremoris*, *Leuconostoc mesenteroides*, *Leuconostoc dextranicum*, *Leuconostoc lactis*, *Lactobacillus sp.* In addition, few others are common contaminants of milk, which may spoil the milk if not chilled after milking of cows. This prompts the need of controlling critical points in the chain from the health of milking animals, milking procedure, health of personnel, general hygiene, and sanitation of udders and immediate chilling of milk after it is drawn from udder.

Milk must be cooled and kept chilled until it either is bottled for use as milk, or arrives at the processor's reception dock for butter, cheese, fermented milk, yoghurt, or cream production. This group needs a different HACCP template to take account of the special requirements for bacterial control, storage, and cooling. Many cheeses rely on identified bacteria to mature properly and the control of good and potentially harmful bacteria is particularly important. Similarly high bacterial counts in milk may interfere in the fermentation process during yoghurt production. Yoghurt bacteria are highly susceptible to bacteriophages. Packaging and transport of these delicate and very time sensitive products is also very important. As with all other sectors of the food supply chain, HACCP plan systems will have to be integrated with those of suppliers and customers to maintain Traceability of milk supply lines.

Animal Drug Residues (ADR) is a factor of concern to consumers. Consumer sensitivity to food safety issues has been heightened by the actions of activists and the media attention they attract. Consumers remain very sensitive to publicity, which suggests milk, and dairy beef may contain violative levels of Animal Drug Residues. The continual development of more sensitive and more rapid residue detection methods, and their use by regulator agencies has led the public to believe that any detectable residue is harmful. Consumers and regulators are more concerned than ever about food safety issues. The food industry is responding to these concerns by implementing Good Manufacturing Practices (GMPs) and Hazard Analysis Critical Control Points (HACCP) programs and by developing faster, more accurate tests to detect pathogen contamination.

The primary concern of consumers, regulatory agencies, and producers in the North American Dairy Industry (NADI) is the Milk and Dairy Beef Quality Assurance Program (MDB-QAP), which is designed to reduce the incidence of violative drug residues in milk and dairy beef by educating producers on proper management techniques, related to the use of drugs. Under the United States

Pasteurized Milk Ordinance (PMO), producers whose Grade "A" permit has been suspended due to violative drug residues in the milk cannot be reinstated until the producer and a licensed veterinarian have completed the Milk & Dairy Beef Drug Residue Prevention (MDB-DRP) and have signed a certificate for display in the milk house. The dairy industry must become proactive in affirming the safety and purity of its products to counteract growing consumer perceptions that milk and meat products may be adulterated. Milk and meat processors are demanding milk and meat free of violative drugs. This is in response to consumer's expectations of milk and meat safety to avoid potential litigation involving product liability.

Water and feed supplies for milk-animal consumption requires a critical overview. A high-producing lactating dairy cow can drink over 150 litres of water on a warm day. An average dairy cow drinks about 110 –125 Lt of water each day depending on atmospheric temperature and nature of feed. However, she will drink less if water quality is poor. In addition, that will limit her milk production and jeopardize her health. Highly contaminated water exposes cattle to disease-causing organisms. A Coliform count over 1/100ml can cause scours in calves. In adult cows, a count of 15-20/100ml can cause diarrhoea and cows may go off-feed. Positive results for faecal Coliform (more than 0 counts/100ml) indicate a pollution problem, which should be investigated and corrected. Microorganisms can contaminate water in wells. However, bacterial contamination is much more likely to occur in the drinking vessel, so keeping water troughs clean is an essential element. Providing a clean water system to milk cows and continual feeding of good quality feed are all factors to be noted in determining critical control points in milk production chain. Ontario producers should contact the Ministry of the Environment (MOE) for help related to taste and odour concerns.

There are seven points considered when assessing water quality, which may include:

1. Organoleptic criteria; Odour and taste

2. Physical and chemical properties

3. Presence of toxic compounds

4. Concentration of mineral compounds

5. Salt imbalance

6. Microbial contamination (e.g. Fungus, bacteria, protozoa, viruses)

7. Pathogenic contamination (e.g. _E. coli_)

For some criteria there is a range of acceptable levels in water but generally a maximum acceptable concentration guideline is given.

Milk and milk products need special care in handling and storage due to their pro bacterial growth medium making them dangerous foods. Dangerous foods are ones that allow for rapid and easy bacterial growth and reproduction e.g. Dairy Products. Hazardous or dangerous is defined as any biological, chemical or physical characteristic that presents an unacceptable consumer health risk. Milk is an excellent medium to grow most of the pathogens and other bacteria under certain growth conditions. Moisture, temperature, growth medium, critical nutrients, aerobic and aerobic conditions jointly contribute to the growth of all microorganisms. Risk to human health starts right from the milking point where mastitis or disease infested milk animal is a CCP risk.

Mastitis Control is critical and needs proper Dry Cow Management (DCM). Dry cow management includes attention to proper procedures for drying-off cows, feeding a special ration, and concern about the cow's environment. Breeding and mastitis problems can result from infections developed during this time. Cows are most susceptible to new mastitis infections during the first two weeks of the dry period, the two weeks before calving, and the two weeks after calving. Bred heifers are prone to new mastitis infections throughout pregnancy, but especially during the last 2 weeks before calving-[99].

Disease control in milk cows is a highly sensible issue and prevention is of high priority. Many animals infected with _Mycobacterium paratuberculosis_ will excrete the bacterium in their milk. This happens most often in cows showing clinical signs of Johne's disease, but also occurs in infected animals that appear healthy. Because no diagnostic test can detect all infected animals on a single herd test, it is better to avoid feeding of raw milk, waste milk, and waste dairy products to vulnerable milk animals in order to eliminate chances of Johne's disease from feeding source and natural nursing should be under controlled conditions. Artificial milk replacers are considered free of _M. paratuberculosis_ because of the way they are processed. A safe and effective alternative to using milk replacers is to pasteurize the waste milk or suitable milk products on the milk farm. Pasteurization kills virtually all _M. paratuberculosis_ that may contaminate raw milk as well as other viral and bacterial agents that could affect the health of dairy heifer replacements. Colostrum, the antibody-rich milk produced by mothers with in the first few days after giving birth, also can contain _M. paratuberculosis_. Because Colostrum is critical to the health and survival of newborns, feeding of Colostrum must be done. However, the risk of transmitting *M. paratuberculosis* infections in Colostrum shall be minimized through qualitative analysis of Colostrum as well as testing of milk animals.

An example of HACCP in a dairy food-processing setting can be found in measures taken at Canadian dairy plants to control outbreaks of *Listeria sp.* There, four areas of possible hazard were delineated: **R**aw material procurement; **P**rocessing technology; **H**ygiene in plant: **C**leaning and **S**anitizing; and **T**esting for quality. These areas were then subjected to a series of control measures, illustrated by the following:

Raw product received must be within a prescribed temperature range, and spills must be cleaned immediately. Footbaths of 200 ppm of residual chlorine should be required of all persons traveling from raw-processing areas to pasteurized-process areas. Processing equipment must be of the proper design and in good working order; there should be no cross-connections between raw product and finished product. Air-circulation systems should flow from processing to receiving, not vice-versa, to prevent admission of airborne bacteria.

Pasteurization at 171 degrees Fahrenheit (77.20 C) instead of 161 degrees Fahrenheit (71.60 C) is recommended when dose loads exceed 4,000 bacteria / gram. Environmental testing for Coliform should be conducted frequently to serve as an indicator of effective cleaning and sanitizing-160. A Total Enterobacteriaceae Count (TEC) is very effective if monitored on a day-to-day basis from the incoming bulk reservoir. *Listeria sp.*, testing should be contracted out unless laboratory facilities are located apart from the plant itself.

During the communist rule in Eastern Europe, few batches of Skimmed Milk were imported in UAE, which contained heat resistant Coliform bacteria. Normal pasteurization temperatures did not eliminate these bacteria. The unpublished study conducted by the author indicated that a 90 C for 16 seconds was needed to destroy those mutant strains of Coliform bacteria. This indicates that where milk powders are the main ingredients, a proper screening of milk powders quality is a QCP (Quality Control Point) as well as a CCP.

Raw Milk quality is an important critical point for the dairy industry. In milk processing, the quality of the product is highly dependent on that of the raw milk used. as in the case of seasonally produced milk, where raw material composition is variable, there are particular advantages in using sensors, which determine the dynamic state of a process on-line, and in real time. However, the complex flow characteristics of typical fluid foods, such as milk, during different stages in processing, call for robust and innovative sensor design.

Once the milk supplied by dairy farms is secured from contaminants, the process of safety continues in the processes of dairy factories where milk is further processed to convert it in to many other dairy products. The products are available in much wider range which may include Table milk, Condensed milk, Evaporated milk, Low fat milk, Long life milk, Powdered milk, Flavoured milk, Goat milk, Sheep milk, Table cream, Crème chantilly, Crème fraiche, Aerosol cream, Canned reduced cream, Clotted cream, Sour cream, Whipping cream, Coffee cream, Long life cream, Yoghurt, Frozen yoghurt, Fruit yoghurts, Cultured buttermilk, Ice cream, Dairy sherbets and many other dairy products.

Pasteurization of milk is a critical factor in quality control of dairy products. Food safety is highly dependent on accurate temperature measurement. Through 'hazard analysis' and a 'critical control system', important temperature control areas are identified and monitored to assure regulatory compliance with the Food Safety. Product cooking and pasteurisation lead to the destruction of pathogenic bacteria and reduction of spoilage organisms to an acceptable level. However, since spores or toxins are not destroyed by this process, cold storage for raw materials and finished goods is vital.

Temperature measurement is also critical to dairy food quality, ensuring product consistency, increasing shelf life, and reducing downgrades. Product heat treatment enables the destruction of pathogenic organisms, reduction of spoilage organisms and the deactivation of enzymes, which influences the setting of coagulum, activity of rennin and maturation of the hard cheese. It also leads to total emulsification of fat, protein, and water, creating a more homogeneous product. Similarly, the prevention of over cooking aids flavour retention in the product. The temperature is also crucial to the process of cooling and slice formation. High product quality manifests itself through the ease of separation of cheese slices from one another, the melting ability of the cheese on the burger and the inhibition of spoilage during shelf life.

Coagulum in cheese making is a critical point to note. In cheese making, the coagulum needs to be cut when it has become sufficiently firm to form discrete particles, which expel whey without fragmenting. For this reason, the moment of curd cutting occurs some time later than the point of gelation. This implies a need to measure the firmness of a gel as it forms and up to the point where it is ready to synerese. At the same time, cutting cheese wire knife shall be free from germs in order to eliminate contamination at this stage of cheese manufacturing. This is to be noted as critical control point.

Curd formation on-line during cheese manufacturing is a critical point for the quality of cheese. As cheese manufacture became increasingly mechanized and food safety issues became more critical, the commercial cheese factory began to operate around a series of quality parameters to assess the gel strength. The scale of operation of modern plants, coupled with ever-increasing demands on quality control, has led to an interest in systems, which monitor curd formation on-line.

Time-based cycle in continuous-cheese-production is a critical factor to cheese safety and quality. Simultaneous operation of a suite of cheese vats requires a time-based cycle with all vats filling and emptying in sequence to assist a continuous flow of milk from the intake/pasteurizing plant. Hence, an on-line device for measuring of curd formation is highly desirable but it would need to be non-intrusive and cleanable-in-place.

From the health of dairy herds to milking – milk receiving in dairy factories – milk processing – dairy manufacturing to packing and preventive measures to control microorganisms involve many critical points which are detrimental to final microorganisms count in cheese. The unripened white cheeses are more critical and require utmost care due to manual manufacturing steps and the low acidic nature of many white cheeses. Middle Eastern white cheeses and Mexican style white cheeses require steps to eliminate pathogens during manufacturing steps, proper heat treatment of milk to destroy pathogens, minimising non-pathogenic microorganisms, controlling growth during processing, personnel hygiene, atmospheric sanitation and packing for acceptable results to satisfy human health and regulatory requirements. A harsh treatment to cheese milk is avoided due to its affect on gel formation. A study conducted by the author concluded that 70 C for a minute is more than sufficient to satisfy all requirements in a white cheese, which is produced from low heat, dried skim milk.

Canada has a very effective food inspection system (CFIA). To maintain and enhance this system, industry and government are continuously incorporating new techniques and methods into food production and inspection to improve food safety. The FSEP is the Canadian Food Inspection Agency's (CFIA) approach to encourage and support the development, implementation, and maintenance of Hazard Analysis Critical Control Point (HACCP) systems in all federally registered establishments of the dairy, and other food manufacturing sectors. Government and food industry developed FSEP jointly in 1991 in consultation with consumer groups.

The Pasteurized Milk Ordinance (PMO), Good Manufacturing Practices (GMPs), and Hazard Analysis Critical Control Points (HACCP) are important controls used by the dairy industry to help provide consumers with a safe milk supply. The PMO is one of the most effective instruments for protecting the quality of Grade A milk in the United States.

National Dairy Council in their comments on Dairy Quality & Safety from Farm to Refrigerator states that the PMO provides a set of requirements for milk and dairy product safety, milk hauling, sanitation, equipment, and labelling. The extensive requirements cover milk from production at the farm to shipment from the processing facility to retail outlets. More than 95% of all the milk produced in the U.S. conforms to Grade A requirements as defined in the PMO. The Grade A raw milk for pasteurization and the Grade A pasteurized milk and milk products must be produced, processed, and pasteurized to conform with specific quality standards, and to sanitation requirements. The National Conference on Interstate Milk Shippers, along with participants from federal, state, and local regulatory agencies, industry, and academia, help to establish standards and regulations related to the PMO-[47].

In 1997, 155.2 billion pounds (70.55 billion Kgs) of raw milk was produced in the U.S. resulting in 1.1 billion pounds (0.5 billion Kgs) of butter, 7.3 billion pounds (3.32 billion Kgs) of cheese, 1.4 billion pounds (0.636 billion Kgs) of dry milk and 1.3 billion gallons of ice cream manufactured. With less than 5% of reported food borne diseases originating from contaminated dairy products, the U.S. dairy industry has an excellent record when considering the amount of dairy products consumed. In-spite of the industry's excellent record, disease-causing bacteria have appeared in dairy-based finished products. Problems associated with the presence of *Listeria monocytogenes*, *Salmonella enteritidis*, *Staphylococcus aureus*, *Escherichia coli* and others have been documented. The products affected have included cheese, ice cream, non-fat dry milk (NFDM), raw and pasteurized milk. Besides microbiological hazards, potential physical hazards include metal, glass, insects, dirt, wood, plastic, and personal effects. Chemical hazards include natural toxins, metals, drug residues, food additives, and inadvertent chemicals-[38].

The U.S. Food and Drug Administration continue a 60-day aging process for raw milk cheese while food technologists still argue the safety of such cheeses. The regulatory agency has expressed some concern over research showing _E. coli_ and other bacteria can survive past the current 60-day holding period. The traditional cheese producers argue that to force pasteurization of all milk used in cheese would spell the end of some of the world's best cheeses. FDA is expected to get closer to issuing its conclusions in coming times [73].

In Netherlands, the Ministry of Agriculture ordered Omni-Kaas u.a. together with the Research Institute for Animal Husbandry and in cooperation with Animal Health Service (GD) and Netherlands Controlling Authority for Milk and Milk Products (COKZ) to develop hygiene protocols, to be used at milking cows and processing of raw milk at the farm. The aim at using these protocols is to decrease the contamination and/or growth of pathogenic bacteria. The use of these hygiene protocols is preferably for people working for farmhouse cheese makers, farmhouse dairy product makers, and dairy farmers. Absence of harmful bacteria before and during preparation of raw milk into farmhouse cheese and other dairy products is very important and it is a sensitive critical factor [145].

In this chapter, we have an overview of the application of HACCP to the Canadian and U.S. dairy industry with some brief comments about other countries experiences. With the importance of Raw Farm Milk (RFM) in determining final product quality, a number of countries are also proposing "cow-to-consumer" systems. We provide a brief overview of the on-farm HACCP components of these programs.

Milk has some unique characteristics in terms of its composition and its potential to be transformed in various ways, enabling it to serve as the basis for numerous dairy products. However milk is also a vulnerable product that must be handled with the greatest care to maintain its quality. For a long time the pollution of milk with undesirable substances has been a specific area of concern.

Some substances that may be found in a cow's feed or that are used as medication are not allowed to enter the milk, or do so in only minute quantities. These are then less of a threat. Such substances include the heavy metals, as demonstrated by the sampling and testing that has already been under way for a considerable time. This has shown that the levels of heavy metals in milk are very low. Other residues or contaminants, including diverse persistent (poorly degradable) environmental pollutants can actually accumulate in milk fat. Because of adequate measures to protect the environment, the levels of these chemicals in milk are low, well under the limits set for these pollutants.

Government policy aims mainly at preventing and controlling the contamination of foodstuffs. By subjecting veterinary drugs and pesticides to strict authorization requirements, undesirable residue accumulation in dairy products is minimised. Dairy cows can for example be exposed to traces of pesticides via the raw materials used in animal feeds, if these chemicals are used to treat the crop. When authorizing these pesticides the possibility that they may end up in milk is taken into consideration. In the case of residues and contaminants that may constitute a danger to public health, the government determines by regulation the maximum residue levels that are permitted in foodstuffs. For pesticides and veterinary drugs the limits are set very comprehensively. The regulations for animal feeds contain limits for environmental contaminants. These limits ensure that there is no undesirable accumulation of these chemicals in milk and that the limits set in the Commodity Act are not exceeded.

The setting of limits for residues and contaminants is increasingly harmonized at an international level. The worldwide harmonisation in the Codex (a co-operative project of the Food and Agriculture Organisation of the United Nations and the World Health Organization) is also of increasing significance. In the event of any trade disputes relating to residue limits, the World Trade Organization (WTO) will take the limits set in the Codex as its starting point.

The example of dairy control can also be seen with on-farm HACCP systems in the Netherlands and in Australia. In Canadian and U.S. applications, the regulatory agencies provide an example of a generic HACCP model designed to control mastitis infections. As with any HACCP system, they also point to the importance of having a program of good management practices being present to complement the HACCP program.

In the United States, voluntary Canadian and mandatory Australian dairy processing HACCP programs have also been outlined. A detailed overview of the International Dairy Food Association's (IDFA) Dairy Product Safety System has been provided. Generic HACCP models for two dairy products have been presented: cheddar cheese and ice cream. Again the importance of having effective prerequisite programs is noted and emphasised. The cost factor involved in planning, implementation, validation, and verification were also taken in to consideration. In an application of the cheddar cheese HACCP model to a large cheese plant, annual validation and verification is estimated to require 600-720 person hours at a cost in the range of $14,000-$18,000. Initial planning and implementation was estimated required 800 person-hours at a cost of slightly less than $20,000.

The dairy industry learned a very valuable lesson from the seafood and meat industries and has taken the initiative to develop their own HACCP / Dairy Product Safety system. This system provides adequate safety control of products and is functional in a practical application. The IDFA program has been officially endorsed by the FDA, and is widely used by the dairy manufacturing industry. If the dairy industry continues to fully implement HACCP at a rapid pace, there will be no need for mandatory HACCP from federal and state agencies. As with most food industry applications of HACCP, an important means of controlling potential hazards in dairy product manufacturing is the use of raw ingredients and materials that are hazard free. If these raw ingredients are hazard free this implies that the only hazards that need to be controlled by a CCP are those that arise within the dairy operation itself. The importance of raw milk in the manufacturing process points to the necessity of having some type of HACCP-based system implemented at the farm level. If adoption of HACCP by the manufacturers/processors and producers does not continue to increase, HACCP should become a mandatory regulatory tool in the United States.

In Canada, the Canadian Food Inspection Agency (CFIA) is responsible for establishing dairy product standards and grades, conducting dairy plant inspections, and regulating packaging and labelling requirements. The CFIA is also responsible for animal health programs and the monitoring of product safety.

The CFIA through their Food Safety Enhancement Program (FSEP) have evolved HACCP generic models for dairy products. Included in the list are butter products e.g. salted, unsalted, light, dairy spreads and blends, Ice Cream; frozen dairy products e.g., light ice cream, ice milk, frozen yoghurt, Soft serve ice cream; frozen dairy product mixes e.g. includes soft serve yoghurt, milk shake mix, UHT milk; ultra-high temperature treated milk products which are aseptically packaged and do not require refrigeration for preservation e.g., UHT cream, UHT milk shakes.

D. Critical Control & Meat Industry:
Humans have hunted animals for meat soon after the arrival of Adam on earth. Meat has played a vital role in human diet since tens and thousands of years before the recorded history of humankind. Though many groups in North America are advocating a vegetable diet in human food, recent scare from mad cow disease prompted many to turn away from beef, the cardiac disease scare also influenced many to be away from juicy beef

stakes but meat market will never scare the majority of humans who rely on meat delicacies for their choice, appetite and nutrition.

Meat and meat products provide proteins, iron, zinc and niacin equivalents. Meat is an important source of vitamin B_{12}. Many countries including Canada are working to produce lean meat. A grading system allows North American customers to make a choice between the range of leanest meat and high fat meat. Health safety plays a vital role in selectivity of such meats. Lean cuts of beef, veal, lamb and goat makes it easy for the consumer to select more healthy lean meat. Beef meat is domesticated many centuries ago and it is obtained from many kinds of cattle including cow, buffalo, etc. Many parts of beef meat like butt, fillets, round, rump and loin, silverside, sirloin, ribs, spare ribs, bacon bones etc., have their own values in terms of taste and nutrition but their safety and risk carries equal weightage to human. Some portions like brain, kidneys, liver tongue, and joints are nutritionally different and may require different process to make it safe for human consumption. Especially joints are given extra heat treatments to destroy microorganisms dangerous to health.

Meat products like sausages and preserved meats go through factory processes where its ingredients selection during raw stage, its processing, chilling, packing and freezing carries many critical stages where special controls are applied to enhance its wholesomeness during the prescribed and regulated shelf lives. The preserved meat includes meats, which have been processed, cured, smoked, frozen so that they can be used later as joints, slices, spreads etc. The important meat products are Bloodwurst, Bockwurst, Black pudding, Bratwurst, Cabanossi, Boudin blanc, Frankfurter, Garlic sausage, Hurka, Haggis, Knackwurst, Mortadella, Plockwurst, Italian salami, Sopressa salami, Turkey salami, Toulouse sausage, Halal Qeema, Halal beef sausage, Turkish Kebabs, Pakistani Kebabs and Weisswurst.

Meat being a rich source of nutrients, it attracts many potential pathogens and spoilage organisms which mainly act on meat proteins. The spoilage organisms like _Clostridium sporogenes_, _Clostridium perfringens_, _Clostridium septicum_, _Pseudomonas sp._, _Achromobacter sp._, _Acinetobacter calcoaceticus_, and many others produce slime, discolouration of meat resulting in souring, putrefaction, and intolerable bad odours. Some of these spoilage organisms are potent pathogens i.e. _Clostridium sp._ Even processed meats will also be affected by _Achromobacter sp._, _Pseudomonas sp._, _Lactobacillus sp._, salt tolerant _Streptococcus faecalis, and Clostridium sp._, and _Micrococcus sp._, if not prevented through critical control measures. The bacterium _Clostridium_ *botulinum* is most notorious in causing food poisoning to humans, which is mostly associated with canned meats. The spores of this bacterium are very heat resistant and need 249.8 °F (121 °C) for three minutes to destroy it in low acid foods. *Clostridium perfringens* is known to sporulate in meat products and produce enterotoxin in foods. The selectivity of critical control points in meat and meat products will depend on the historical evidence, possible contamination points, and microorganism destructive treatments, which will destroy such, and similar organisms and preventive measures which will eliminate the production of toxins during transition to processing and consumption.

Chemical food poisoning and safety from it, requires intense attention in the meat industry. Chemical additives used in meat industry go under rigorous evaluations to pass safety parameters in order to be allowed as additives in meat. However, their rate of addition is a critical control point, which should be adequately administered according to the formulation and regulatory guidance. Nitrates and nitrites are added to meat products to inhibit the growth of *Clostridium perfringens* and *Clostridium botulinum* and to produce desirable meat oriented colour. These products are carcinogenic and shall be strictly used as per the regulatory limits. Similarly additives are to be added with caution, as there added quantities should reflect its purpose not its blind usage to replace risk preventive processing.

Packaging materials for meat, packaging machines, packaging temperatures, and subsequent meat storage are the generic critical factors. A proper labelling covering all aspects of consumer safety and product perseverance suffice the need of postproduction transitional measures.

Inspection of meat processing and distributing units is part of food safety drive. In 1998, after two years of negotiation between the meat industry, consumer groups, and Congress, the U.S. Department of Agriculture (USDA) introduced HACCP system of meat inspection. "Hazard Analysis and Critical Control Point," or HACCP, was the first major meat inspection overhaul in America since the early 1900s. Under the aegis of the USDA, the "poke and sniff" method has been in application as the first comprehensive American meat-inspection system employed in slaughterhouses around the country.

USDA inspectors were given the authority to physically monitor all carcasses and cuts of meat as they moved down the slaughter line. Inspectors would literally touch, smell, and prod the meat to test its wholesomeness. The "poke and sniff" system was designed to prevent rotten, blemished, or damaged meat from entering the food supply. The inspectors, who used their sense of smell and touch to distinguish contaminated meat from clean cuts, routed out cuts of meat with lesions, growths, and abrasions. However, the "poke and sniff" system had its drawbacks, most troubling of which was the inability of the system to detect invisible pathogens and microbes-104.

After the 1993 Jack in the Box _E. coli_ outbreak, in which four children died and 700 people fell ill, both consumers and politicians lobbied for a revised system that would pay greater attention to microbiology. The common consensus in food safety was that invisible germs posed as great a danger to consumer health as visible contamination such as legions and diseased parts, and that the "poke and sniff" system was neither stringent nor scientific enough to ensure the safety of American meat.

CCPs are the realistic steps in food safety. The USDA made plans to analyze all of the critical control points where germs could enter the system, and in order to monitor contamination, they introduced a science-based program of microbial testing. Instead of just conducting a physical "poke and sniff" test, under the new HACCP system, inspectors were mandated to make sure meat plants tested carcasses for invisible pathogens such as _E. coli_ and _Salmonella_. This was a major change in the philosophy of meat inspection: Meat plants were ordered to conduct their own microbial testing, and the responsibility shifted from USDA inspectors to the meat plant owners and operators. The meat industry was for the first time legally obligated to actively participate in food-safety and inspection programs.

Under the HACCP system, there is no single way to inspect a plant, no pre-ordained template to ensure the wholesomeness of meat. Instead, each meatpacking and processing plant is required to create and implement their own HACCP system, which they submit to the USDA for approval. Once approved, USDA inspectors on the ground, monitor this plan. Instead of the old "poke and sniff" method, inspectors now make sure that meat plants follow their HACCP plan.

According to figures gathered by the Centers for Disease Control (CDC), the incidence of _Salmonella sp._, in the U.S. is slightly lower under the HACCP system than it was under the old system. Elsa Murano, undersecretary of food safety at USDA, said that HACCP "brings the system up to the 21st century. It was what we needed to do. It's improved food safety in meat and poultry." Salmonella is a group of bacteria that live in the intestinal tracts of humans and animals, including birds. Humans can acquire Salmonellosis after they consume foods that have been contaminated by animal feces that contain salmonella bacteria.

However, critics argue that the CDC figures show a decline in _Salmonella Sp._, emerging before the full implementation of HACCP occurred. They argue that the meat industry cannot be trusted to test and regulate itself. According to former meat inspector Patsy McKee, "In theory, HACCP is great. However, these plants are not going to regulate themselves. Plants are not effectively implementing their HACCP programs."

International importance of Food safety geared momentum from American concept. HACCP invention in the United States showed a path of safety for meat producers internationally. Since January 1997, all Australian abattoirs have been required to operate under a new Australian Standard (ARMCANZ National Standards), which includes a mandatory HACCP plan. Abattoirs exporting to the United States have also implemented the US Mega Regs-88.

All Australian plants are required to operate under an Australian standard with a HACCP program. Each processing facility has a unique Meat Safety Quality Assurance (MSQA) program. The Australian beef and sheep meat industries have integrated HACCP into a Total Quality Management (TQM) system that incorporates Good Manufacturing Practices (GMP), HACCP, and Standard Operating Procedures. The program is called Meat Safety Quality Assurance (MSQA). It is the responsibility of each participating Australian establishment to develop and implement an MSQA system specific to the company-201.

These individualized programs are extensive – they are HACCP-based, comply with United States Department of Agriculture's (USDA) Mega Regs, and are audited by the Australian Quarantine and Inspection Service (AQIS) which is the agent for the USDA and the Canadian Food Inspection Agency (CFIA) certifying compliance to North American standards.

Mega Regs played an important role in food safety. The New US regulations, the so-called "Mega Regs" took affect on January 26, 1998. The Mega Regs set new standards for control of _E. coli_ and _Salmonella sp._, bacteria on poultry carcasses and offered consequences for companies unable to meet the new standards. Mega Regs actually states that there will be "zero milk and faecal material" on the carcases. This means cattle are much easier to process without contamination, if they have: clean hides, dry udders, empty stomachs and are calm- not stressed by dogs, transport and other cattle etc.

TQM is one of the basis in HACCP management. J. M. Juran (1993) in his Quality Planning and Analysis book defines "TQM as the system of activities directed at achieving delighted customers, empowered employees, higher revenues and lower costs"-127. HACCP could be incorporated in any quality system e.g. ISO-9001: 2000.

GMP's deal with what we do before we produce a product. The six HACCP prerequisite programs focus on premises, transportation, & storage, equipment, personnel, sanitation & pest control, and recalls. HACCP prerequisite programs are actually GMP's. An effective prerequisite program will actually decrease the number of critical control points during the hazard analysis of the product/process.

A unique producer of Beef in the United States refused to use Bovine Growth Hormones (BGH). Mel Coleman Sr.'s story starts at a meeting of leading beef producers in 1979. Mel Coleman first brings up the idea of producing beef without using antibiotics and hormones. As per him, fundamentally, it is wrong to use medicine for the sake of production. We have a HACCP system in place right from conception to consumption. For instance, in his system when a calf is born it is critical that he gets that first milk from his mother called Colostrum, which is full of antibodies. That is a critical control point for a live animal. When the calf is weaned, that is a critical control point because it is stressful for that young animal to be taken away from his mother-146.

Culling out the diseased animal from slaughtering is a major priority and an important critical control point. Beef animals having higher antibiotic levels than permitted should be culled out, this a controlling point for all the animals. Similarly, in a meat plant or in a slaughtering plant, it is the critical control requirement that when the animal is eviscerated that a gut is not split and the insides of the viscera is scattered through the meat because it would contaminate it. That is very critical not only safeguarding the meat from spoilage but mainly to eliminate multiplication of pathogens after contamination.

He went clear on to the critical control point of a cold store and lay down the procedure for storekeeper to keep meat frozen or chilled as recommended. It is critical that incharge keep the meat cold enough as recommended and keep the surrounding clean. The two main things in the meat store are temperature and cleanliness. On industrial level he talked about critical control points from birth clear through to the kitchen, conception to consumption. Meat professional and technologist always believe that there needs to be control from conception to consumption.

Adhesion of bacteria to surfaces in meat processing environments can result in biofilm formation on meat contact surfaces or other areas such as floors, walls, and drains. It has been shown that microorganisms can remain on equipment surfaces after standard cleaning practices. Thus cleaning and sanitization is to be religiously followed, verified and record maintained.

Biofilms have been recognized as a potential source of contamination, which may lead to product spoilage (reduced shelf life) and/or disease transmission. As bacterial attachment to a surface is one of the first steps in biofilm formation, any surface that can inhibit adhesion would decrease the potential for biofilm development.

Ground meat including hamburger, pork patties, and ground lamb and ground poultry products such as chicken patties or ground turkey receive more handling than roasts, chops, and other cuts or parts. More handling, especially grinding and mixing, means a greater likelihood of contamination by bacteria such as _Salmonella sp._, _Campylobacter sp._, Listeria _sp._, and _E. coli_ _0157:H7_. So grinding process of meat is a major critical control point.

Keep ground meat and poultry in the refrigerator or freezer and use it within one or two days. To prevent ground beef from premature browning, it should be tightly wrapped and frozen, or stored for no more than two days at 40 °F (4.40 °C). The purple-brown colour that sometimes develops in ground beef is due to oxidation, which does not affect the safety of the meat. However, a colour parameter is a quality issue and can be included critical control point for quality matter.

For best quality, frozen raw meats should be used within 3 to 4 months. Defrost frozen ground meats in the refrigerator, never at room temperature. If microwave defrosting is committed, cook immediately. Defrosting and thawing are critical to meat and meat products safety.

Over all hygiene of the plant and home kitchens dealing meat and meat products are critical to meat safety. A proper cleaning and sanitization system based on Good Cleaning Practices (GCPs) shall be used.

Processing of meat to manufacture meat products is for the purpose of enhancing keeping quality and developing organoleptic taste as per the parameters. To destroy any bacteria that might be present, one must cook ground meat or poultry thoroughly. The Food Safety and Inspection Service (FSIS) of the USDA recommend the use of a meat thermometer when cooking meat and poultry. Check ground beef patties with a thermometer to be sure they are cooked to an internal temperature of 160 °F (71.20 °C). Ground poultry should be cooked to 165 °F (73.90 °C) measured by a meat thermometer, which has been inserted into the thickest part of the patty. If a beef patty is not thick enough to check from the top, insert the meat thermometer sideways into the patty. The thermometer shall be calibrated and sanitized before inserting in to the products. These are the noted critical factors to control as CCPs.

Cross contamination points should be properly listed and prevention steps taken to avoid contamination. Keep everything clean and sanitized– personnel uniforms, production environment, hands, utensils, counters, cutting boards and sinks to avoid cross contamination. Do not let raw meat or poultry juices touch ready-to-eat foods either in the refrigerator or during preparation and processing.

Packing of meat products in right and acceptable material and keeping it at recommended storage temperatures would suffice the critical safety requirements. The foreign body contamination precaution would be similar to any automated food filling and packing systems except the temperature variance.

In Canada, CFIA developed HACCP Generic Models for Meat and Poultry products. These generic models were developed through pilot projects or expert committees, to be used as examples or guidelines for various processes/product types. Specific generic models can be used as a starting point upon selection or template for further customization to reflect a particular plant environment and specific product. Generic models are designed for use in a plant after needed modifications from plant to plant and product to product. They must be adapted to reflect the specific conditions of a given plant.

In Canada, list of Meat and poultry meat products includes: Beef Slaughter; slaughter operations for all red meat species, (except hog), Boneless Beef; red meat boning operations, Cooked Sausage; cooked, cured, ready-to-eat meat products e.g., wieners, bologna, Meat spread (Cretons); cooked, pasteurized meat products requiring refrigeration for preservation e.g., head cheese, Cretons, Fermented Smoked Sausage; dry fermented meat products sausages e.g., salami and some types of pepperoni, Assembled (Pizza); multi commodity food products with or without meat e.g. pizza, submarines, sandwiches, Dried Meat (Beef Jerky) non-fermented dried cured meat products e.g., beef jerky, Cooked/Sliced Ham; cooked, sliced meat packaged after heat treatment e.g., luncheon meats, Ready to Eat Poultry Products: (Fully Cooked Chicken Wings); cooked, ready-to-eat poultry products e.g., chicken wings, drumsticks, (Chicken Breast Fillets); raw or partially cooked, may be cured e.g., seasoned or breaded breasts, fingers, Chinese Style Dried Sausage; cured, dried/ sausages (not ready to eat) , Mechanically Separated Meat (Chicken); mechanically separated or deboned meat products , Poultry slaughter (Chilled Ready to Cook Whole Chicken); poultry slaughter operations e.g., turkey, Cornish hens, fowl , Hog slaughter; hog slaughter operations , Ready to Cook Poultry Products (Seasoned Formed, Breaded Chicken Burger); poultry products such as burgers, nuggets , Prosciutto (Salted Ham); Cured hind leg of pork, prepared in accordance with a variety of traditions Fresh/Frozen Stored Products (Meat, Non-meat, Food, Non-food).

E. Critical Control & Seafood:

Humans even before the advent of written history have consumed seafoods and in modern times certain regions are significantly dependent on fish and fisheries products. In Canada, fish remains a staple food for people of minority groups like Inuit, American Indian tribes and social groups living in fishing belt. In western countries, the comparative consumption of fish is lower than that of meat and poultry. Fish are considered healthy to heart because of its polyunsaturated omega-3 fatty acids, eicosapentaenoic acid, and decosahexaenoic acid. These fatty acids are believed to be converted in to prostaglandin, which lower the triglycerides in the blood of the fish-consuming individual. Which in turn strengthen immune system, lowers the risk to heart attacks and improves arthritic ailment?

The fish and fisheries products are mostly consumed fresh. To store fish for 2-3 days period, its fins, scales, gills, and guts are removed and packed in anaerobic clean container under refrigeration temperatures of < 39.2 °F (4 °C). The frozen fish are kept for a maximum period of six months at deep frozen temperatures. The consumers should look for freezer burn when buying frozen fish to avoid health risks, avoid rancid smell when buying smoked fish and buy only fresh looking raw fish whose gills are still fresh enough to attract appetite. The best examples of edible fish are Barramundi (*Lates calcarifer*), Australian bass (*Macquaria novemaculeata*), Black fish (*Girella tricuspidata*), Carp (Cyprinus *carpio*) and Coral trout (*Plectropoma maculatum*) etc. Examples of other products are shellfish; Abalone (*Haliotis ruber*), Cockle (Katylesia *sp.*), Crabs; *Scylla serrata, Charybdis cruciata, Macrochira Kaempferi, Cherax destructor*, American Lobster *Homarus americanus*, Blue leg prawn *Penaeus latisulcatus* and School prawn *Metapenaeus bennettae* etc.

Preserved seafoods necessitate the importance of eliminating health risks during the given shelf life of fish and fish products. Canned anchovy, Caviar, Cod dried and salted, Smoked cod, Kamaboko, Canned pilchard, Canned salmon, Salmon roe, Canned sardine, Smoked trout and Canned tuna etc., are the best example of preserved seafoods. The normal principles in food preservation require scientifically proven preventive measures, which require implementation through HACCP food safety system.

While the seafoods are good source of nutrition, dietary benefits, and therapeutic value, these products are not risks free to human health. Naturally, these products are excellent for human nutrition; the conditions under which they are harvested, processed, packed, stored, and consumed carry certain risk factors, which shall be prevented to maintain wholesomeness of this delicate food. Microbiological contaminants are prevalent in fish and fisheries products. *Vibrio parahaemolyticus* has been the cause of commonest food poisoning in Far East and Japan among prawn and crab eaters. *Aeromonas hydrophila* is associated with diarrhoea to humans when ingested through fish consumption. Scombrotoxic fish poisoning is caused by toxins produced during the storage of fish and may cause vomiting, stomach crams and diarrhoea to consumers. Ciguatera poisoning is common to pacific and Caribbean consumers of fish such as barracudas, sea basses, etc. The toxin may be entrapped in the livers of such fish and it will organoleptically appear sound.

In December 1995, the United States Food and Drug Administration (US-FDA) issued seafood regulations based on the principles of Hazard Analysis and Critical Control Point (HACCP). A Critical control step means a point, step, or procedure in a seafood process at which control can be applied, and a seafood safety hazard can as a result, be prevented, eliminated, or reduced to acceptable levels. Any missing link in seafood safety results in someone's misery.

A tender tuna steak lightly seasoned with lemon pepper and grilled over a charcoal fire is one way to please a seafood lover's palate. However, blue marlin served up with a dose of scombroid poisoning or steamed oysters with a touch of Norwalk-like virus are more likely to turn the stomach nasty, instead of treating the palate. Generally, seafood is very safe to eat, but no food is completely safe, and problems do occur. HACCP system is meant to prevent such an occurrence.

Phillip Spiller; director of the U.S. Food and Drug Administration's (US-FDA) Office of Seafood; pointed out that while FDA has regulated seafood for decades, a new FDA program that went into effect in December 1997 aims to further ensure seafood's safety. This program requires seafood processors, repackers and warehouses in both domestic and foreign exporters to this country, to follow a modern food safety system that is Hazard Analysis and Critical Control Point, or HACCP. Seafood safety could be further ensured if seafood retailers integrate HACCP in their operations. Consumers are expected to continue their role, too, choosing seafood retailers and products carefully, handling and serving their products with care in the home. "Consumers are a step along the way to ensuring that only safe seafood goes in the mouth," says Mary Snyder, director of programs and enforcement policy in FDA's Office of Seafood. The consumers have to know what they are eating, where they are eating and what they are doing about any suspected hazard-[41].

How to identify an acceptable Sea Food Handler who would provide safe seafood is another criteria to consider. Anyone who has ever smelled rotting seafood at the fish counter has a good idea of what a poorly run seafood market smells like. However, the absence of any strong odour does not necessarily mean that the seller is practicing safe food handling techniques. Based on FDA's Food Code, here are some other points to consider Employees should be in clean clothing and wearing hair coverings. They should not be smoking, eating, or playing with their hair. They should not be sick or have any open wounds. Employees should be wearing disposable food grade gloves when handling food and change gloves after doing non-food tasks and after handling any raw seafood. Fish should be displayed on a thick bed of fresh, not melting ice, preferably in a case or under some type of cover. Fish should be arranged with the bellies down so that the melting ice drains away from the fish, thus reducing the chances of spoilage.

Any normal consumer must evaluate general impression of the facility, it should look clean, it should smell clean without any putrefying odour, and it should be free from of roaches, flies, and other bugs. A well-maintained facility can indicate that the vendor is following good sanitation practices. The seafood employee should be knowledgeable about different types of seafood and its preservation. He or she should be able to tell you how old the products are and explain why their seafood is fresh. If they cannot, you should take your business elsewhere and satisfy your requirements so that you entertain your confidence.

There are four types of contamination commonly found in all foods variably, namely Microorganisms, Chemical, Physical and natural Toxins which will generate strings of critical control points (CCPs) during farming, catching, processing, packing, and storage of fish and fish products:

Bacteria, parasites, viruses, and microbial toxins cause microorganism's hazards. Bacterial Pathogens associated with raw and processed seafood are *Salmonella sp., C. botulinum, Listeria monocytogenes, Vibrio cholera* O1, *Vibrio cholerae non-Ol, Vibrio parahaemolyticus,* and *Vibrio vulnificus* etc. Parasites that are sometimes found in raw seafood are: *Anisakis sp.* and related worms, *Diphyllobothrium sp., Nanophyetus sp., Eustrongylides sp., Acanthamoeba sp.,* and other free-living amoebae, *Ascaris lumbricoides* and *Trichuris trichiura* etc. Viruses that sometimes contaminate raw seafood are: Hepatitis A virus, Hepatitis E virus, Rotavirus, Norwalk virus groups, and other viral agents.

Chemical contaminants are either from naturally occurring toxins and/or polluted environments or from human error in not rinsing, storing or diluting chemicals correctly and sometimes due to cross contamination. Sea borne spill of oil is the major hazard for edible fish.

Physical contaminants are foreign bodies, which find their way into the edible product. These may be such things as glass, metal, plastic, jewellery, hair, insects, dust, or others.

Natural Toxins found in seafoods are critical risks related to human health hazards that are: Ciguatera poisoning, Shellfish toxins (PSP, DSP, NSP, ASP), Scombroid Tetrodotoxin (Pufferfish) etc.

Critical Control and Food Allergen:

Food allergy is one of the major forms of adverse reaction to foods. A food allergy is an immune response to a food, which is normally a protein or glyco-protein present in a food naturally, or by contamination, or produced by processing, cooking, or digestion. Food allergy is now recognised as an important food safety issue. The preventive measures shall be taken by all food manufacturers in formulating foods so as to avoid, wherever possible, inclusion of unnecessary major allergens as ingredients.

The food operators shall organize raw material supplies, production, production schedules, and cleaning procedures so as to prevent cross-contamination of products by foreign allergens. It is a necessity to train all food ingredient formulation, weighing, recombining and processing personnel in an understanding of necessary measures and the reasons for them to provide appropriate warning, to potential purchasers, of the presence or possible presence of a major allergen in a product.

A HACCP system will place an appropriate system for recall of any product found contaminated with allergens, at the same time if a product is composed of one or more allergen ingredients it shall be declared on the label as a warning. There are few foods or food ingredients to which someone, somewhere, is not allergic, in some cases in very small quantities, but the risk should be treated seriously and safeguarded against by all food manufacturers, retailers, and caterers. Over 170 foods have been documented in the scientific literature as causing allergic reactions. The food manufacturer should concentrate on food allergens declared by regulatory agencies in Canada and the United States.

The three different critical points by which an allergen could end up in a food are cross-contamination of an ingredient before it is received or after the receipt, accidental wrong formulation and cross-contamination by an allergen from a different product in the system. Appropriate preventive controls in the food processing and production and label warnings to the potential purchasers are necessary. Food products containing milk proteins, milk sugar, egg proteins, Soya protein, gluten, certain preservatives, sodium salt and other known allergens should be labelled with clear indication of their presence. For more information, please refer Food Safety Risks in Chapter: 04 of this book.

HACCP and Retail Food Operations:

HACCP plans and operating procedures are adaptable to any food production, processing, or distribution activity. The food industry began realizing a number of years ago that the lack of proper food-handling procedures could lead to very drastic situations concerning food-borne microorganisms, toxic chemicals, and physical contaminants. The United States Center for Disease Control and Prevention (CDC) reported that they in the United States experience 4 to 7 million cases of food-borne illnesses resulting in 5,000 deaths and $3 billion to $6 billion in costs annually. The U.S. food distribution and marketing system is a potential source for these causative agents-[10].

Federal, state, and local food regulatory agencies, along with other food educational and organizational groups are working to implement the HACCP Food Safety Program in the entire food chain — from producers and growers to processors, and on to the marketing and distribution channels.

The operating principles of HACCP system are applicable to any of the food chain activities and to any size of business. The critical areas within supermarkets and other food sales and marketing areas that have a potential to cause consumer harm are essentially the same whether the operation is a large, multifunctional store or a small mom-and-pop grocery and/or deli.

The entire concept of the HACCP program is to provide the consumer with a safe consumable product. The responsibility for producing and marketing these safe products rests with the food industry. Workers in retail food establishments must be imparted with understanding about the hazards that are present and the effects these hazards might have on anyone consuming the products.

People in the United States and Canada do not go to the supermarket with any fear concerning the safety of the food that they purchase and take home. Majority of the food-borne illnesses related to retail food operations are not created in the food stores. They are created at home or in a restaurant where people frequently dine on foods of their choice. A Guide for Retail Food Establishments could be obtained from US-FDA.

Food allergens are the critical factor in retail food business where unknowingly consumers end up consuming foods where added ingredients could be an allergen for vulnerable consumers. The United States Food and Drug Administration have identified eight foods or food ingredients that are responsible for 90 percent of the food allergic reactions. Those foods are milk and milk products, eggs, legumes (peanuts and soy), tree nuts, wheat, crustaceans, fish, and shellfish. Allergen risk assessment and control is not an easy task at the manufacturing level, let alone at the retail level. Nevertheless, retail food establishments also need to evaluate their operations to determine where allergen hazards might occur and establish methods for managing those hazards. All aspects and stages of the operation must be part of the risk evaluation.

Ingredient purchasing and subsequent storage are important steps where screening of raw materials and processed ingredients that could cause allergy and possible contaminants could be checked, and prevention taken in time. Such preventive steps could include obtaining a fully disclosed ingredient list from the supplier including details on sub-ingredients, protecting raw ingredients in storage to avert contamination, labelling raw material to indicate allergen content and taking preventive measures while substituting raw materials verifying that substitution material have the same allergen profile as the original material. A complete control would require preventive steps during Preparation, Recombination, Production, Packaging, Labelling, Sanitation, Display/Service, and Staff Training/Education.

During the production, make all products with allergenic ingredients at one time or at the end of a production run, then perform a complete clean up before running other products. Do not allow reuse of single service articles such as tray liners. Dedicate separate utensils or equipment to allergenic products whenever possible. Protect work-in-process from cross contact with allergenic products/ingredients in use at other work areas. Discourage rework or carry-over product; if necessary only use like into like product. Use standardized recipes so that ingredients are the same from one batch or serving to the next.

For Packaging and Labelling, verify label accuracy; update to reflect current formula, ensure compliance with labelling regulations which generally require declaration of all ingredients; exception to this include spices, some colours, flavours, processing aids and incidental additives at insignificant levels or that have no technical function or effect. Allergenic ingredients are never exceptions, they must be declared at any level - there is no 'insignificant level'. Check labels on incoming ingredients; supplier may have sent the wrong product or may have used the wrong label. Limit use of precautionary labelling (such as 'may contain') in lieu of good manufacturing practices. Do not list ingredients that are not in the formula. Consider cross-contact potential on packaging/portioning utensils. Consider using terms for ingredients that explain from where they are derived and what source.

Nevertheless, because of the large complex distribution system that we use to deliver our food from the supplier to the consumer, any situation that arises concerning the safety of the food product can result in literally hundreds of people becoming ill. The Critical Control Points (CCPs) can range from the bacteria spread on the knife or slicers in the meat department to an improper use of chemical sanitizer used in the deli to a light bulb that inadvertently falls into the mixer in the bakery. The incidence of dead fly falling in to cheese vat from the insect killer lamp due to air blowing from air conditioning unit or a roach crawling under the mechanical box of a food packing machine should not be a surprise but pre-emptive actions should be taken to prevent such discontentment.

Process approach to HACCP is new to many regulators. It is better designed for use in retail and food service settings than traditional HACCP approaches because it eliminates lengthy flow-charting and hazard analysis for every type of food product. It is practical to identify possible hazards associated with retail and food service operations and the control measures available to prevent, reduce, or eliminate the risks of these hazards. Application of the "process approach" of HACCP to routine inspections of retail and food service operations is easier and motivating to accomplish. In the process approach, desired and planned results are achieved more efficiently when activities and related resources are managed systematically as a critical process. Thus hazards and risks involved are easily identified, understood, and prevented.

The HACCP program is designed so that we are aware of the Critical Control Points (CCPs) that we have within our establishment, and that we ensure that these critical factors are monitored in such a way as to produce a safe food supply.

HACCP & Catering Industry:

Food safety should be a primary concern when buying food from outside caterers. Epidemiological data show that many outbreaks of food poisoning are caused by food produced in mass catering. Large-scale catering operations are particularly hazardous because of the way the food is stored and handled. Outbreaks can involve large number of dining people. A Person fed through mass catering is especially vulnerable - for instance children, the elderly, and hospital patients, especially those who are immuno-compromised.

The Hazard Analysis Critical Control Point (HACCP) system can be applied to the Catering Industry, which will consist of, an assessment of hazards associated with growing, harvesting, processing or manufacturing, storage, marketing, preparation and/or use of a given raw material or food product. Determination of the critical control points is required for controlling any identified hazards and establishment of procedure to monitor critical control points. All seven principles shall apply no matter what type of food segment is adopting the HACCP process. Food handlers prepare many different types of foods in many different types of business. It does not matter what type of food is prepared, caterer's goal is to provide food to the customer that is maintained at required temperatures, looks good, smells good, tastes good and is safe to eat.

Catering establishments such as restaurants, cafes and canteens are a major source of food poisoning outbreaks. This fact is borne out in the epidemiological data available for food-borne associated illnesses. Current food safety knowledge and management practices among caterers are clearly inadequate and new flexible, process based systems are required which take into account the highly variable nature of catering operations i.e. changing products and procedures, diverse employee capabilities and inconsistent product volumes etc. Such flexible, efficient, and robust systems are best achieved through the application and integration of Hazard Analysis and Critical Control Point (HACCP) systems within normal catering operations.

First attention is to legislative changes, which will place the onus on food operators, including caterers, to fully implement food safety management systems through implementation of HACCP principles. The principle objective of this proposal is to carry out the research, development and dissemination work that will be essential to ensure that appropriate, specific, detailed and applicable HACCP systems are available to caterers. The free availability of such a knowledge-based expert system would be invaluable in promoting the consistent delivery of safe food to consumers and would facilitate nation-wide compliance with the existing and proposed national and trans-national legislation.

The United States Food and Drug Administration (US-FDA) publishes the Food Code, which provides guidance on food safety, sanitation and fair dealing that can be uniformly adopted by jurisdictions for regulating the retail segment of the food industry. The model Food Code is the cumulative result of the efforts and recommendations of many contributing individuals, agencies, and organizations. Section 3-301.11 of the 1999 Food Code, entitled "Preventing Contamination from Hands" was added to the code in response to outbreaks of food borne illnesses caused by food that had been contaminated with pathogens transmitted by food preparation workers. FDA believes that the considerable number of illnesses transmitted by food worker contamination of food demands rigorous intervention measures. Three major intervention areas are addressed: exclusion of ill food workers from the workplace, removal of pathogens from the hands of food workers, and the use of barriers to prevent bare-hand contact with ready-to-eat foods-[121].

Health Canada has taken steps in collaboration with the aircraft catering services industry to improve public health standards for all travelling Canadians and non-Canadians. Health Canada's Occupational Health and Safety Agency (OHSA) have signed an agreement with Cara Operations Limited, LSG Sky Chefs and CLS Catering for voluntary compliance with established public health regulations. The regulations relate to the food standards for caterers/flight kitchens providing meals on aircraft flights originating in Canada. The role of Health Canada's OHSA is to ensure that public health requirements and standards for food are consistently met, given the ongoing changes in food science and food safety. Health Canada is a signatory of World Health Organization's International Health Regulations. In addition, harmonization efforts with the United States Center for Disease Control (CDC) in the cruise ship inspection program have been successful in promoting safe food handling, sanitation and effective outbreak investigations on cruise ships in Canadian waters.

Microbial testing is an essential element in inspection and auditing of catering facilities, and is an absolute requirement in the validation of critical limits and the verification of HACCP. Generally microbiological sampling is used in pursuit of specific monitoring; individual premises or group of similar operations, rather than the longer-term strategic aims associated with the development of an integrated food safety management system.

Professional catering companies of today have their own laboratories where microbiological analyses of ingredients, ready - to - cook articles and prepared meals are carried out, as also are bacteriological tests of surfaces coming into contact with food. Other meal samples are sent to officially accredit testing laboratories to check for the absence of pathogens. Computers are used to record the important phases of the manufacturing process, liquid nitrogen may be used to cool hot meals and the entire process of cooling, and completed hot meals are also computer-monitored. Special purpose built machines are used in the preparation of hot dishes. They can prepare meat - based dishes according to pre-set parameters, and consistently do so while keeping the same quality. The machine could be programmed to carefully monitor the preparation process and informs staff that the meat is ready to serve. Hygienic conditions normally comply with all CFIA and FDA requirements. All production premises remain air-conditioned and are cooled at a temperature of around 15 °C. Critically, the Hazard Critical Control Point (HACCP) system is being introduced to ensure easier observance of hygienic regulations and food safety.

Trends in Canada show that consumers are interested in nutrition and that they want to eat foods that are best for their health and safe. People of Chinese origin are frequent visitor to restaurants; people from Indian subcontinent are the least bothered of outside eating. At the same time, the average Canadian eats out almost 5 times per week, so it makes sense to promote healthy eating in restaurants. Inspections, complaint investigations, food recalls, legal and educational programs are carried out by public health inspectors in all food establishments in order to reduce the incidence of food-borne illness.

Eat Smart Ontario's Healthy Restaurant Program (ESOHRP) goal is to contribute to the reduction of chronic diseases such as heart disease, cancer, and food borne illnesses in Ontario. In addition to establishing and maintaining the program standards at restaurants, "Eat Smart" will achieve its goal through social marketing, education, training, and the support of all sectors of society.

The Canadian Food Safety Adaptation Program (CFSAP) provides an opportunity for Food Caterers, National Associations or groups who are involved directly or indirectly in the food production, marketing, distribution and preparation of food to develop risk management strategies, tools and systems to enhance food safety throughout the total food chain. In order to be eligible, these activities must use the Hazard Analysis Critical Control Point (HACCP) definitions and principles as defined by the Codex Alimentarius Commission-18.

In the United States, Food safety is one of the most important educational initiatives in the restaurant and foodservice industry, and the National Restaurant Association Educational Foundation (NRAEF) has done its part to make it a top priority once again in September 2002. The NRAEF's International Food Safety Council, (IFSC), created National Food Safety Education Month (NFSEM) to focus on the importance of food-safety education for the restaurants and foodservice industry and raises awareness of the industry's commitment to food safety. Each year, the IFSC supplies the restaurant and foodservice industry with a training and promotion guide filled with weekly training activities and promotional pieces to help industry professionals take part in this national awareness campaign.

In one of the survey conducted in Ireland where catering industry suffered *Salmonella sp.,* scare found that 80% source their eggs from *Salmonella sp.,* controlled flocks. However, in light of the survey it is evident that there is a genuine awareness of this risk but equally a genuine reluctance by caterers to use pasteurized egg in these high-risk dishes. Some caterers were even willing to remove these high-risk products from their menus rather than use pasteurized egg. The Food Safety Authority of Ireland aims to ensure that food complies with legal requirements or appropriate recognised codes of practice. Therefore, in the interests of consumer protection and in keeping with the findings of the survey, caterers are advised to source their fresh shell eggs from reputable suppliers with *Salmonella sp.,* controls in place, such as suppliers implementing the Board Bias code of practice for eggs-55.

Breaking the chain of unsafe practices that can cause food borne illness in catering is the most appropriate step. Food operators throughout the food chain bear responsibility for the hygiene of foodstuffs during the preparation, processing, manufacture, packaging, storage, transport, distribution, handling, sale and supply of foodstuffs. All food and food ingredients must be traceable to its source. Owners of food premises are responsible for guaranteeing that food handled in their premises is controlled and safe. They are also required to keep all documentation, which should be made available to the authorities whenever the documents are required for the purpose of verification. Consumers should be able to assume that all food offered for sale is safe for its intended use and consumer should also bear the responsibility for the proper storage and handling of food until its consumption. The main task of the *supervisory authorities* in catering is to lay down food safety standards and to ensure that the internal control systems operated by food manufacturers, processors and food services are appropriate and operated in such a way that the prescribed standards of a jurisdiction are genuinely met.

Chapter: 02
<u>Valuing Food Safety Risks</u>

<u>Overview:</u>

Investors will risk capital in an industry only if they believe that the future rewards outweigh the risk. Investors considering projects in the food industry are concerned about how a food safety problem might affect future cash flows from the investment. While food borne disease outbreaks may be rare events, a few incidents in recent years have dramatically reduced the revenues of the firms associated with the problem. The research has been done which provides a first attempt to link food safety risks to investment decisions, using the real option method of valuing the effects of uncertainty. The concern in the frequency of problems is often ignored that becomes a prelude to a large-scale problem in food safety. The form of a model; Exponential Hazard Rate Parameter (EHRP) may be used to account for food safety risks by adding the possibility of a discrete drop in future cash flows to the stochastic process for future returns[-29].

The results are constrained by the lack of data on the value of revenues lost as a result of food safety problems. The Food Safety and Inspection Service data on meat products recalled for bacterial contamination provides information on quantity; further investigation would be required to estimate values. In a hypothetical investment project and various levels of the food safety risk parameters in the model, option values range from 39% to 59% of sunk costs of the project. Option values are interpreted as the opportunity cost of immediate investment, or the value of waiting until some uncertainty is resolved. These outcomes suggest that there are significant incentives to postpone investments due to uncertain future cash flows.

The probability of occurrence of a problem; the Exponential Hazard Rate Parameter (EHRP) is the dominant food safety parameter in determining real option values in the model. *Exponential model* is associated with the name of Thomas Robert Malthus (1766-1834) who first realized that any species could potentially increase in numbers according to a geometric series. This model structure is appropriate if business decision-makers believe that the probability of a food safety event occurring is more important than the size of the event, in terms of the decrease in cash flows for the firm. If further inquiry reveals that decision-makers are less concerned with frequency of problems than with scale of the problem, then an alternative model structure must be considered.

While it is clear that the chance of occurrence is the main determinant of option values, the direction of its effect is ambiguous. A decrease in the probability of occurrence of food safety problems can either raise or reduce real option values. One would expect that a decrease in risk would reduce option values. If a specific investment project falls in the range at which reduction in the probability parameter increases option values, then HACCP would not stimulate more rapid investment in food industry modernization. Researchers need to understand this ambiguity and its driving forces. The unexpected results occur when projects are smaller and when the probability of occurrence of a problem is very low.

The numerical experiments also revealed a range of parameters in which reductions in both the probability of occurrence and in the scale of the food safety problem reduced option values. If HACCP program significantly affects the probability of an outbreak, then HACCP has overall and long-term financial implications for firms and for the food industry, through the linkage to investment decisions. Cost of food safety should be understood by all food-manufacturing organizations. Cost of food safety should never be valued as an obscure expense but as an indispensable element for the success of food business and profitability. Risk reduction accomplished through HACCP would be an incentive for more rapid investment, which would enhance efficiency and could offset some costs of HACCP implementation.

This examination of financial decisions under uncertainty points out some specific data needs for evaluating business risks related to food safety. According to this research, understanding what factors determine the hazard rate parameter is the first target. The probability of a drop in cash flows resulting from a food safety event may be defined at the firm level, and could perhaps be understood by surveys or interviews to elicit subjective probabilities or tolerances. It is also possible that food safety events in firm affect cash flow industry-wide. Such spill over effects can be estimated from commodity market data or stock price data.

A. <u>Valuing Bakery Food Safety</u>:

Bakery products in Canada include the baker's delicacies of Italy, French, English, Chinese, lately from Indian subcontinent and many other countries. Questions to be explored are whether these diversified bakery resources and products authenticate both a cosmopolitan 'sense of Canadian place' and an associated egalitarian ethos, and whether these aspects of various food characteristics are incorporated, derived from, adopted or appropriated by mainstream Canadian food control and safety system. At the same time we should not forget our own ethnic Indian bakers, who originate from baking potato to Indian delicacies of this day. The variety of Canadian Aboriginal foods is as diverse as the many regions and tribes across the continent. Corn was, and continues to be, a very important crop and used in bakery products such as corn bread. There are many aspects in bakery manufacturing which are important to safety and social obligations. Right ingredients, right manufacturing, decorating, and bakery packaging may all be included in baking skills to create a value in bakery products. Multicultural foods are appreciated in Canada, at the same time we have to value the importance of safety to entertain our ethnic and diverse food values. Key decisions should be made based on accounting principles that recognize the concept of the cost of food safety in terms of human health.

Bakeries can be found in foodservice operations (restaurants etc.) or operating as wholesalers and/or retailers. Bakeries in North America manufacture, from raw ingredients, one or more of the following types of baked goods: breads, cakes and icings, cookies, pies and tarts, donuts, Danish pastries, bread and rolls, frozen dough, cookie dough, biscuits and a variety of other products. Retail bakeries make products and sell on the same property.

Knowledge and Competencies define what a baker must know and be able to produce a saleable safe product for the consumer. The quality of bakery products normally originates from wheat trait and quality specifications. Bakery products require that flours utilized to produce them, meet certain specifications. However, even though primary characteristics such as protein and ash may be comparable in flours derived from various fields, hundreds of secondary characteristics working in combination can produce huge variations in the ways flours work, the products baked from them and its affect on consumers' safety and quality perceptions.

Valuing the best waffles is one interest of consumers, which are obtained by using yeast for the dough. We can also use self-raising flour or baking powder, but the result is not as tasty. Waffles with yeast cannot be stored for longer than one or two days. One should eat them during the baking or as soon as possible afterwards; warm them up in the iron, which was used for the baking.

Labelling like in all other foods, manufacturers must list ingredients in descending order of predominance by weight, from most to least. Under the new requirements, the ingredient list must declare: Source of protein hydrolysates e.g., hydrolyzed wheat gluten and hydrolyzed soy protein, which are used in many foods as flavourings and flavour enhancers. Caseinate as a milk derivative in the ingredient list of foods that claim to be non-dairy, such as coffee whiteners should be highlighted as a milk derivative to indicate and warn allergic consumers.

Vegetables are also very well valued in bakery products and full line of dehydrated, roller dried and freeze dried products are added to enhance veggies bakery food. Indian Samosas with stuffed potato is an item enjoyed by all. Many fruit preparations add colour, flavour, and texture enhancing stabilizers to muffins, pancakes, waffles, cakes, cookies, and quick breads.

Different flavours and colours in natural and artificial edible forms add value to many products of individual choice. Examples of standard flavours are fruit derived essence like apple, apricot, banana, blueberry, cherry, cranberry, grape, huckleberry, lemon, lime, orange, peach, pineapple, raisin, raspberry and strawberry etc. Other popular flavours are like brown sugar, caramel, chocolate, cinnamon, honey, and maple etc. The Novelty flavours used are bubble gum, marshmallow, molasses, peppermint, and rootbeer etc. This list of flavours and colours shall conform to FDA in North America.

Yeast based natural flavour enhancers are adding value in terms of typical bakers' choice. Romano and Parsley bread uses natural flavour enhancers to improve aroma and flavour. The enhancers also increase salt perception and especially improve the dairy/buttery notes. In other bakery products, one of the enhancers used is to mask bitterness in high fibre breads. Cheese flavour enhancer is used to increase cheese flavour in cheese crackers and cheese bacon muffins. Studies have indicated that enhancers can increase sweet, grain and salt perceptions, and decrease sour notes in traditional white bread.

Milk, one of the nature's most complete food, is yielding secrets to researchers that promise a bright future for a new family of fractionated functional ingredients for bakery food formulators.

The first is high-value milk protein fractions - separated milk components with specific functional properties. By separating milk into different fractions, formulators can select the specific functional and nutritional qualities needed for a particular bakery product replacing egg if it is to be replaced. Whey-based thickeners can replace more expensive gums with a reliable, locally available, economical ingredient option in bakery foods. An allergen alert is required on the label. There is a long list of bakery products, which are available in the Canadian and US markets. All these products are rich in carbohydrates and added fat thus vulnerable to many spoilage and pathogenic microorganisms.

One critical point, which is most important in post-processed bakery products, is their storage temperatures. Value of bakery products and shelf life are enhanced if appropriate storage temperatures are maintained. Table: 2(1) – Bakery Food Storage and Risk of Spoilage, is indicative of its value to the bakery industry.

The 21st century has brought many changes in the bakery industry, which can be seen in the shifting of technical and production knowledge from the manufacturer to the ingredient's supplier, faster development times for new products through research, health and nutritional concerns due to diversity of bakery products and requirement for healthy food, new channels of distribution like catering to airlines, cruisers, defence forces and famine prone Afro-Asian regions, continued company restructuring to cut cost of production and plant consolidation for increased productivity. New snack products are replacing meals when consumers are looking for convenience and "good-for-you" products. These major changes are merging product line and distribution methods for major snack manufacturers and wholesale bakers. Bakery food safety is as important as any other food product though it may not require that sensitive handling as milk and meat. Bakery products containing milk and meat ingredients require same preventive conditions as other dairy or meat products. Cakes and pastries are very much valued by the combined society of Canadian populace.

These products remain in the limelight because of their vulnerability to microbial pathogens like _S. enteritidis, E. coli,_ and other enterogenic bacteria.

Baked items are normally safe because of intensive oven temperatures, which destroy microorganisms. However, post-processing conditions may bring undesirable changes. When the embers are first removed from the oven, the oven is around 850 °F (454 °C), perfect for pizza, but too hot for bread. When the temperature has dropped to around 450 °F (232 °C), then it is time to put in the bread. The ideal temperature for pizza is when the wall of the oven is around 850 °F and the floor is around 750 °F. This cooks a pizza in about 90 seconds. Under these temperatures none of the organisms commonly known as spoilage or pathogenic could survive. Since such bakery foods are kept aerobic, much of them have a limited shelf life under ambient temperature.

Majority of the outbreaks, it is not the baked food item, which causes problem of microbial contamination but the additive ingredients, which are used, in the unpasteurized form. When twelve chocolate mousse cakes had been delivered to the hospital by a bakery no one questioned the sanitation, manufacturing process and products safety. The bakery had prepared the fillings of the cakes using raw shell eggs. Environmental investigations at the bakery revealed severe defects in structural and operational hygiene. Why such bakeries are functional? Where are the regulations to control such operations? Are there any quality checks and preventive processes in such bakeries? The answers will lead to Hazard analysis Critical Control Points (HACCP) as a solution-205.

On August 10-2000, serotyping by the British Columbia Centre for Disease Control Society (BCCDCS) Laboratory Services identified four *Salmonella enteritidis* (SE) cases. A 3-day food history was completed for 15 cases to identify common foods consumed by this group. The bakery was closed in the morning of September 08-2000 and a public advisory was initiated to prevent further illness from consumption of the baked products. Samples of the implicated products, including the egg base made from raw shell eggs, were submitted for analysis. Reportedly, raw shell eggs were found to be contaminants. On September 09-2000, baking resumed on site using pasteurized liquid egg products only -92.

In Canada, We hardly hear any outbreak from bakery products though use of allergen products has been a burning issue in the country. Peanuts, Soya bean, lactose, casein, and other allergy related products, when used shall be declared so that the people who have allergic tendencies could take absence.

Table: 2(1) – Bakery Food Storage and Risk of Spoilage

No.	Food	Temp.	Shelf Life	Spoilage organism	Changes	Prevention
1	Bread	25 °C	< 3 days	Fungi, Yeast & Bacteria	Stale	Long Preservation at 4 °C
2	Bagel	25 °C	<3 days	Fungi, Yeast & Bacteria	Stale	Long Preservation at 4 °C
3	Chapatti	25 °C	< 1 day	Fungi, Yeast	Stale	Eaten warm & Fresh
4	Croissant	25 °C	< 4 days	Pseudomonas Bacteria	Musty, Rancid, sour	Freeze up to six months
5	Danish Pastry	25 °C	< 3 days	Fungi, *Pseudomonas sp.*, *Streptococcus sp.*	Musty, Rancid, sour	Freeze up to two months

6	Hot Cross Buns	25 °C	<4 days	Fungi, Yeast & Bacteria	Sour,	Freeze up to six months
7	Muffins	25 °C	< 7 days	Fungi, Yeast & Bacteria	Musty, Rancid, sour	Chilled 7 days Frozen six months
8	Nan	25 °C	Eaten warm	Fungi, Yeast & Bacteria	Stale	Freezing is not advised
9	Paratha	25 °C	Eaten warm	*Pseudomonas Sp.*	Stale, dried	Half cooked frozen up to two months
10	Pita Bread	25 °C	< 2 days	Fungi	Mouldy	Freeze up to two months
11	Sourdough Bread	25 °C	< 2 days	Fungi & *Lactobacillus plantarum*	Stale	Freezing not advisable
12	Angel cake	25 °C	Eaten same day	Fungi, Yeast & Bacteria	Oxidized, Sour, & Rancid	Freezing not advisable
13	Chocolate Cake	4 °C	< 5 days	Fungi, Yeast & Bacteria	Sour, Rancid & Moldy	Freezing not advisable
14	Christmas Cake	4 °C	< 30 days	Fungi, Yeast & Bacteria	Sour, Rancid & Moldy	Freezing not advisable
15	Fruit Pudding	25 °C	Eaten fresh	Fungi, Yeast & *Escherichia coli*	Sour, Rancid & Moldy	Chilled 2 days

The root cause of any hazard in food manufacturing is supposed to be at the bottom of whatever problem is revealed in the observance of non-conformity. Unfortunately, it is found only by performance of a process, the HACCP eyes must look before and beyond the immediate situation. That is how the HACCP is a hazard preventive system best encouraged for the bakery industry, which rarely relies on non-conformities but solely relies on identification of hazards and its preventive solutions before the commercial production.

B. Valuing Beverage Safety:

When it comes to beverage safety value, consumers believe the beverages offer the biggest bang for their buck. As convenience and flavour become paramount considerations for consumers and processors alike, the phrase "innovate or die" could very well become the rallying cry for refrigerated and frozen food manufacturers seeking to capture increased share of stomach.

Search for a more safe, nutritional, and thirst-quenching beverage by consumers will always attract manufacturers to innovate and step ahead in competence. The launch of fitness water; an enhanced water beverage featuring essential vitamins, minerals, and electrolytes by Vancouver based Canadian manufacturers are an example to quote. Reebok Fitness Water will compete in the Alternative Beverage category and will help pioneer a new concept within the bottled water segment: enhanced water beverages.

The Canadian refreshment beverage industry has already introduced a new class of fortified beverages, everything from waters and juices to sports and dairy-based drinks in to Canada. These so-called "functional beverages" are products fortified with minerals, vitamins or herbs that allow consumers to bolster their diets with the nutrients they need, in a healthy and convenient way. Functional beverages respond to the needs and the priorities of today's active individuals and families. The Canadian refreshment beverage industry points to experience in other markets that shows that these products are in high demand and that people understand how they fit into their daily diet and nutritional programs. Total sales of functional beverages are expected to reach approximately $500 million dollars per year. The refreshment beverage industry currently accounts for 12,000 jobs in Canada, and pays more than $100 million in capital, property, and payroll taxes annually to various levels of government across the country. The federal government collects an additional $175 million in goods and services tax (GST) revenues on non-alcoholic liquid refreshment sales in Canada.

Tea has been consumed by significant percentage of people in Canada and it is considered as a healthy beverage. People value tea because of less caffeine in tea. Those who often avoid coffee and prefer tea must know that tea offers a great hot beverage alternative to coffee because it has two to three times less caffeine than coffee. However, a recent survey suggests 36 per cent of Canadians believe tea has more caffeine than coffee. It also showed that 22 per cent of Canadians say they are drinking more tea now than two years ago. As with green tea, studies have touted for its antioxidant properties? However, fresh tea with milk may give some benefits while same tea kept longer and consumed later may lead to hyperacidity to susceptible consumers. Canadians drink more than seven billion cups of tea a year. Annual sales in 2001 were $269.5 million-203.

Contrary to the belief that heavy tea consumption may lead to digestive disorder, it has been also studied and found that tea consumption leads to heart health and reducing the risk of cancer.

Major research developments reveal that tea may reduce Low Density Lipoprotein (LDL, or "bad" cholesterol) levels by 10 percent, consumption of as little as four cups of tea per day may contribute to cardiovascular health by improving endothelial function. As seen in clinical studies, tea may reduce oxidative stress, as indicated by decreases in DNA damage in smokers, and tea consumption is linked with a 60 percent decrease in rectal cancer among women-13.

The food and beverage-processing sector is Canada's third largest manufacturing sector. Food and beverage processing accounted for 14% of Canadian manufacturing GDP in 1998. Approximately 2,800 establishments produced shipments valued at $52 billion in 1998 and provided approximately 240,000 jobs. About 16% of the value of shipments is exported, and of this amount, 73% is exported to the US-215.

The Canadian processed food and beverage industry has grown significantly. The Canadian non-alcoholic beverage sector represents the largest single category within grocery outlets with retail sales of over £ 1.6 billion in 1998. The biggest movers are flavoured soft drinks and health choices such as Soya drinks, bottled water, tomato and rice drinks, as well as instant breakfasts-214.

The Canadian Food and Drug Regulations strictly prescribe the labelling of all pre-packaged food, beverages including alcoholic beverages, requirements for ingredient labelling, durable life dates, nutrient content claims, mandatory nutrients declarations, and foods for special dietary needs. The Consumer Packaging and Labelling Act provides for a uniform method of labelling and packaging of consumer goods (products sold at retail). It prevents fraud and deception by providing for factual label information from which consumers can make an informed choice. It also requires the use of metric units of measurement and bilingual labelling. Canadian government already regulates its food thus valuing food products and its safety from fraud.

The Canadian Food and Drugs Act prohibits the labelling, packaging, treating, processing, selling or advertising of any food (at all levels of trade) in a manner that would mislead or deceive consumers as to the character, value, quantity, composition, merit or safety of the product. As well, it prohibits health claims that might suggest that a food is a treatment, preventative, or cure for specified diseases or health conditions. It also requires bilingual labelling-103.

Packagings for beverages play a marketing and safety role. Aluminium, glass, plastic, and bi-metal containers, gable top paperboard, Tetra bricks and even plastic cups all have variable impact in the beverage safety and shelf life. Recycling of these packaging materials contributes to environmental safety.

Let us review few of the common safety problems with beverages all over the world. On March 02-2000, an outbreak of food poisoning affected several students of a secondary school. A total of 269 students came down with food poisoning. Food borne outbreak traced to the consumption of contaminated iced drink made from non-food-grade ice. The presence of *Staphylococcus aureus* in a sample of ice block as well as the detection of both *Staphylococcus aureus* and *E. coli* in the water container indicated that contamination could have occurred in the factory and during preparation of the iced drink. Now The Ministry of the Environment in Singapore has further tightened its control over the production and sale of food-grade ice. Ice for consumption is required to be properly packed and labelled to indicate its intended use-[79].

In the summer of 1987, seven persons living in Westchester County, New York, developed lead poisoning after ingesting a homemade beverage stored in a ceramic bean jug. Excessive absorption of lead is one of the most prevalent and preventable childhood environmental health problems in the United States -[60].

The November 4th edition of the Journal of American Medical Association reports that 62 people from 21 states contracted *Salmonella sp.*, poisoning by drinking unpasteurized orange juice served at Walt Disney World. None had traveled to Florida together. Seven Disney guests were hospitalized-[130].

It is safer to drink directly from a labelled and sealed can or bottle of a beverage than from a questionable unlabelled container. Wet cans or bottles should be dried before opening, and surfaces, which are contacted directly by the mouth in drinking, should first be wiped clean. Water that has been adequately chlorinated will provide significant protection against viral and bacterial waterborne diseases.

In Ontario, before water is pumped for drinking purpose it goes many safety procedures to ensure safe drinking. The processes of rapid mixing of chemicals known as coagulants and coagulant aids to make the small physical particles in the water clump together (coagulation), and then the gentle mixing to form larger groups of particles known as floc (flocculation). Alum (aluminium sulphate), polyaluminum chloride, and a group of chemicals known as polyelectrolyte are the material currently used for the purpose of flocculation. This thicker, denser floc floats down and settles out of the water in large tanks (sedimentation) or is removed during the next stage, filtration. In this stage, the remaining floc, other chemical and physical impurities, and most of the biological impurities (bacteria, etc.) are removed. The water flows by gravity through filters called dual media filters and is then collected via an under drain system. Dual media filters are made up of layers of sand and anthracite, a coal-like mineral.

When tap water flows from a reservoir to local community it under goes a final chlorination treatment before the supplies are permitted. Chlorine gas is injected into the potable water pipeline to maintain chlorine content at a set point usually 1.5-2.00 ppm. In Canada, the destruction of disease-causing organisms in the raw and treated water through the addition of the chemical chlorine is the most important step in the water treatment process. When chlorine is added to the raw water as it enters the plant, the process is known as pre-chlorination. When chlorine is added to the water after the filtration stage it is known as post-chlorination. Additional chlorine can be added through a process known as super chlorination when the levels of bacteria are high. By the time chlorinated water reaches to the city consumers, the chlorine content remains to a level of 0.75 – 1.00 ppm that is expected to be safe for human health.

However, chlorine treatment alone may not kill some viruses and the parasites that cause giardiasis, ameobiasis, and cryptosporidiosis. Sulphur dioxide is then added to the water and combines with the excess chlorine to reduce the chlorine residual (remaining chlorine) to an acceptable level before the ammonisation stage.

In 1963, Toronto Council decided to add fluoride to our treated water supply. Lake Ontario water, like many natural sources, already has some fluoride present in low concentration, so our water treatment plants add additional fluoride after the filtration stage to raise the level to 1.2 mg/l. Ammonia is added at the end of the treatment process and combines with the remaining chlorine. This stabilizes the chlorine so that it remains dissolved in the treated water for longer periods of time, keeping the water safe during its long trip through the distribution system. Ammonisation also prevents minute amounts of chlorine from evaporating out of your drinking water causing smells and associated tastes. When the water has passed through all these processes, it is then pumped to an extensive distribution system serving the City of Toronto and parts of the Region of York. Typical water in Ontario would read the parameters as mentioned in Table: 2(2) Exemplary Water Analysis Report on Ontario water supply.

In areas where chlorinated tap water is not available, or where hygiene and sanitation are poor, travelers should be advised that only the following may be safe to drink: Beverages, such as tea and coffee, made with boiled water, canned or bottled carbonated beverages, including carbonated bottled water, soft drinks, Beer and wine.

Table: 2(2) - <u>Exemplary Water Analysis Report on Ontario water supply</u>-217

Characteristics of South Peel Water (Average values)	
Hardness	130 mg/l or 8.9 grains/Imp.gal.
PH	7.4
Fluoride	0.70 mg/l
Iron	0.01 mg/l
Alkalinity	99.3 mg/l
Turbidity	0.07 NTU
Colour	<5 TCU
Water Characteristics	
Specific Gravity:	1.00 Water reaches its highest density at 4 degrees Celsius. It becomes less dense at higher and lower temperatures.
Water weights:	1 kg/l, 1000 kg/m^3, 10 lb / imperial gallon 62.4 lb/ft^3 at 4°C
Pressure:	1 psi = 2.31 ft of water 1 ft of water = 0.433 psi 1 m of water = 1.42 psi 1 psi = 6.895 Kilopascals
Water boils at:	100°C / 212°F
Freezes at:	0°C / 32°F

Summary of Analytical Results for Jan - March 2003

Americans this year will consume more than 2 billion gallons of juice -- much of it consumed by young children. The good news is that more than 98 percent of the juice sold in this country is completely safe, because it is pasteurized -- that is heated to a high enough temperature and held at it for a sufficient duration to kill dangerous pathogens such as *E. coli* 0157:H7 and *Salmonella sp*. However, nearly 40 million gallons of juice that will be consumed this year will be unpasteurized. The Food and Drug Administration (US-FDA) estimates that more than 6,000 consumers could be sickened this year by the consumption of tainted, unpasteurized juice.

Canadian and US industry took a strong position in favour of requiring that all juices be pasteurized or receive an equivalent treatment just as is done for milk today. Governments around the world, consumer groups and the industry have long recognized that pasteurization or a process that ensures the same degree of safety is the best way to kill the most dangerous pathogens that make people sick. The food technologists in North America, the Canadian and US FDAs, should follow suit and commit to the pasteurization of all juices they regulate, US-FDA did not yet proposed such a measure. In April, they proposed two new regulations, including a warning label for juices that are not pasteurized, which we believe should be viewed as an acceptable interim step only. Instead of requiring pasteurization as soon as possible, they have chosen to expand the regulatory requirements for all processors -- including those that pasteurize their juice -- even though the source of the problem falls within just two percent of the juice supply and a fraction of processors. Furthermore, they have proposed to exempt all juice sold in restaurants, juice bars and many retail establishments, where some 15% of unpasteurized juice is sold. That is more than 5 million gallons -- 85 million servings -- that will not be covered by the new regulations.

The Canadian and United States food regulators should clearly enforce, the foolproof way of erasing food borne illnesses carried by juices is to simply require pasteurization of all juices and fruit drinks, or use of an equivalent process. This is the approach the food industry in the United States will strongly support. The freshly crushed or squeezed juices ready for immediate consumption could be exempted as such a food safety threat vaguely applies there.

1. Juice Safety Status in Canada:

Unpasteurized fruit juice and cider products have been involved in several recent foods borne outbreaks of bacterial origin. The most likely means of contamination identified has been fruit and/or juice becoming contaminated through direct contact with animal/human faeces or through indirect contact by water, food handlers, or soiled equipments. Even Freshly squeezed juices would require satisfactory hygiene to eliminate cross contamination.

Four million (4,000,000) litres of unpasteurized apple juice/cider are sold every year in Canada, representing 6% of the total apple juice production in Canada. In addition, an estimated 2% of the Canadian population consumes unpasteurized juice and cider.

These products are usually sold to consumers at orchards, cider mills, farmers markets, roadside stands, country fairs, and juice bars. Some unpasteurized fruit juices/cider is also sold in refrigerated display cases or produce sections of stores that carries some degree of risk.

Traditionally, unpasteurized fruit juices / cider have been considered non-hazardous due to their relatively low pH level. However, as a result of several recent outbreaks of food poisoning in North America involving unpasteurized fruit juices, it has become clear that certain harmful bacteria can survive these acidic conditions.

A risk assessment entitled "Qualitative Risk Assessment: Unpasteurized Fruit Juice/Cider" was prepared by Health Canada in collaboration with the Canadian Food Inspection Agency (CFIA) and was finalized on May 10, 2000. This risk assessment, which was qualitative rather than quantitative, was prepared using information from current publications and documents. The development of this document involved extensive literature and Internet searches, as well as consultation with industry, Provincial/Territorial agencies, and CFIA. It was used as the basis for deriving appropriate risk management options that could minimize the contamination of unpasteurized juices.

The risk assessment concluded that present controls during processing of unpasteurized juices/ciders could not completely guarantee the absence of harmful bacteria (pathogens) from fruits or their juices. Illness associated with exposure to the contaminating bacteria, which represent the hazards in these products, can be severe or fatal, particularly with children, the elderly, and persons with weakened immune system.

The prominent pathogens involved in these cases have been identified as _Escherichia coli_ O157:H7 and _Salmonella SP_. The infectious dose for _E. coli_ O157:H7 is not yet known. However, based on the relatively high attack rates during outbreaks, it appears that the number of bacteria required to cause illness is very low. _E. coli_ O157:H7 can cause severe damage to the lining of the intestine resulting in a condition called haemorrhagic colitis, the symptoms of which can include stomach cramps, vomiting, fever, and bloody diarrhoea. Patients are given fluids to prevent dehydration from diarrhoea. In a small percentage of people, haemolytic uremic syndrome (HUS) can develop, which may require patients to undergo blood transfusions and kidney dialysis. The disease can lead to permanent loss of kidney function and can be fatal in some cases (Doyle and Cliver, 1990; Doyle and Padhye,

1989). Children, the elderly, and persons with weakened immune systems are considered to be at the highest risk.

Salmonella sp. is commonly found in the intestinal tract of humans and animals. Environmental sources of the organism include but are not limited to water, soil, insects, animal feces, raw meats, raw poultry, and raw seafoods. All known species of _Salmonella sp._ are pathogenic to humans (Doyle and Cliver, 1990). The _Salmonella sp._ infection that has been most associated with juice outbreaks is the gastroenteritic syndrome that is caused by non-typhoid strains of _Salmonella sp_. The severity of non-typhoid salmonella infection (known as Salmonellosis) varies with the number of bacteria ingested and the susceptibility of the individual. Incubation is 8 to 72 hours before symptoms occur (D'Aoust, 1989; D'Aoust, 1997). Principal symptoms are nausea, vomiting, abdominal pain, dehydration, and non-bloody diarrhoea that can appear suddenly. Duration of the illness is usually from 1- 4 days. Human infections resulting in Enterocolitis from non-typhoid salmonellae are generally self-limiting. The successful treatment of uncomplicated cases of Enterocolitis may require only supportive therapy such as fluid and electrolyte replacement (D'Aoust, 1997).

The percentage of the Canadian population that consumes these products is estimated to be 2%, but the actual incidence of illness as a result of consumption of juices in the Canadian population is unknown. In addition, the incidences of foodborne pathogens of concern in unpasteurized fruit juices, as well as data on infectious doses that will cause illness, are not yet available.

This risk assessment demonstrated that the risk of infection by food borne pathogens such as _E. coli_ O157:H7 and _Salmonella sp_. as a result of drinking unpasteurized juices/cider, is considered to be low, but the potential health consequences of infection can be severe.

One of the methods commonly used by the juice industry to control pathogens is the application of heat. This process is most often referred to as "pasteurization". There is presently no standard for the "pasteurization" of juice in Canada – only milk and raw eggs have pasteurization standards. When a standard is developed and prescribed in regulation, the recommendations for the production and distribution of juice in Canada should be revised to include this standard[175].

2. Juice Safety Status in the United States:
In the United States of America, 98% of all juices are pasteurized or subjected to equivalent "kill steps," making them safe for consumption – just like pasteurized milk. 98% of juices – over 2

billion gallons – pose no health risk to consumers because they are heat-treated.

Out of total juice consumption in the United States, 2% of all juices are not pasteurized and are not safe from contamination by disease-causing organisms like *E. coli* O150:H7, *Salmonella sp.*, and *Cryptosporidium parvum*. These 2% of juices – which is about 38 million gallons or more than 600 million servings – are responsible for an estimated 6,000 – 6,200 illnesses per year because they are not pasteurized.

Although US-FDA's proposed labelling requirement for unpasteurized juices is finalized and enforced, 84% - 95% of these 6,000 + attacks will continue to occur annually (US-FDA estimates a 5 – 16% reduction with a mandated warning statement). Since pasteurized juices are not responsible for any illnesses in a given year, mandating the Hazard Analysis and Critical Control Point (HACCP) program for processors of pasteurized juices will not affect much to public safety but it would further guarantee the safety of pasteurized juices produced and packed in industrial and commercial environment.

Of the 900 juice processors in US-FDA's Official Establishment Inventory, all but a very few utilize pasteurization, so a substantial number of companies and their employees may face tough times as they struggle to meet HACCP's positive burdens. The FDA estimates the annual economic savings of requiring unpasteurized juices to be pasteurized at $174 - $251 million – and no illnesses. The FDA estimates the savings of labelling unpasteurized juices at $1 million to $6 million – with little change in the number of illnesses. Under US-FDA's proposal, all restaurants, juice bars, and other retail processors selling juice on-site for immediate consumption will be exempted from the labelling and HACCP requirements. This accounts for over 15% of unpasteurized juices and over 4,000 establishments -72.

C. Valuing Dairy Food Safety:

The quality and safety of market milk begins with the milk producer. Milk and other dairy products, currently available to the consuming public, reach a level of quality and safety far superior to 50, 25 or even 10 years ago. New technology and practices by the milk producer have been major factors in improved milk quality and safety. Next to grains and livestock's, dairy is Canada's most important sector with net farm cash receipts of $4.10 billion in 2000. Canada exports butter, milk powders, condensed milk, and evaporated milk to developing countries. In the year 2000-2001 dairy years export totalled close to $395 million. Canada also imports dairy products worth $ 510 million mainly cheeses from EU, New Zealand and the United States.

Even with higher levels of quality, some consumer groups challenge and question the safety of the milk supply. These challenges can -- justifiably or unjustifiably -- affect the milk producer's profits and staying power. A continued search for excellence is the best strategy to offset any challenge. To reach higher levels of excellence, the dairyman must recognize the potential issues and know the interrelationship of the issues to milk production. Dairymen are faced with seven basic food safety issues relating to milk and milk products:

- **P**athogenic microorganisms
- **M**ycotoxins
- **N**aturally occurring allergens
- **C**hemical residues
- **D**rug residues (Antibiotics)
- **H**ormones
- **D**airy Hygiene

Of the seven food safety issues, the public views chemical residues (particularly pesticides) as the leading health threat. However, scientific experts rank pathogenic microorganisms as the No. 1 potential risk to public health.

The scientific ranking of pathogens as the top potential health risk is based on historical information from investigated food borne illnesses. Through the investigation of food borne illness and deaths, the Centers for Disease Control (US-CDC) have developed a substantial database. In 1990, a CDC publication reported that the greatest percentage of food borne illness cases, 87 percent for a 15-year period, was caused by pathogens. The same report identified chemicals of non-farm sources as being responsible for only 4 percent of the cases. Farm sources of food borne illness were not specifically identified in the report.

The value of milk and milk products come from special carbohydrate (CHO) lactose, which forms the basis of its conversion in to many products like yoghurt, buttermilk, and flavoured milks. At the same time, if correct manufacturing technology and safety measures are not enforced, milk carbohydrates become a source of microbial growth, which is evident from the Table: 2(3) - The Bacterial Spoilage & Pathogenic Risks From Few of The Carbohydrates. In formulating and evolving any manufacturing procedure, valuing milk constituents is an important and critical aspect of the quality assurance and food safety.

Although many cases are unreported, the US-CDC and the Food and Drug Administration (US-FDA) estimated that 3-14 percent of the U.S. population become ill each year as a result of pathogenic bacterial contamination of food. These illnesses result in around 9,000 deaths per year. U.S. food-related illness from Mycotoxins, drug residues, Agricultural chemicals, and hormones is either nonexistent or limited. However, underdeveloped countries have reported problems where excessive doses of these products can be more common.

Milk and dairy foods derived from milk are among the safest, highest quality foods in Canada and the United States. The stringent government regulations and dairy industry programs, along with continued vigilance at every stage of production, processing, and distribution contribute to the safety and quality of milk and milk products. By taking a proactive approach, the dairy industry, working with government agencies, can effectively meet new food safety challenges as they may arise and continue to provide consumers with safe and high quality dairy products. Good Manufacturing Practices (GMPs), code of behaviour established by the dairy industry and FDA are indispensable part of protecting milk's quality. The practices relate to methods and control procedures used in dairy plants for the processing, packaging, and storage of milk and milk products. Hazard Analysis Critical Control Points (HACCP) is a voluntary, well structured, and scientifically proved approach to dairy food safety, and it is being adopted by the dairy industry not only in North America but in GCC (Gulf Cooperation Council) countries, EU and most of the Asian countries.

Milk producers must continue with farm practices, which protect the public from food, associated hazards even though few illnesses can be traced to the farm. At the same time, producers must be aware of public perceptions of possible hazards and risks so they can strengthen current quality practices and prevent adverse circumstances. Negative consumer perceptions erode the per capita consumption of dairy products.

Consumers rightly expect that the milk products they purchase be of high quality. The two most visible food safety issues related to animal-derived dairy foods are microbial and chemical contaminants. Livestock producers, veterinarians, and feed producers recognize residue avoidance as the key to consumer confidence, and are enhancing and formalizing programs which will permeate every facet of the production system.

Table: 2(3) - The Bacterial Spoilage & Pathogenic Risks From Few of The Carbohydrates

No	CHO	End Result	Spoilage Organisms	Pathogenic Organisms
1	Lactose	Produce gas and acids, some may not produce gas	*Lactobacillus* sp., *Streptococcus* sp., *Leuconostoc* sp.	*Escherichia coli*, *Salmonella* sp., *Shigella* sp., *Klebsiella* sp., *Staphylococcus* sp. *Enterobacter aerogenes* *Listeria monocytogenes* *Clostridium* sp.
2	Glucose	-Produce gas and acids -Few species may not produce acids	*Lactobacillus fermentum* *Leuconostoc* sp. *Streptococcus* sp., *Bacillus sp.* *Pseudomonas mallei*, *Spirillum lunatum*	*Escherichia coli*, *Salmonella typhimurium*, *Citrobacter freundii*, *Enterobacter cloacae Hafnia alvei* etc., *Staphylococcus aureus*, *Clostridium sphenoides*, *Clostridium botulinum*
3	Sorbitol	Produce acids and may be associated with gas	*Lactobacillus casei*, *Pseudomonas fluorescens*,	*Escherichia coli*, etc., *Citrobacter freundii* etc., *Salmonella typhimurium* *Klebsiella pneumoniae* *Enterobacter cloacae* etc., *Yersinia* sp., *Erwinia salicis* etc.
3	Xylose	Some may produce H2S, Produce acids	*Lactobacillus xylosus*, *Leuconostoc* sp. (10% positive)	*Citrobacter freundii* etc., *Salmonella typhimurium* etc. *Klebsiella pneumoniae*

| 4 | Sucrose | Produce gas and acids | *Lactobacillus lactis,* *Lactobacillus delbrueckii* *Leuconostoc sp.,* *Pseudomonas fluorescens* | *Klebsiella pneumoniae* *Enterobacter aerogenes* *Serratia marcescens* *Enterobacter aerogenes* etc., *Hafnia alvei* etc., *Proteus sp.,* *Yersinia* sp., |
| 5 | Maltose | Produce acids | *Lactobacillus jensenii,* *Leuconostoc sp.* | *Escherichia coli,* *Edwardsiella tarda,* *Citrobacter freundii* *Salmonella typhimurium,* *Shigella dysenteriae,* *Klebsiella pneumoniae,* *Enterobacter cloacae,* *Hafnia alvei,* *Serratia marcescens,* *Proteus sp.,* *Yersinia enterocolitica,* *Clostridium sphenoides* |

The US Food and Drug Administration (US-FDA), which must approve all drugs meant to be marketed for use in animals, establishes tolerances for drug residues (similar to speed limits) to insure food safety. The US-FDA also establishes "withdrawal times" or "withholding periods" which are times after drug treatment when milk is not to be used for manufacturing or human consumption, and during which animals are not to be slaughtered. This allows time to the animals to eliminate the drug residues.

Food Animal Residue Avoidance Databank (FARAD) offers the means to provide access to a vast array of information on effective residue avoidance and quality assurance programs. Provide livestock producers, Extension specialists, and veterinarians with practical information on how to avoid drug, pesticide and environmental contaminant residue problems. The drugs and pesticides used in modern animal Agriculture improve animal health and thereby promote more efficient and humane production.

Johne's disease, pronounced YO-knees, was identified more than a century ago, yet remains a common and sometimes costly infectious disease of dairy cattle. In spite of this, many U.S. dairy producers are unfamiliar with Johne's disease. One information from the National Animal Health Monitoring System (NAHMS) Dairy '96 Study, a national study of dairy health issues conducted by USDA-APHIS-VS in 1996, estimates that the cost of Johne's disease can be quite high. The study found that, in infected herds where at least 10 percent of the culled cows showed clinical signs like those of Johne's disease, the average cost to those producers was $245 for each cow in the herd per year. In other words, the cost for a 100-cow dairy with at least this number of Johne's culled cows with clinical disease would be about $24,000 each year. The majority of this loss was due to reduced milk production, this lost productivity costs the U.S. dairy industry $200-$250 million annually [42].

Canada has been free of Foot and Mouth Disease (FMD) since 1952. FMD is an extremely serious livestock illness and it is one of the most contagious of animal diseases. Meat or animal products infected with the virus or raw or improperly cooked food waste containing infected meat or animal products are never fed to susceptible animals. The CFIA prohibits importation of susceptible animals and animal products from countries infected by FMD or Johne's disease. The CFIA suspends the issuance of import permits for live animals, semen, embryos, and animal products from susceptible animals. As a precaution, the CFIA investigates whether there are any import permits that have been issued but not used, and traces of any infected products that may have entered Canada.

A proper dairy hygiene system exists in the industry to tackle all issues related to food safety during processing and packing. The Canadian National Committee of the International Dairy Federation (FIL-IDF Canada) groups the different partners of the Canadian dairy sector. FIL-IDF Canada is the only national forum where all partners of the Canadian dairy industry discuss issues relevant to the sector in a non-political way (e.g. the National Dairy Code). There are various benefits of being members of FIL-IDF Canada. It provides a forum for all sectors of the industry to meet, discuss, and develop practices, guidelines and standards, which are beneficial to the Canadian dairy industry as a whole. Canada has one national industrial hygiene organization -- the Canadian Registration Board of Occupational Hygiene (CRBOH). It seeks to advance the profession by accreditation of qualified practitioners and establishing a standard of ethical practice. CRBOH is also Canada's representative in the International Occupational Hygiene Association (IOHA).

As the marketing of safe dairy foods have developed manifold since the advent of HACCP in 1960, many countries have formed special boards, institutions, and commissions to deal with safe and wholesome dairy food business. These institutions are industry regulators, charged with directing the operations of the sector from the farm to marketing, specifically to promote development of the sector and the consumption of safe milk and milk products. Their operational activities differ from country to country. In every country, the meaning, and the actions, of such dairy institutions are different, even because the interpretation of the "translated words" is not the same in all the countries. For example the Irish Dairy Board Co-operative is a commercial co-operative. Its function is to market and export the products of its member manufacturing co-operatives, dairy companies and to generating a satisfactory return for the primary producers or dairy farmers. In UK: Milk Marketing Board (MOB), Milk Development Council (MDB), in New Zealand: New Zealand Dairy Board (NZDB), in India: National Development Dairy Board (NDDB), in Canada: Canadian Dairy Commission (CDC) and in the United States: U.S. Dairy Export Council (USDEC), National Conference on Interstate Milk Shipments (NCIMS), World Dairy Expo and USDA are such examples which value the milk and milk products for its nutritional, beneficial, safety and commercial worth.

In Canada, Canadian Dairy Commission (CDC) is such an agency which was created in 1966 through the Canadian Dairy Commission Act to provide efficient Canadian producers of milk and cream with the opportunity to obtain a fair return for their labour and investment; and to provide consumers of dairy products in national and international markets with a continuous and adequate supply of safe and wholesome dairy products of high quality. The commission is a central facilitator for the multi-billion dollar Canadian dairy industry; it works closely with industry stakeholders represented by organizations such as the Dairy Farmers of Canada, the Consumers Association of Canada, and provincial boards and agencies.

D. Valuing Meat Safety:

Valuing meat safety is a public good like other food products. The perishable nature of meat and its sensitive vulnerability to major diseases makes this food more critical to human health and its safety. Demand and willingness to pay for food safety are strictly related to the concerned market and consumers. In North America, a clear economic and national interest rationale exists for governmental involvement in meat food safety. By providing the regulation, technology to accurately and consistently grade, process, preserve, improve yield determination, and meet exact customer specifications, the Canadian and United States meat industry adds to the overall profitability.

Figures for 1997 show that the red meat industry as the largest sector, $10.4 billion, of Canada's food processing industry and the third largest of all manufacturing industries in the country. It employed directly about 35,500 Canadians and was the second largest Agri-food exporting commodity, about $3.00 billion in 1997, following grains / oilseeds. Figures for 1998 indicate growth in output, employment, and exports.

The National Animal Health Program (CFIA-NAHP) protects Canadian livestock and poultry from serious diseases that could restrict trade or pose a risk to human health. By avoiding production losses due to defects, the stability and competitiveness of livestock and poultry production are assured. The international marketability of live animals and meat products is enhanced because of Canada's reputation for being free of certain serious diseases. However, recent identification of BSE in one of the slaughtered cow in Alberta almost maimed Canadian beef export to USA and Japan. It was slaughtered and no part of it entered the human food chain. At stake was the sterling reputation of Alberta's $3.8-billion beef industry. In 2002, Alberta's beef exports to the U.S. were worth $1.9 billion - $1.3 billion in processed beef and veal, the remainder in live on-the-hoof sales. The ban of beef export to international market would cost $550 million per month. At the same time it also left a credibility note to the international market that Canadian regulatory agencies and the meat industry alike believe in safety and never hide any such incident for commercial gain. Any factor, which relates to food safety and human health, is given stringent and critical attention. This is good in the long run of the Canadian Beef Export and Canadian meat consumption.

The importation of animals and animal products from foreign countries is controlled to reduce the risk of introducing serious animal diseases. The Meat Hygiene Program (CFIA-MHP) ensures that meat and poultry products leaving federally inspected establishments for interprovincial and export trade or being imported into Canada are safe and wholesome. It also monitors registered and non-registered establishments for labelling to avoid fraud and audits the delivery of a grading program based on objective standards of meat quality and retail yield to facilitate the marketing of meats from producer to consumer.

Beside governmental control, many organizations value the meat industry and incorporate programs to monitor and research safety standards. The Canadian Meat Science Association (CMSA) was created in 1985 and now includes representatives from all sectors of the Canadian meat industry, from academia and from government. The CMSA strives to help its membership in professional development by providing a forum for the exchange and dissemination of new developments in meat science research, teaching and application of new technology in the meat industry.

The Canadian Meat Council (CMC) serves as the vehicle to express the collective views of the membership and to speak for the meat packing/processing industry in Canada and to contribute to the competitiveness of the industry domestically and internationally. Canada Beef Export Federation (CANADA BEEF) was established in 1989. They are an independent non-profit organization committed to improving export results for the Canadian cattle and beef industry. Canada Pork International (CPI) is the export promotion agency of the Canadian pork industry. The Canadian Pork Council (CPC) provides a national leadership role for hog producers in achieving a dynamic and prosperous pork industry in Canada. It is a joint initiative of the Canadian Meat Council, representing the pork packers and trading companies, and of the Canadian Pork Council, which is the national hog producer organization.

Canadian Cattlemen's Association (CCA) is the only national association representing the interests of Canada's 90,000 beef producers. The CCA provides the leadership and unity necessary to speak as one voice for the beef industry. This includes assisting in its development, adaptation to new ideas and technologies, and in its prosperity. The CCA is structured to represent every phase of the production system the purebred, cow/calf, and back grounding and feedlot sectors.

According to TRENDS-1996, the top food selection concerns and the percentages of the shopping public that considered these factors "Very Important" in food selection were as follows:

    (1) Taste, 88%;
    (2) Nutrition, 78%;
    (3) Product Safety, 75%;
    (4) Price, 66%;
    (5) Storability, 43%;
    (6) Food Preparation Time, 38%;
    (7) Ease of Preparation, 36%;
    (8) Recyclables of Packaging; 34%.

Interestingly, worry about product (food) safety has not changed much in the past six years; this issue ranked third in importance in food selection concerns in 1991 (72%) and fourth in importance in food selection in 1992 (71%), 1993 (72%), 1994 (69%) and 1995 (69%) in TRENDS reports for those respective years (Food Marketing Institute, 1991, 1992, 1993, 1994, 1995) -193.

Possible food-safety concerns about beef (Smith et al., 1994b) include:

(**a**) The presence on meat of food-borne pathogens; most important would be *Salmonella sp.*, *Listeria monocytogenes*, *Campylobacter jejuni* and *Escherichia coli* O157:H7),

(**b**) Residues, in meat, of pesticides (of either or both of the types--chlorinated hydrocarbons and organophosphates),

(**c**) Antibiotics (fear of residues of the antibiotics, in meat, and/or of development and presence, on meat, of antibiotic-resistant strains of human pathogens because of continued exposure of human pathogens--that have livestock vectors--to feed-grade antibiotics) and

(**d**) Residues of livestock growth promoting compounds in meat; concern is about the presence, in beef, of residues of naturally occurring growth-promotant (the hormones--estrogens, testosterone, progesterone) as well as of the chemically synthesized growth-promotant (the xenobiotics--trenbolone acetate, melengestrol acetate, zeranol).

In another interesting survey the number following each item is the percentage of supermarket shoppers who identified that item as a "serious health hazard".

(**a**) Contamination by bacteria or germs, 77%;
(**b**) Residues, such as pesticides and herbicides, 66%;
(**c**) Product tampering, 66%;
(**d**) Antibiotics and hormones in poultry and livestock, 42%;
(**e**) Food handling in supermarkets, 41%;
(**f**) Irradiated foods, 29%;
(**g**) Nitrites in food, 24%;
(**h**) Additives and preservatives, 20%; and
(**i**) Food produced by biotechnology, 16%.

Critics who question the safety of red meat (beef, veal, pork, lamb, mutton) do so by emphasizing concerns about residues of hormones, antibiotics and pesticides, in red meat, and about presence, in and on red meat, of bacteria--especially food-borne pathogens. The critics are correct in stating that consumers are concerned about presence of bacteria on red meat; "Spoilage," "Freshness," Bacteria/contamination," "Quality control" and "Unsanitary store workers" are top-of-mind concerns ranked first, second, third, fifth and sixth in TRENDS-1996.

"Pesticides/residues/insecticides/herbicides" are also top-of-mind food-safety threats and ranked fourth in TRENDS-1996. However, critics are not absolutely right about residues of "Antibiotics" or "Hormones" being top-of-mind concerns as food-safety threats because of "Antibiotics/Hormones" ranked 17th in unaided-response queries in TRENDS—1996-[193].

In January 1993 an outbreak of Haemorrhagic colitis caused by the O157:H7 serigraph of *Escherichia coli* occurred in the western part of the United States. Epidemiological investigations indicated that the most probable cause of the outbreak was undercooked ground beef consumed at several "Jack In The Box" restaurants in Washington, California, Idaho and Nevada (Sofos and Smith, 1993). It is believed that 1 to 4 people died and that 350 to 500 people were made sick by the *E. coli* O157:H7 in "Jack In The Box" hamburgers (Sofos and Smith, 1993)-[196].

US-Centers For Disease Control (1994)-[139] released a summarization of their data for "Location Of Food Mishandling" in relation to outbreaks of food-borne illness. The latter report attributed 77% of food mishandling to mistakes made at food-service sites (including restaurants and deli's), 20% of food mishandling to errors made in the home and 3% of food mishandling to problems generated at processing plants. At food-service sites and in the home, the biggest problems of food mishandling are:

(**a**) Cross-contamination,
(**b**) Temperature abuse, and
(**c**) Undercooking

Because it is so difficult and so extraordinarily expensive to try to find food-borne pathogens on or in beef by use of sampling protocols, the only rational approach to lowering incidence of, and lessening the odds of encountering, food-borne pathogens like *E coli* O157:H7, is to use every piece of science and technology that we can muster to "intervene" to kill food-borne pathogens in some sequential, multiple-hurdle application of bacteriostatic / bactericidal technology-[194].

E. <u>Valuing Seafood Safety:</u>

Most current major health risks associated with seafood safety originate in the environment and should be dealt with by control of harvest or at the point of capture. With minor exceptions, risks cannot be identified by an organoleptic inspection system. Inspection at the processing level is important to maintain the safety of seafood, but there is little evidence that increased inspection activities at this level would effectively reduce the incidence of seafood-borne disease-03. However, when quality considerations are taken into account, seafood inspection, and training and process monitoring programmes from producer to consumer can be expected to reduce the number of illnesses resulting from seafood.

In the United States, the major sources of information on seafood-borne disease and illness are the Centers for Disease Control (CDC), Food-borne Disease Outbreak Surveillance Program, and a database on shellfish-associated food-borne cases maintained by the Food and Drug Administration (FDA) and Northeast Technical Support Unit. The CDC data are derived from reports of food-borne outbreaks submitted by state health departments to the CDC.

The FDA data come from books, news accounts, CDC reports, city and state health department files, Public Health Service regional files, case histories, and archival reports −03.

The Fish Inspection Directorate, Canadian Food Inspection Agency, and Government of Canada collect data for Canada. The data report annually the cause of illness, description of product causing the illness, product type, country of origin, and the numbers of incidents and cases. Table: 2 (4) is indicative of sea-born illnesses in Canada.

Seafood products causing illnesses in Canada from 1991 to 1997 came from 13 different countries or groups of countries. A total of 29 different species of fish and shellfish and or seafood products are implicated in seafood-borne illnesses. The top six in number of outbreaks were mussels, clams, tuna, barracuda, and marlin.

These six represented 56 percent of the outbreaks. The top seven in number of cases were tuna, mussels, clams, barracuda, lobster tails, marlin and oysters, representing 76 percent of all outbreaks. All other species or products implicated were whelk, Mahi mahi, mackerel, swordfish, crabmeat, salmon, and oysters/quahogs. Clams and dips, haddock and clams, halibut, sole fillets, sharks, scallops, salmon/shrimp/scallops, Pollock, chicken, shrimp, quahogs, kippers and parrotfish/doctor fish were also found to be implicated with illnesses.

The top three countries in products causing outbreaks were Canada and the United States representing 76 percent of the outbreaks. Other countries implicated in one to four outbreaks and/or one to six cases were Singapore, Ecuador, Thailand, China, Canada/United States, Peru, India, Cuba, Fiji, Guyana, and Trinidad/Tobago. Four outbreaks (six cases) could not be traced to the product source.

Table: 2 (4). Summary of the number of seafood-borne illnesses and cases in Canada by causative agents during 1991 to 1997

Causative agent	Outbreaks	Cases
Histamine	19	55
Fecal Coliform	15	15
Decomposition	14	26
Paralytic shellfish	6	21
Ciguatera toxin	6	14
DSP	4	4
**S**taphylococcus	2	2
High bacteria count	2	2
**E**scherichia coli	2	3
**V**ibrio	2	2
Tetramine	1	2
Salmonella	1	12
**E**. coli and	1	1
**S**almonella and _S._	1	4
Allergy to	1	1
Parasites	1	5
Total	**78**	**169**

Source: Derived from (Andruczyk 1998) Andruczyk, Maria. 1998. Ottawa, Canada

While the economic theory, which guides the estimates for valuing seafood safety, still needs major development, at the same time it is necessary to proceed with practical estimates needed to evaluate current programmes and practices. First, the health risks of various diseases must be converted to a common monetary value, with these costs, or the amount they are reduced, representing the benefits of disease reduction. Second, the costs and effectiveness of control strategies must be determined. Third, the costs of disease must be compared to the costs of controlling it to determine worthiness to society of implementing the control.

Costs in valuing food safety are expenses directly related to manufacturing products, or services being incorporated; like the cost of raw materials, processing, laboratory monitoring and evaluation, salaries of persons turning raw materials into sellable safe food, depreciation of equipment and cost of controlled transportation to consumers etc. Costs must be defined at three levels.

Society Level Costs (SLC): SLC is defined as hospital and medical costs, loss of productive output, disease surveillance and investigation costs and loss of life.

Private Level Costs (PLC): PLC is specific to the affected individual; include absence from job, loss of leisure time, and travel of caretakers to hospital, willingness-to-pay, pain, and suffering.

Firm Level Costs (FLC): FLC items measure loss of sales and consumption, cost of reputation loss, product recall, or discarding and legal costs and settlements. In order to be useful, all these costs must be translated into monetary values, which is a very difficult task. The interested reader can follow this technique using _Salmonella sp_. and the Canadian poultry industry (Curtin and Krystynak 1991).

To define costs and benefits at all levels, it is useful to demonstrate an example of a regulation imposed by a country for the purpose of improving the safety of a fish product caught and processed by industry in that country. Within the country of the regulation, input suppliers, fishermen, fish processors, fish distributors, consumers and government incur costs and benefits. In other countries, fishermen, fish processors, fish distributors, consumers, governments of the countries, and any relevant union of governments incur costs and benefits.

One major problem in using any estimation technique is the identification and measurement of risks of contracting a food-borne disease (Roberts and Foegeding 1991). Another major problem is that it is difficult to make a direct connection between the econometric model using actual data and the theoretical base on which the model is built. Several consumer demand models for food safety exist and many economists are working hard to overcome the data problems in current studies (Smallwood and Blaylock 1991).

An excellent summary of the theoretical considerations of valuing food safety and comparison of the Cost-Of-Illness (COI) and Willingness-to-Pay (WTP) methods exist as summarized here (Roberts and Marks 1995). Cost-of-illness (COI) method includes the value of lost leisure time, the opportunity costs of lost household production and other measures associated with the illness. This move towards evaluation estimates the means society will save by avoiding the food-borne illness. In most cases this technique uses actuarial data and observations data, which reflect the actual actions of individuals on which to base the cost saving estimates.

Social costs include costs to individuals, industry costs and public health surveillance costs. Costs to folks falling sick due to consumed contaminated food can be measured through documenting medical costs, income loss, productivity loss, degree of disease, type of disease, pain and distress, leisure time costs, child care costs, risk aversion costs, travel costs, vocational and physical rehabilitation costs etc. In the midst of these costs, the losses incurred due a product failure due to safety issues increases Industry costs and could include product recalls, plant closings and cleanups, product liability costs, reduced product demand, defamation cost and insurance administration. Public health surveillance costs include disease surveillance costs, costs of investigating outbreaks, measures to eliminate recurrence and costs of cleanup.

COI can be taken to mean as measuring the cost of an illness to a specified economy (e.g. jurisdiction of a municipality or a country) in the form of its effects on the current and future value of foods and food services produced by the market of that region or country. The important analysis of what the individual will actually pay to avoid the illness should be included in the COI.

The most theoretically correct measure to use is the willingness-to-pay technique (van Ravenswaay 1995). This involves the knowledge of a possible risk and taking measures to reduce the risk or eliminate the risk so that illness is pre-empted to occur. This actually measures peoples' willingness-to-pay for the reduced risk of death or illness from consuming food in a specified population of people. Contingent valuation (CV) in a marketing situation observes the results of the experiment conducted which forms the basis of this technique. Hedonic scale has been used to evaluate a food product thus valuing food attributes could base the pricing accordingly. Such method is called Hedonic Pricing (HP). This technique is normally used to estimate the value that consumers place on various attributes of a food commodity. An example would be the value one processor, consumer or distributor places on the dairy fat content, specific gravity and total solids content of milk. This estimation method differs from CV in that the estimation function uses observed market price and qualitative data. Hedonic pricing provides an objective valuation of food attributes such as nutrition and fat content while CV deals with subjective valuation of food attributes such as food safety -136.

The gurus of the valuing system believe that WTP method is the most theoretically correct based on economic theory, its use has not been free from disputes. The United States Office of Management and Budget (OMB) has issued guidelines that establish a preference for using observational or behavioural data in benefit cost estimates (BCE) that measure the impact of major rules such as the benefits and costs of seafood safety programmes or regulations. OMB mandates that when benefits come from risk estimates and an agency chooses to estimate benefits with point estimates, then the expected values of the risk estimates must be used. The OMB guidelines acknowledge that it is difficult to estimate the WTP of an individual for commodities (e.g. food safety) not traded in the market because it is impossible to use observational data and methods. However, OMB also indicates that using CV methods warrants an additional burden of analytical rigor. The same is true regarding CV used to evaluate food safety regulations and benefits and costs-15. CV critics argue that its problems are insurmountable and its use should be abandoned. OMB does not take this position, but it does impose an extra burden on deriving estimates not based on real world behavioural data.

Comprehensively, they maintain that theory that evaluates social preferences for food safety should contain six elements:

(1)   Preferences for collective action as well as preferences for self-protection by industry and consumers, including the cost of choices avoided;

(2)   Determination of the optimal level of food safety and the demand for governmental intervention to administer and enforce the "optimal" level of food safety;

(3)   The costs of all participants in the marketplace and regulatory agencies to keep informed of the latest

scientific developments linking diseases with food, identifying high risk individuals and high risk consumption practices, and identifying high risk food production and marketing practices;

(4) The benefits to society of reduced human illness costs at the current level of food safety for microbial contaminants;

(5) The willingness of high-risk and risk-averse individuals to pay for safer food as well as risk neutral consumers;

(6) The willingness of society to pay for the safety of others.

Probably the greatest amount of activity by economists concerned with food safety economics in recent years has dealt with improving the various methods of estimating the benefits resulting from reducing the health risks from food, instead of estimating the actual costs and benefits. Until all theoretical questions can be adequately answered, backed with data sources and techniques that make WTP questions reliable, then the COI is the best method of evaluating the value to society of food safety-[183]. COI estimates are also usually lower than WTP estimates, and are more conservative estimates. The interested reader is referred to the article for detailed comparisons of the uses of COI and WTP at the government, industry, and individual levels.

Data sources and reliability create major problems in the estimation of the value of food safety. Statistics on food-borne disease in developed countries represent only a small amount of the actual numbers of illnesses resulting from food. In developing countries, food-borne illness is recognized as a widespread problem with estimates of unreported cases that approach 90 percent in non-industrialized countries-[01]. Data problems can be summarized into three areas -[198].

First, it must be assumed that food-borne illness can be distinguished from other types of illness and the transmission method of contracting the disease. Second, it must be assumed that the types of food-borne illnesses are known which then provides the basis for counting the persons contracting the disease. Third, no database exists which contains all cases of food-borne illness. The available data sources and the way they are categorized in the United States are available (Steahr 1995). In addition to these costs, it is usually necessary to collect primary data from the fishing, processing, and distribution level private firms in order to estimate the costs incurred by those firms. These data are time-consuming and expensive to collect.

Four aspects of food safety relate to data used to inform public policy -126. First, food safety data present a news problem, which are not freely shared. In the short run, emphasis is to share freely "bad news" and it must be endured for the purpose of reference and improvement rather than for the punitive actions while data should be collected to document the severity of the problem and for preventive actions. In the long run, data can document that food safety improvements are being made. Second, complete, and well-integrated information bases on which to make food safety public policy decisions do not exist. Third, the costs of acquiring food safety data are high and detrimental to one's food business. Fourth, resource distribution among producers and consumers is practically non-existence. Cutting through all these issues is the situation that academic and agency structures do not always foster cooperation to solve these issues, not only within countries, but also among them. The academicians, agencies, and the industry should cooperate for preventive actions.

F. Valuing Environmental Protection:

Environmental Protection reflects the concern for our natural resources and the implementation of programs to protect these natural resources. The growth of intensive animal Agriculture systems and urban encroachment into rural areas has led to increased concerns about air, water and odour quality. The 1998 U.S. National Water Quality Inventory (NWQI) reported that Agriculture sources are responsible for 60 percent of the pollution in contaminated rivers and streams and 45 percent of the pollution in contaminated lakes. In March 1999, the EPA and the US Department of Agriculture developed the Unified Strategy for Animal Feeding Operations which has a goal that all Animal Feeding Operations (AFO's) should develop and implement technically sound, economically feasible, and site-specific Comprehensive Nutrient Management Plans (CNMP's) to minimize impact on water quality and public health".

1. Environmental Stewardship:

Environmental stewardship is an important aspect of the dairy industry because people working together with the environment will protect the natural resources and help prevent further degeneration of the soil, water, and air. This will ensure the safe supply of Agriculture products while maintaining the natural environment. Many programs are available to assist the dairyman in implementing environmentally conscious facilities that are cost effective, environmentally sound and adhere to federal, state, and local regulations. These practices are sometimes referred to as Best Management Practices (BMPs). Federal, state and local laws stipulate necessary guidelines that must be followed in order to construct or expand a confined livestock system. These guidelines are designed to help protect our natural resources. Proper management of wastewater by the dairyman allows the maximum utilization of the nutrients available in manure for fertilizer, bedding, etc. and it aids in the overall contribution to the health of the environment for the dairyman's family, livestock, neighbours, and community.

2. Water: Livestock wastes that are improperly transported or disposed off can be a potential hazard to the surrounding environment and community. Nutrient and bacterial contamination of water resources can be a concern when manure wastes are not managed properly. If people come into contact with livestock waste runoff, their health can be adversely affected due to the bacteria, protozoa, and viruses that may be present in the manure. Waste in surface waters reduces the oxygen in the water, damaging aquatic life. If the waste enters the ground water, then drinking water for the surrounding community is affected.

3. Odour: When livestock manure is improperly handled and stored it can produce strong gases and odours. These odours can be irritating to livestock, dairy employees, and surrounding communities. Waste in surface water can lead to excessive algae growth that can result in unpleasant odours and taste. Some gases commonly associated with livestock manure include:

1. Carbon Dioxide
2. Ammonia
3. Hydrogen Sulphide
4. Methane
5. Carbon Monoxide

4. Air: The improper management of barn manure affects air quality of the surrounding food-manufacturing units. Methane is a gas that contributes to smog and global warming. Ruminant animals are large producers of methane gas; the proper management of livestock waste can help to reduce the amount of methane released into the air and increase the producer's profits.

Animals belonging to the suborder Ruminantia (order Artiodactyla) include antelope, camels, cattle, deer, giraffes, goats, okapis, pronghorn, and sheep. Most ruminants have a four-chambered stomach, two-toed feet, and small or absent upper incisors. Camels and chevrotains have three-chambered stomachs. Ruminants eat quickly, storing masses of grass (grazers) or foliage (browsers) in the first stomach chamber, the rumen, where it softens. They later regurgitate the material, called cud, and chew it again to further break down the indigestible cellulose. The chewed cud goes directly to the other chambers, the second chamber reticulum; omasum is the third stomach serving as a muscular stomach, in that it assists the movement of digesta into the final stomach, the abomasum, where various microrganisms help in the digestion of food.

Future generations will benefit from efforts made now to sustain and conserve natural resources. There are local, state, and federal regulations that need to be followed in order to comply with the laws regarding the construction of Agricultural facilities. Many types of permits are necessary to meet the standards set forth in environmental policies.

The future will bring increased demands on the dairyman to meet specific regulations concerning water, air, and environment. Informed veterinarians that are aware of regulatory changes can act as mediators between the dairyman and the community. Many of the environmental programs available are currently voluntary, but the dairyman that takes the initiative to put these programs into effect now will be prepared for future laws that will be passed. Many resources are available to the livestock operator to assist in implementing environmental protection programs into his/her operation. This will help to guarantee future generations the use of our natural resources.

Food Safety Protection Needed:

Center for Science in the Public Interest (CSPI) the database of food borne-illness outbreaks, documents more than 1,600 outbreaks over the last decade. Even so, the database includes only a small fraction of the outbreaks that actually have occurred, because outbreaks so often go unreported. Foods regulated by the FDA, such as vegetables, eggs, and seafood, account for almost 80 percent of the outbreaks in the database. The FDA has about 770 food inspectors for its 57,000 plants, so, on average, a single FDA inspector has responsibility for 74 food plants. By contrast, USDA has approximately 7,600 inspection personnel for about 6,500 meat, poultry, and processed-egg plants. That imbalance between risk and resources led CSPI and other consumer organizations to call on Congress and the President to develop a single, coherent food-safety statute that is implemented by a single, independent food-safety agency. Such an agency could allocate its resources according to risk. In contrast, USDA's meat and poultry inspectors cannot be assigned to inspect plants that produce fish, shell eggs, or other FDA-regulated foods, even in the face of documented health problems or new health risks-[147].

With the increased movement of people, movement of consumer goods around the globe, multinational ventures in investments, guaranteed food security, access to adequate food supplies, sustainable food resources, conflicts in Africa and Middle East, GM organisms, biotechnology products, persistent effects on biogeochemical cycles, and terrorist threats against western interest, food safety has become a topic of widespread international interest. A clear economic and health rationale exists for governmental involvement in food safety; both consumers and industry would be better served by standards and SOPs that are well understood. Because of the quality of Canadian and U.S. food production and the governmental standards that are in place, most food safety hazards today are fairly modest in scope and severity.

As much as possible, the government's aim of safeguarding the health and safety of Canadians must be balanced against the freedom of individuals to make personal choices on food and beverages they wish to consume. It is wisdom to apply whenever these two interests are at odds, Health Canada's actions, given the Department's mandate, must always favour the former over the latter. The goal of harmonizing global standards on food safety through intergovernmental co-operation and academicians all over the world is needed for the global food safety. Health Canada should pursue mutual recognition agreements with other countries to harmonize food safety standards and SOPs based on factual science.

Minister of Agriculture and Agri-Food, Lyle Vanclief clearly elaborated the importance of food safety in Canada and emphasised that "Canada needs to remain on the leading edge of new scientific developments, so that our food supply continues to be one of the safest in the world". Under the *Food and Drugs Act*, Health Canada conducts a thorough safety assessment of each new product before it can be sold in Canada. Under the new *Canadian Environmental Protection Act* (CEPA), Environment Canada and Health Canada conduct risk assessments of new substances including biotechnology products, to determine if there are adverse effects to the environment or human health, prior to their import into or manufacture in Canada.

Customers Safety Concerns: Satisfying customers are the slogan of today's quality perception. The food industry has responded to this demand with creative attractions to many organoleptic and nutritional innovations to satisfy customers and simultaneously improving safety. Nevertheless, simply letting the market determine food safety might not protect all consumers, especially those susceptible to food borne illness, such as the elderly and small children. Unregulated economic markets could fail to provide a satisfactory level of safety from the consumer's and regulatory standpoints.

Food security and safety are tightly linked. On one hand, transgenic technology may hold the greatest potential to increase food production, reduce the use of harmful chemical pesticides, and provide nutritional foods. On the other hand, some argue that the technology, rather than being a hope, represents a new threat to both the environment and human health safety. North American food safety regulatory structure is the best in the world and ensures the safety of both the domestic and export food supply. Critics and health watch groups say that as good as this structure is, even more food product labelling is needed to let consumers know which products include or exclude genetically engineered foods and ingredients. Food safety is ongoing program where improvements are continual.

A risk assessment approach to the design of food safety regulation looking at where hazards enter food during production and where it is easiest to control them has been advocated by the National Academy of Sciences (NAS) and used by USDA and FDA in their most recent regulations.

Let us review the impending concerns on the food safety issues from the technologies being developed for better usage. Concerns against irradiated food; microbiological parameters, BGH, GE, and terrorism are on the horizon with uncertainties for the curious ones and breakthrough for the optimistic ones awaiting experiences to highlight their point of view. Majority of the consumers in Canada are expected to trust their governments and regulatory authorities for their safe food supplies by keeping a watch on outbreaks of Creutzfeldt - Jakob Disease (CJD), Severe Acute Respiratory Syndrome (SARS), Bovine Spongiform Encephalopathy (BSE), and West Nile Virus (WNV) Infection.

(1) Irradiated Food Safety Concerns: Food Irradiation is a preservation process, similar to the principles involved in the pasteurization process. The first patent to irradiate food was filed a century ago sometimes during the year 1905, as a tool to preserve perishable foods at the time. While pasteurization uses heat energy to kill all pathogenic Microorganisms and partially destroy spoilage Microorganisms, irradiation uses a form of energy called "Ionizing radiation" destroying microorganism according to the intensity of radiation dosage. Since the irradiation process kills the same Microorganisms that cause both spoilage and food borne illness, it did work to make some selected food safer. Since 1971 some of the foods that US astronauts consume have been irradiated. Since the anthrax attacks in late 2001, irradiation is being used to remove pathogens from US mail, medical equipments, health care apparatus, and hygiene products. The ionizing radiation provides energy sufficient to break DNA molecule of a cell thus killing the organism instantly. The good thing to feel good about irradiated food is that irradiation process does not make the food radioactive.

Irradiated food safety to public health has been in question. Two public interest organizations; Public Citizen and the Center for Food Safety submitted 11 pages of comments in response to the U.S. Department of Agriculture's (USDA) call last November-2002 for comments on whether irradiated food should be permitted to feed the 25.4 million children who sign up for the federal program each year. These organizations asserted that Children who participate in the National School Lunch Program should not be fed irradiated food because there are no long-term health studies on children who eat such food -35.

Irradiation is also known to destroy various nutrients. It is understood that irradiation does alter nutritional values of food due to breakdown of enzymes, vitamins and other substances of the food itself. The most affected is thiamine but not at levels significantly different from other processing technologies like pasteurization, UHT, and evaporation etc. Because of such suspected disruptions, flavour and palatability of food remains a question. The high moisture foods like cheese; fresh fruits and vegetables have miserably failed with their organoleptic evaluations. Some low moisture foods like meat products and some fruits like berries could be treated with lower level of irradiation to enhance their shelf lives farther than the normal.

While Irradiation of food gives protection against bacteria belonging to family Enterobacteriaceae _E. coli_, _Shigella sp_. _Salmonella sp_. etc., the concern against radiolytic products of food irradiation is increasing with unending sight. It is argued that Irradiation produces radiolytic products, some of which are unique to food irradiation (so called Unique Radiolytic Products (URPs). These chemicals entail a health risk for consumers (for example, formaldehyde, benzene and lipid peroxides are carcinogenic, others, such as formic acids and quinines are toxic). Extremely low levels of benzopyrenes and formaldehyde are formed during food irradiation but it is their presence due to the process of irradiation is causing stir rather than its adverse effect, which is yet to be proved.

After years of debate and discussion, Health Canada has released a draft proposal to approve the irradiation of ground beef, poultry, shrimp, and mangoes while considering its usage for other foods. Companies have been reluctant to market irradiated products, even though the processes has been approved since the 1960s in Canada for wheat, flour, whole wheat flour, potatoes, onions, spices and seasoning mixes. Irradiation causes minor chemical modifications, similar to cooking, which may make some foods taste slightly different. Food irradiation, at permitted levels, does not diminish the nutritional value of the food. Any living cells in the food, including potentially harmful bacteria, are killed or damaged.

Sceptic Canadians will oppose food irradiation even more strongly when they understand the potential health risks and nutrition problems with irradiated food. There are speculations that Irradiation will cause induced radiation resistance in microbes through mutation. If the population of harmful microorganisms is high they might produce toxins, which are a bigger health risk than the dead microorganisms in the irradiated food. It is of a concern that Irradiation may kill microbes, but toxic chemicals already produced will not be affected, the same is applicable with any heat-treated food. Some bacteria such as *Clostridium botulinum* (botulism) are highly radiation resistant.

Another concern is the corner cutting by the food processors that may take undue advantage of this technology. It is believed that the Canadian CFIA would not sit aside to allow such fear materialise in the Canadian food industry where food irradiation may be permitted. Food producers who are permitted to use irradiation must still meet all food hygiene and sanitation rules and regulatory guidelines. Definitely the foods with high moisture content like milk and most of the milk products will be independent of such concerns as FSEPs regulatory directives, GMPs and PMOs requirements will render the milk and milk products completely safe.

The least could be done to satisfy the sceptic consumers to label the irradiated foods, as it is unacceptable that consumers will receive NO notice of irradiated foods used by restaurants or food servers such as hospitals or other institutions. The idea or recommendations that irradiated foods do not require labelling if they comprise less than 10% of another food. It should be unacceptable to satisfy and safe guard the interest of concerned consumers.

As far as the World Health Organization (WHO) is concerned, irradiated food does not pose a health risk because of the irradiation process itself but the microorganisms left behind or get entry after treatment will still cause problems to human health as do the untreated foods. Thus all standard food safety measures like SOPs, GMPs and SLPs embedded with in a HACCP system will give maximum possible protection to food and consuming humans.

(2) Chemical Food Safety: Many food additives, sweeteners, stabilizers and colorants have been found to cause gridlock risks to consuming food customers. For example Cyclamate is artificial sweetener suspected of carcinogenic actions to human health. Saccharin already approved in North America causes bladder cancer when given extra dosages to male rats. Aspartame is another sweetener, which is linked with complications of Phenylketonoria (PUK) and causes to some consumer's nausea, headaches, and seizures etc. However, their recommended usage is considered safe by the government agencies, its long-term effect and quantity consumed remains a risk factor. Therefore, moderation and prevention is up to the choice of users. All the products containing such artificial sweeteners are labelled for the knowledge of consumers.

Sodium nitrite is an important food preservative, which is used to inhibit the growth of *Clostridium botulinum* in meat and meat products. At the same time it is carcinogenic and it is associated with many health complications if used beyond ADI. Similarly other additives like potassium nitrate, sodium nitrate, sodium propionate (may cause migraine headaches) Butylated hydroxyanisole (BHA); not for children etc., and many others are linked with one complication or the other when used in excess amounts than ADI.

The Stabilizer additives like Agar agar (associated with constipation) Carrageenan (associated with induced ulcerative colitis), Guar gum (associated with nausea and abdominal cramps) and many others such permitted additives are associated with some sort of health complications to vulnerable individuals. A generalized reaction is rare unless consumed beyond ADI. Therefore, moderation and prevention is up to the choice of users. All the products containing such artificial stabilizers are labelled for the knowledge of consumers. It is worth noting that it is possible to omit many additives, which may be present in a food and could cause reactions to certain consumers. The Food and Drugs Act and Regulations of Canada lists components of ingredients or classes of ingredients set out in the table under clause B.01.009 do not require to be shown on a label. Some products like lard, gelatine, and bourbon whisky, which are religiously offensive to Muslims and Jews, may cause interference in to their religious beliefs. Products like soy flour, whole-wheat flour, sweetening agents and animal fats may cause allergic reactions to certain groups of people, which they cannot identify or trace back to their ordeal.

It is not hidden from the eyes of human health watchdogs that the addition of so many diverse materials in our daily food supplies does pose toxic risks. The Food and Drugs Act and Regulations of

Canada needs revision to reclassify certain additives, which need labelling, and violators reprimanded with heavy penalties. This is one step, which may help safeguard consumers and pre-empt producers of illegal and adulterated foods.

(3) Microbiological Food Safety: Beside technological concerns in food safety issues, food safety in the United States and Canada has been continuing to be very good. Occasional outbreaks of food borne illness and deaths attributable to such illnesses have caught the attention of the public, the media, and governmental agencies internationally. The perception that such outbreaks are increasingly frequent and serious is prompting queries into the best means of reducing their frequency and extent. Question of comparative safety issues with imported and domestically produced foods have impacted re-thinking of legislation, which betters the food safety.

Senator Richard Durbin in his speech to re-introduce legislation on food safety stated that the General Accounting Office (GAO) estimates that as many as 81 million people will suffer food poisoning this year (1999) and more than 9,000 will die. Children and the elderly are especially vulnerable. In terms of medical costs and productivity losses, food borne illness costs the nation up to $37 billion annually. The situation is not likely to improve without decisive action. The Department of Health and Human Services predicts that food borne illnesses and deaths will increase 10-15 percent over the next decade if uncontrolled. He emphasised effort to consolidate the food safety and inspection functions of numerous agencies and offices into a single, independent food safety agency[180].

Twelve different government agencies have authority over different aspects of food safety in the United States, with the Food and Drug Administration (FDA) and the USDA carrying the brunt of the burden. Primary responsibility for food safety in meat and poultry rests with the USDA; the FDA has primary responsibility for all other foods. Similarly Health Canada, Agri-food Canada, and CFIA share the responsibilities in Canadian federal jurisdictions while provincial and territorial governments also play enforcement and coordinating role with in their jurisdiction.

Microbiology is an important science in food safety. This science can trace many food-borne illnesses to specific pathogens found in food. As consumers live longer and become more affluent, they demand higher levels of quality and safety standards. Changes in production practices, diversified ingredients resourcing and new sources of food, introduce new risks into the food system. In addition, more foods are purchased away from home or in prepared form, the less control by consumers. Diversity in food consumption and manufacturing systems opens new chapter in food safety measures.

However, sometime back a U.S. Court of Appeals decision upholding a Texas court's decision blocking the USDA from closing a beef processing plant that failed a series of tests for control of *Salmonella sp*. raises questions about standards and its impact on public food safety. Today, food safety is receiving a great deal of attention from the public and government for several reasons.

Let us review the safety issues related to meat industry. Since the early years of the 20th Century, USDA has relied on meat carcass inspection at the point of slaughter. While this system removed diseased animals from the food supply and ensured sanitation procedures, it was not designed to address microbial pathogens and other spoilage microflora, such as *E. coli* and *Salmonella sp*.

Both of these are enterogenic bacteria and can live in the gastrointestinal track of animals without harming them, and may enter meat during slaughter and processing. It may not be a material issue to the consumers but the diseases spread by these bacteria have several things in common. All of them pass to human consumers through daily food intakes. Most of these bacteria cause familiar, similar, and common symptoms like headache, diarrhoea, bloat, stomach cramps, nausea, vomiting and alleviated fevers. Imagine what sort of effect these germs cause to the infants, seniors, and immune compromised individuals of the society who rely on such a food for their nourishments.

Let us briefly discuss some of the microorganisms, which are transmitted through food and cause illnesses in humans. The most common bacteria are *Campylobacter sp.*, *Clostridium sp.*, *Escherichia coli*, *Listeria monocytogenes*, *Mycobacterium paratuberculosis*, *Salmonella sp.*, *Staphylococcus aureus,* and *Shigella sp*.

Campylobacters are bacteria that are a major cause of diarrhoeal illness in humans and are generally regarded as the most common bacterial cause of gastroenteritis worldwide. In developed and developing countries, they cause more cases of diarrhoea than, for example, food borne *Salmonella sp.*, bacteria. In developing countries, *Campylobacter sp.*, infections in children under the age of two years are especially frequent, sometimes resulting in death. Campylobacters are mainly spiral-shaped, S-shaped, or curved, rod-shaped bacteria.

There are 16 species and six subspecies assigned to the genus *Campylobacter sp.*, of which the most frequently reported in human disease are *C. jejuni* (subspecies *jejuni*) and *C. coli*, *C.*

laridis and *C. upsaliensis* is also regarded as primary pathogens. Foods implicated with *Campylobacter sp.*, infections are water, raw poultry, rarely on red meat, raw milk, offal, and frozen foods.

Food borne botulism is the name of the disease (actually a food borne intoxication) caused by the consumption of foods containing the neurotoxin produced by *C. botulinum*. This type of botulism is caused by the ingestion of *C. botulinum* spores, which colonize and produce toxin in the intestinal tract of infants (intestinal toxaemia botulism). Almost any type of food that is not very acidic (pH above 4.6) can support growth and toxin production by *C. botulinum*. Botulinal toxin has been demonstrated in a considerable variety of foods. Foods implicated are canned corn, green beans, soups, beets, asparagus, mushrooms, ripe olives, spinach, tuna fish, chicken, chicken livers liver pate, luncheon meats, ham, sausage, stuffed eggplant, lobster, and smoked and salted fish.

Perfringens food poisoning is the term used to describe the common food borne illness caused by *C. perfringens*. Ingesting food contaminated with Type C strains also causes a more serious but rare illness. *Clostridium perfringens* is characterized by intense abdominal cramps and diarrhoea, which begin 8-22 hours after consumption of foods containing large numbers of those *C. perfringens* bacteria capable of producing the food poisoning toxin. The illness is usually over within 24 hours but less severe symptoms may persist in some individuals for 1 or 2 weeks. A few deaths have been reported as a result of dehydration and other complications. Foods implicated are meat, gravies, and meat joints.

Table: 2(5) – Risk of Spoilage from Water Activity of Foods

Aw	Related	Food Products
0.03-0.50	No bacterial and mycological growth	Noodles, Whole Egg Powder, Cookies, Crackers, bread crusts, Whole milk powder (WMP), Skimmed Milk Powder (SMP), Butter Milk Powder (BMP), Dried Casein etc.
0.60-0.65	Osmophilic yeasts, few molds, Xerophilic molds, *Saccharomyces bisporus*	Dried fruits, Rolled oats
0.75	Most halophilic bacteria, Mycotoxigenic aspergilli	Jam, marmalade, glace fruits, marzipan, marshmallows
0.80	Most molds, most *Saccharomyces sp.*, Debaryomyces, *Staphylococcus aureus*	Most fruit juice concentrates, condensed milk, syrup, flour, high-sugar cakes, pulses containing 15-17% moisture

.87	Most halophilic bacteria, Mycotoxigenic aspergilli, Many yeasts, Candida, Torulopsis, *Hansenula micrococcus*	Fermented sausage, sponge cakes, dry cheese, margarine, foods with 65% sucrose or 15% NaCl
0.80-0.91	Most molds (Mycotoxigenic penicillia), most Saccharomyces (bailii) species, Debaromyces, *Salmonella sp.*, *Vibrio parahaemolyticus*, *C. botulinum*, *Lactobacillus*, *Clostridium perfringens* Some molds	Some cheese (Cheddar, Swiss, Provolone), cured meat, fruit juice concentrates with 55% sucrose or 12% NaCl
0.91-0.95	Many yeasts (Candida, Torulopsis, Hansenula), Micrococcus *Staphylococcus aureus*,	Fresh and canned fruits, vegetables, meat, fish, milk, cooked sausages, breads, foods with up to 4 oz sucrose or 7% NaCl, Brined white cheeses
0.95-1.00	*Salmonella sp. E.coli Vibrio parahaemolyticus*, *C. botulinum*, *Serratia sp.*, *Shigella sp.*, *C. jejuni Lactobacillus sp.*, *Listeria monocytogenes*, *M. paratuberculosis*, *Pediococcus sp.*, some molds, yeasts (*Rhodotorula sp.*, *Pichia sp.*) *Pseudomonas sp.*, *Escherichia sp.*, *Proteus sp.*, *Shigella sp.*, *Klebsiella sp.*, *Bacillus sp.*, *Clostridium perfringens*, some yeast.	All fresh foods with succulence including milk and milk products, meat and meat products, fruits and fruit products, cereal products where moisture content is high enough to attract microbial growth under favourable state, chicken, poultry products etc.

Infection due to Enterohaemorrhagic (causing intestinal bleeding) *E. coli*, e.g. *E.coli* O157 is an important food borne disease. Although their incidence is relatively low, their severe and sometimes fatal health consequences, particularly among infants, children and the elderly, make them among the most serious food borne infections. Pathogenic *Escherichia coli* strains, such as *E. coli* O157, which produce a potent (vero-) toxin cause haemorrhagic infections in the colon, result in bloody diarrhoea or life-threatening complications such as kidney failure. Foods implicated with *E. coli* O157 outbreaks are mainly related to beef, sprouts, lettuce but juices have also caused outbreaks. Water is the most identified source of *E. coli* as one can refer to Walkerton water crisis in Canada.

Listeria monocytogenes is the cause of Listeriosis, which has a fatality rate of up to 30%. The most frequent effects are meningitis and miscarriage or meningitis of the foetus or newborn. Many types of foods have been implicated in Listeriosis cases. Often a long refrigeration period seems to have contributed to outbreaks. Foods implicated are coleslaw, Vacherie Mont d, soft cheeses, raw meat, poultry, turkey frankfurters, dried mushrooms, and salami etc.

The disease caused by *M. paratuberculosis*, known as Johne's disease or paratuberculosis, is an incurable, chronic, infectious, Granulomatous enteritis of ruminants, characterised clinically by diarrhoea, weight loss, debilitation and, ultimately, death. Johne's disease is one of the most widespread bacterial diseases of domestic animals throughout the world. It is most common in cattle and to a lesser extent in sheep and goats. Asymptomatic carriers also exist. As the causative organism of Johne's disease, *M. paratuberculosis* may be found in dairy animals. *M. paratuberculosis* contamination of commercial raw milk supplies must therefore be assumed to occur. Relatively little is known about the incidence and survival characteristics of *M. paratuberculosis* during the processing of milk and manufacture of dairy products. Because *M. paratuberculosis* can occur in the milk of cattle and goats with Johne's disease as well as in the milk of asymptomatic carriers, and since a possible association exists between *M. paratuberculosis* and Crohn's disease, interest in the thermal inactivation of this organism in milk at pasteurisation temperatures has arisen. Foods implicated are mainly milk and meat from infected herd.

Salmonellae are ubiquitous human and animal pathogens, and Salmonellosis, a disease that affects an estimated 2 million Americans each year, is common throughout the world. Pathogenic *Salmonella sp.*, ingested in food survives passage through the gastric acid barrier and invades the mucosa of the small and large intestine and produce toxins. Invasion of epithelial cells stimulates the release of proinflammatory cytokines, which induce an inflammatory reaction. The acute inflammatory response causes diarrhoea and may lead to ulceration and destruction of the mucosa. The bacteria can disseminate from the intestines to cause systemic disease. Non-typhoidal Salmonellosis is a worldwide disease of humans and animals. Salmonellosis includes several syndromes (gastroenteritis, enteric fevers, septicaemia, focal infections, and an asymptomatic carrier state). Contaminated food is the major mode of transmission for non-typhoidal salmonellae because Salmonellosis is a Zoonosis and has an enormous animal reservoir. *Salmonella typhi* and *Salmonella paratyphi* cause enteric fever including symptoms of malaise, slow pulse, spleen enlargement and constipation. Foods implicated are water supplies, milk, ice cream, raw shellfish, and unwashed fruits from warm countries.

Staphylococcus aureus leads to the release of exotoxin. This organism is salt tolerant making its pathogenicity through white cheeses, which are brined. The best defence against this organism is pasteurization of milk and application of GMPs, SOPs, and strict adherence to HACCP principles.

Shigella sp. is enteric and food personnel who do not wash their hands may contaminate plant, machinery, outfits, and food materials in the recombination, processing, or packaging systems. Food borne carriers have been known in meat, fish vegetables, milk and milk products and poultry. Deaths may occur with Shigella infections though if treated in time the epidemic is controllable.

The water activity in food products is a detrimental factor, which should be kept in mind when we seek to preserve our foods against spoilage and pathogenic organism. Table: 2(5) – Risk of Spoilage from Water Activity of Foods may not list all microorganism but the list represent important groups which would help prescribing a treatment to suppress their growth.

The policy of sniffing and rejecting the meat cannot detect microbes and their potential risk to human health. It was an attempt to address this gap that led to the Texas suit against USDA. More than 90 percent of federally inspected plants met that standard on *Salmonella sp*. However, after the Texas plant in question failed salmonella tests three times over eight months, USDA moved to shut it down-157. The Texas beef plant appealed, contending that because *Salmonella sp*. is not an adulterant and because it is destroyed during normal cooking, its presence is not a public safety issue. While the beef processor in question eventually went out of business, its court victory left confusion about the role of standards in the future. Now, *Salmonella sp*., *tests* must be used in conjunction with other information to shut down a plant, and can no longer be the sole basis for that decision.

This leaves several issues in how food safety is regulated not fully resolved. These include USDA's legal authority under current meat inspection laws as well as the scientific validity of sampling and testing procedures. One question that might be asked is if it makes economic sense to set a microbial pathogen standard for meat and poultry plants.

The appeals court decision said that historically, responsibility for reducing food pathogens rested with the final food preparers. Professor Laurian J. Unnevehr of University of Illinois Department of Agricultural and Consumer Economics; believes that changing habits and products have complicated that assumption. Food preparation methods have changed with the advent of more fresh foods and use of new technologies such as microwave ovens, and food preparation has increasingly moved outside the home. Clearly, consumer protection in this changing food system means shifting more responsibility to the food industry for food safety. Both consumers and industry would be better served by standards that are well understood. "Because of the quality of U.S. food production and the governmental standards that are in place, most food safety hazards today are fairly modest in scope and severity."

However, she adds, a U.S. Court of Appeals decision upholding a Texas court's decision blocking the USDA from closing a beef processing plant that failed a series of tests for control of salmonella raises questions about standards-157.

The question becomes, developing standards that are most effective and least burdensome to the food industry for achieving improved food safety. Standards can be based on outcomes, such as the prevalence estimate 7.5 percent _Salmonella sp._, standard, or on processes used in production, such as requiring specific sanitation procedures. The prevalence estimate is the number of positive samples divided by the total number of samples analyzed, expressed as a percentage. The percentages of sample sets meeting the _Salmonella sp._, performance standards are based on "A" sets that were completed during the specified year, as defined by the collect date of the last sample in the sample set. Code "A" sample sets is collected at randomly selected establishments. "B" and "C" represent sample sets collected from establishments targeted for follow-up testing following a failed set -169.

Food safety from microbiological reasons could also be attained by the technique, which has been practiced by ancient people. The basic principles of water activity (Aw) apply to microbiological growth in all foods. Risks to food come from the amount of water available for the metabolic activity of microbiological foes (pathogenic and spoilage microorganisms) of human food. For a longer shelf life, the selectivity of moisture percentage in food products could be best adjusted, which meets its safety, demands. The Table: 2(5) – Risk of Spoilage from Water Activity of Foods; indicates the importance of lower moisture contents to different food products, its safety and its perseverance.

Mad Cow Disease: The first human form of mad cow disease called Creutzfeldt Jakob Disease (CJD) was identified in British men. This disease inflicts human when Bovine Spongiform Encephalopathy (BSE) infested meat is consumed unknowingly. It results in spongy plaque build-up in human brain similar to those of people who die of Alzheimer and Parkinson diseases.

Elimination by monitoring the dairy and meat herds for BSE is the best prevention. Isolation and quarantine of suspected animals and eventual destruction has lead to eradication of this disease in Great Britain and Japan. The screening should be done right in the farm rather than in factories, otherwise it will result in proliferation. In 2003, BSE scare devastated Canadian Beef industry though it was more of a publicity outcry than any noted material damage to human health.

(4) Bioterrorism and Food Safety: Bioterrorism is just the latest example of the problem with relying on old laws to regulate new hazards. The latest development of chemical and biological terrorism has alerted the public to the possibility that we may be confronted with intentional contamination of food, water, or air. While every effort must be made to prevent those acts in the first place, it is clear that better food inspection offers a critical avenue to protect our food supply from both intentional and unintentional contamination.

On June 12 President George W. Bush signed into law the Public Health Security and Bioterrorism Preparedness and Response Act of 2002 (the Bioterrorism Act) which includes a large number of provisions to help ensure the safety of the U.S. from Bioterrorism, including new authority for the Secretary of Health and Human Services (HHS) to take action to protect the nation's food supply against the threat of intentional contamination. The Food and Drug Administration (FDA), as the food regulatory arm of HHS, is responsible for developing and implementing these food safety measures, including four major regulations.

A stronger, federal food-safety system is an essential component of a defence against terrorist attacks on the food supply and also would help to prevent food borne illnesses due to unintentional product contamination. Consumers have become sensitized to the issue of microbiological contamination of food, in part, because of much better reporting of food-poisoning outbreaks. Several years ago, Center for Science in the Public Interest (CSPI), began tracking food-poisoning outbreaks, so we could better identify which foods were actually making people sick.

Today the U.S. federal government spends over one billion dollars a year to support the numerous agencies and multiple bureaucracies that have a food-safety role. Senator Durbin's Safe Food Act of 1999 offered a much-needed strategy during this time of crisis to correct some of the deficiencies in US federal food-safety system that have left consumers to wander and the food industry itself—vulnerable. Today, for example, the Food and Drug Administration (FDA) must ensure the safety of nearly four million food shipments entering the US from more than 100 different countries. However, the FDA has been understaffed who are rarely available to conduct those inspections. Not surprisingly, less than one percent of those four million shipments are inspected.

(5) BGH Safety Concerns: Bovine Growth Hormone (BGH) as a food controversy of historic proportions has been under debate in the United States. At stake is the quality and safety of America's food supply, the health of tens of millions of consumers, the survival of the family farm, the suffering of millions of animals and the future direction of US farming and Agricultural system. In November 1993, the US Food and Drug Administration (USFDA) approved the sale of genetically engineered bovine growth hormone (BGH) for use in dairy cows. Milk and dairy products derived from BGH-treated cows are now on sale nationwide-[11].

The Center for Food Safety (CFS) project has been established by the International Center for Technology Assessment (CTA). It was established to carry out vital and historic initiatives in food safety, environmental protection, and sustainable Agriculture. The goal of the CFS is to preserve organic food; ensure the testing and labelling of genetically engineered foods; and to carry out litigation efforts when the U.S. government fails to act appropriately. Center for Food Safety's mission is accomplished by using grassroots, public education, media outreach, and litigation. Currently, there are many important reasons to safeguard and monitor current food supply and production means.

Bovine somatotropin (BST or BGH) is a natural protein hormone that stimulates the production of milk. Dairy farmers have found that by injecting BST identical to cows own BST hormone increase milk production, efficiency of feed utilization, and less manure per cow. The researchers have found no evidence of any health risks with BST treated cows' milk. Animal fat contained in meat is also modified by the use of Hormones specific to the purpose.

(6) GE Safety Concerns: Genetically Engineered (GE) foods as a gap in our food-safety protection remain to be tackled. Genetically engineered (GE) foods require immediate attention. The FDA, which shares with the Environmental Protection Agency (EPA) and the U.S. Department of Agriculture (USDA) the regulation of GE plants that are used for human food, does not approve them or even require a safety review before they are sold to consumers. Nor does FDA give the public an opportunity to comment on GE foods before they are introduced into the food supply. The FDA says that, to date, all biotech companies have voluntarily consulted with the agency before marketing their foods. However, that "behind-closed-doors" system does little to instil public confidence in the safety of this powerful and potentially valuable new technology.

On May 18, 1994, the FDA approved Calgene's genetically engineered tomato, the Flavr Savr. Over the last three years, the FDA has Okayed at least seventeen more genetically engineered foods, including corn, potatoes, canola, and squash. Presently, there are 36 genetically engineered whole foods on the market. Soon hundreds of genetically engineered foods will be introduced to the marketplace.

This year (2001), the FDA proposed to mandate that companies notify the agency of their intent to market GE foods and to submit specific information for agency review. That was a step in the right direction, but Center for Science in the Public Interest (CSPI) has urged FDA to both review and actually approve the safety of every genetically engineered crop before it is marketed.

The majority of people in North America feel that they should have the right to know if their food is genetically engineered, as is the case with the citizens in the European Union, Japan, Australia, and many other countries. A more precise method of transferring specific genes from one species to another is Genetic Engineering (GE). An example of a genetically engineered food is Bt sweet corn. This type of corn was developed by inserting a gene from a soil bacterium, _Bacillus thuringiensis_, into the genome of a corn variety to protect it from the European corn borer, a devastating pest to field crops. The transfer of a required gene to a valuable fruit genome to enhance the required characteristics is considered a technological breakthrough at the same time its side effects are left to germinate without any food safety guarantees. It seems trial and error still continues with our science advancement, which is extraordinarily expensive when it applies to human lives.

Genetically Modified Foods (GMF) are not considered as precise as advocates would like to convince the curious consumers. To create a transgenic food, desired trait gene is spliced in to the target genome while guarantees for the proper functioning of the genome may not be available thus unexpected and surprises could be in store. That is why contention against GMF is growing. WHO recommends precise safety measures in the development GMF, as risks are considered genuine? It is also possible that allergen list could expand the periphery to an extent that health related matters would need extra resources to consumers. It is yet to be seen how economics expert analyse the cost difference between the cost effective GMF and cost provocative health risks.

The EU requires labelling to declare GMF; it should be done in Canada and the United States. A complete elimination of GMF in our daily food is a rare possibility while we continue to consume unknown amounts of GMF portions; a negative effect is yet to be identified. Still it is a right of consumer to know its source as we do in milk of cow, goat, camel or sheep, further down on the line of identification we label pasteurized or unpasteurized product issues.

(7) Antibiotic Concerns: The human health watch groups are on continual watch of antibiotics traces, which may end up in our milk and milk products, beef and beef products, poultry and poultry products, fish and fish products etc. The microorganisms secrete chemicals, which are lethal to competing microorganisms in a host or substrate. That is advantageous where a treatment is on course to eliminate identified competing bacteria. That chemical which eliminates the non-desirable bacteria is called antibiotic. The possibility that bacterium develops a resistance to a particular antibiotic alarms the health conscious people as the resistant bacterium may severely damage one's immune system and treatment drugs may become useless. Proliferation of resistant strain in our food system is a serious issue.

One such example could be taken from penicillin, which is an antibiotic to _Staphylococcus aureus_. After the Korean war of early fifties, this bacteria developed resistance to penicillin resulting in health disaster and deaths. An alternative drug Methicillin was developed to counter _S. aureus_. By the end of Vietnam War, this drug was also found to have lost its antibiotic property against _S. aureus_ because of bacterial resistance. Then came Vancomycin and lately Linezolid is on line to treat the _Staphylococcus aureus_. So is the case with many other microorganisms, which develop resistance in zoonotic system and land on human plates. There are at least thirty-seven veterinary drugs listed in division 15 of The Food and Drugs Act and Regulations of Canada, which list common name, active substance and their maximum residue limit in ppm for different foods, which may be inherited from food animals. A strict enforcement of the limit is vital for the safety of consumers in the continual consumption.

In Canada, regulatory agencies are ever watchful of any release of such antibiotics to milk or meat. The manufacturers of foods like milk, meat, and poultry are equipped with SOPs and regulatory advice, which will not let such contaminants, end up in our Canadian foods. Consumers in home based food supplies should be aware of such dangers and should respond appropriately so that they or their hosts do not end up consuming tainted products.

For a further study on the risks factors involved with food safety please refer Chapter: 04 - HACCP Evolution.

(8) Sub-Standard Processing Concerns: There are incidences when production of food lends itself to abuses within the industry, as costs are cut to generate huge profits for the owners of the few food businesses. Whether it is the production of white cheeses from unpasteurized milk manufactured in unregistered home locations, or production of fruit juices from unregistered small businesses, it all contribute to human health hazards in a society like Canada and United States. One may ask how and why we are exposed to this level of pathogenic risk, given the number of local, state, and federal regulations and agencies that govern and oversee our food production and processing. The answer is simple; some consumers who are the customers of such unhygienic products help operate such businesses because of low price, individual choice, or aloofness of health impacts. It also puts pressure on governmental agencies and lawmakers who need public cooperation to identify and notify the agencies against such vendors or sub standard food manufacturers.

Under mandated Canadian and US federal HACCP regulations, food processors in Canada and the United States must develop written plans that detail every step within their respective food preparation processes, which must eliminate or reduce the number of microbes insufficient to cause illness. The effort should be to exceed regulatory laws in minimising harmful microorganisms. In these plans, they must identify critical steps where contamination can occur, then keep written logs with initialled checkpoints for each step. This paper log supposedly ensures all steps in the process were followed. Government inspectors then check these written logs, instead of inspecting the plant or the food itself.

The Federal government regulate meats such as beef, bison, pork, poultry, seafood, ham, lamb, sausages, and veal. Nonetheless, each year there are numerous incidents of food poisoning and even deaths attributed to poorly processed meat products. In cheese prepared from milk contaminated with _Listeria monocytogenes_, growth of the pathogen is possible if the pH is higher than 5.5. The number of _Listeria monocytogenes_ in soft cheeses may increase by a factor of 10 following storage for 25 to 30 days. On the other hand, the number of _Listeria sp._, decreases in hard cheeses like Cheddar, feta, and blue mould cheese during the course of ripening. Those who advocate no-pasteurization for cheese milk should resort to alternative technologies, which will eliminate pathogens from cheese milk. Heat treatment of milk is not the only technological solution available to ensure the microbiological safety of cheese. An attractive alternative to pasteurization uses microfiltration to assist in the removal of bacteria from raw milk. This technique has the potential for meeting both legislators' and consumers' requirements.

The bottom line is to eliminate chances of health risks from the food, which are manufactured by employing SOPs, GMPs, SHPs, and HACCP system. No food should be allowed in the Canadian and US markets that is from unregistered, non-standard, and sub-standard manufacturers.

Measuring the benefits of safer food:

Economic Research Service (ERS) USDA; established a new, extramural research program to measure the benefits of safer food with the help of a special appropriation in 1999. ERS used a competitive selection process to award funding for two cooperative agreements in food safety research, one with Harvard University and the other with the University of Wyoming to apply state-of-the-art economic analysis to estimate the benefits of improving the safety of the Nation's food supply:

"Valuing Reductions in Food borne Risk Associated with Bacterial Pathogens" James Hammitt and Kip Viscusi, Harvard University

"Estimating Consumer Benefits of Improving Food Safety" Jason Shogren, University of Wyoming

These research projects will apply state-of-the-art valuation methodologies to measure consumers' willingness to pay for reductions in food safety risks from microbial pathogens in foods. Using such techniques as contingent valuation, experimental auction markets, and retail sales experiments, researchers will develop estimates of consumers' willingness to pay for safer food.

Firms invest financial and human resources to prevent microbial pathogens, carcinogenic chemicals, and other harmful additives from entering their food products. Many firms invest only in resources mandated through regulation, but many others choose an investment level that exceeds the regulated standard. ERS research examines the costs of regulatory compliance and private food safety investments and assesses the types of technologies adopted. Much ERS research focuses on the incentives for making food safety investments. These incentives include: genuine concern for producing pathogen-free products, fear of a lost reputation for selling pathogen-free products, contractual requirements with customers and suppliers, fear of lawsuits arising from the sale of contaminated products, and State, local, and Federal government regulatory requirements-54.

ERS provides analyses of the economic issues affecting the safety of the U.S. food supply, including the effectiveness and equity of alternative policies and programs designed to protect consumers from unsafe food: ERS estimates the human illness costs of food borne disease at $6.9 billion per year for five food borne pathogens. These estimates, continually updated and expanded by ERS, have helped policymakers identify the magnitude of the societal impact of food borne disease. Benefit/cost analyses of programs for improving food safety provide insight into the least-cost interventions at locations throughout the food continuum.

Risk assessment provides information on the relative risks of pesticides versus pathogens, as well as information on how much reduction in human illness can be achieved by various interventions from the farm to the table. Coupling economics with risk assessment is an integral part of benefit/cost analyses.

To estimate the costs of illness from different valuation methods used by different Federal agencies make it difficult to compare programs adopted by these agencies. Risk management could be more readily comparable if the different agencies' programs have a consensus approach to assigning values to risk reductions and each agency accepted the commonality of the program. Such comparisons could provide risk managers with information to help them choose food safety programs that reduce both food borne illness and public costs. As a first step toward generating a consensus on the current state of knowledge and deciding on a common approach, several agencies planned a conference, held September 14-15, 2000, at the University of Maryland, College Park, Maryland, USA. The outcome of the conference is serving as guidance for a consensus approach.

U.S. companies offer insurance to protect businesses against losses due to food borne pathogens from product recalls, disease outbreaks, sales losses, or other business disruptions. To receive low insurance premiums, firms have an incentive to disclose their maximum food safety efforts. In contrast, under HACCP regulations, firms have an incentive to identify the minimum number of critical control points for monitoring by regulators-129.

In other countries too organizations are striving to measure the benefits. The forces escalating food safety in the United Kingdom (UK) are better crisis management and restoration of consumer confidence, whereas in Canada and Australia risk management and prevention of trade-threatening food safety issues are key. Within the UK and Australia, food companies are increasing vertical alliances, partly in response to the UK 1990 Food Safety Act that requires "due diligence" and increases legal liability for contaminated incoming products-125.

Food safety presents a double moral hazard problem, since neither consumers nor producers can accurately detect the other's efforts and both share the losses if illness that occurs. Given this sub-optimal outcome, government regulation could increase social assistance, especially if it increases information and causes changes in behaviour to improve food safety-206.

FOOD SAFETY AND LEGAL SYSTEM:

Studies conducted on Incentives that arise from food poisoning cases in the U.S. legal system focuses on the U.S. product liability system for food poisoning cases and make six key points.

First, current legal incentives to produce safer food are weak, though slightly stronger in outbreak situations and in markets where food borne illness can be more easily traced to individual firms. Far less than 0.01 percent of cases are litigated and even fewer are paid compensation.

Second, even if potential plaintiffs can overcome the high information and transaction costs necessary to file lawsuits, monetary compensation provides only weak incentives to pursue litigation. Firms paid compensation in 56 percent of the 294 cases examined in this study and the median compensation was only $2,000 before legal fees.

Third, indirect incentives for firms may be important and deserve more research. For example, firms may be influenced by costly settlements and decisions against other firms in the same industry.

Fourth, confidential settlements, health insurance, and product liability insurance distort legal incentives to produce safer food. The settlements should be separated from the committed act. A committed act should be considered as a violation and should be dealt by enforcement authorities separately while claims of civil damage could be dealt either by court or out of court settlements.

Fifth is the ambiguity about whether microbial contamination is "natural" or an "adulterant" hinders the legal system from effectively dealing with the food safety issues. Microbial contamination is either due to negligence of raw material supplier or due to errors connected to processor or related to abuse by handler, vendor or due to intentional acts, all are harmful to human health. For litigation purpose, the source should be identified and a control at all level imposed by regulators. The violators should be accountable for their part of responsibilities. The consumer is always a victim and reading the product labels to accommodate required conditions should be the responsibility of the consumer. There may not be a punitive action against consumer but a moral obligation to protect him.

Sixth, a brief comparison of the incentives from U.S. and English legal systems suggests that more research is needed to understand the strengths, weaknesses, and relative impact of each country's legal system on the incentives to produce safer food-[82].

1. Mode of Lawsuits Success: **I**n the United States, it has been noted that Food borne illness lawsuits, though usually unsuccessful, help food industry focus on safety. Less than a third of the jury verdicts tracked by ERS from 1988-97 awarded compensation to plaintiffs in food borne illness cases. Even though firms responsible for microbial contamination compensate relatively few food borne illnesses, such firms cannot ignore the potential legal consequences and catastrophic losses of making or distributing contaminated food products that might cause illness or death.

The median award to winning plaintiffs was $25,560, while a few much higher awards raised the mean to $133,280 (1998). Plaintiffs were more likely to win if they could link the illness to a specific pathogen, and more severe illnesses tended to result in higher awards.

Both food firms and consumers make food-handling errors that lead to food borne illness, but the proportion of illnesses due to each is unknown due to data limitations.

Feature Food borne illness jury trials have better chance of success, higher awards by identifying specific pathogens. Less than a third of the jury verdicts tracked by ERS from 1988-97 awarded compensation to plaintiffs in Food borne illness cases. Plaintiffs who alleged illness from a specific pathogen were more likely to receive compensation (42 percent) than Plaintiffs, who did not, and the expected award was far higher when specific pathogen or illness was alleged ($82,333 vs. $4,554).

Salmonella sp. was the most frequently cited pathogen, followed by hepatitis (any type). Food Safety Efforts accelerated in the 1990's. The developments in food safety Policy during the last decade have helped the Nation make progress in the Goal of ensuring the safest possible food supply. Changes in regulations Governing food production and responses by producers have helped control and reduce risks from microbial pathogens. New research and surveillance efforts have helped us better determine the extent of food borne illness in the United States and the most important sources of food safety risks. Educational efforts have increased public awareness and enabled consumers to protect themselves from food borne diseases.

2. Legal System & Limited Incentives: Legal observers suspect that most food borne illness claims, perhaps as many as 95 percent, are settled confidentially out of court. Analogies with other types of product liability cases suggest that those settled out of court may have the strongest claims, while those that go to trial may have serious disputes about the causation of the illness or the amount of damages to be awarded. With confidential settlements, direct economic signals from the legal system about the costs of producing pathogen-contaminated food are usually restricted to the responsible firm and its insurer.

Because jury verdicts find firms responsible for microbial contamination in relatively few cases, the legal system provides only limited feedback to firms about the need for greater food safety. Nonetheless, such firms cannot ignore the potential legal consequences and catastrophic losses of making or distributing contaminated food products that might cause illness or death.

The small percentage of food borne illness lawsuits that are resolved in the public view may indirectly influence the behaviour of other firms. This is particularly true for lawsuits that attract adverse media attention. Other firms may decide to increase investments in food safety after observing the economic costs to defendant firm's accused of producing contaminated food products that caused illness. For example, an effective, industry-generated, food safety reform occurred after the large 1993 outbreak from hamburgers contaminated with *E. coli* O157:H7 and subsequent litigation. The restaurant chain revamped its food safety program and significantly altered the practices of the fast food industry with respect to meat products. As we are increasingly able to identify the source of a food borne illness, the power of litigation to shape industry behaviour about food safety will increase.

3. Legal Incentives in Outbreak Situations: Incentives for firms to avoid large outbreaks of food borne illness are probably stronger than the incentives to avoid isolated, sporadic cases of illness because outbreaks have greater potential to damage firms. Public health authorities are also more likely to become involved in outbreaks, and technological advances have improved the chances that widely scattered cases will be traced back to a source and linked to each other. For example, CDC traced the 1998 Listeriosis outbreak (80 illnesses, 21 deaths) to hot dogs and luncheon meats produced and sold by specific companies.

According to one attorney experienced in food borne illness litigation, it is primarily the business disruption and negative publicity of the catastrophic food borne illness or outbreaks that cost firms' money, so it is these extraordinary, nonrecurring illnesses or outbreaks that have the potential to substantively shape corporate behaviour. In the rare instances where food borne disease outbreaks are linked to particular firms, the impact on those firms can be large i.e. the restaurant chain involved in *E. coli* O157:H7 outbreak in 1993 lost an estimated $160 million in the first 18 months of the outbreak.

In Los Angeles Superior Court the American Environmental Safety Institute filed a lawsuit against Hershey Food Company and Nestle USA, Inc, saying that chocolate has a deadly amount of lead in it. The Institute wants to have the chocolate companies put warning labels that chocolate contains lead-[28].

4. Class Action Lawsuits for Similar Outbreaks: Food borne illness and the reasons for litigation may decrease if firms continue to improve quality control practices to ensure safer food. In contrast, improvements in pathogen detection and identification techniques (including DNA fingerprinting and more rapid microbial tests) may increase the chances that Food borne illnesses (particularly outbreaks) will be detected and linked to specific food products and firms.

Several law and consulting firms now specialize in food borne illness lawsuits. Class action or "mass" lawsuits may be more frequently used in the case of outbreaks resulting in many similar, mild illnesses, particularly as identification and documentation of outbreaks improves, as legal expertise in this area grows, and as media coverage of successful class action suits involving consumer products accumulates.

In Canada, a class action suit could be filed in case of food poisoning or food consumption leading to illnesses. A class action lawsuit has been filed in the Supreme Court of British Columbia against Alfalfa's Canada Inc., carrying on business as Capers Community Markets, on behalf of all persons who were infected or exposed to Hepatitis A after eating Capers food products. The unnamed person who became ill after consuming food purchased from Capers in February and March 2002 and was subsequently diagnosed as having been infected with Hepatitis A [-89].

Roughly 55 per cent of Canadians say they want more information on healthy food choices. Restaurants do not advertise that eating a typical hamburger combo means eating all the fat you need in a whole day. Some American and Canadian lawyers say that could make for the next wave of lawsuits. However, as long as the food is safe, let customers decide what they seek or like to feed themselves. Canada is leading the world in efforts to snuff out smoking through advertising. However, whether French fry boxes will come with warnings of clogged arteries and heart disease in the near future remains to be seen [-70].

In January 2000, some people in Ottawa had filed a class action lawsuit against the company that processed the pasta salad that made them sick. The Canadian Food Inspection Agency issued a recall as more people in Ottawa fell ill. Federal food inspectors have been investigating the plant to locate areas where the contamination may have occurred. The salad was shipped to stores in Ontario, Quebec, and the Maritimes. More than 600 people, mostly in Ontario, fell ill after eating tainted Greek pasta salad. The salad was contaminated with the Shigella bacteria. The victims claiming more than $50 million in damages for lost wages, pain and suffering have launched at least two class-action lawsuits [-137].

While the threat of a lawsuit filed by a consumer affected by food borne illness provides an incentive for food manufacturers and retailers to supply safer food, recent research suggests these incentives are limited. The vast majority of consumers who experience a food borne illness do not file a legal claim. Most food borne illnesses are short-lived and do not entail significant consequences. Even in more serious cases it is often impossible to identify the food associated with the illness.

The incubation period of some food borne illnesses may last a few days or even weeks, hindering the identification of linkages. Samples of the contaminated food may no longer be available by the time the illness occurs. Genetic fingerprinting can sometimes be used to link a pathogen identified in the patient to a pathogen in a food source at the store where it was purchased or the facility where it was processed, but this is expensive, when it succeeds at all. Thus, the information costs and transaction costs of litigation are high relative to the expected award.

Furthermore, legal observers suspect that most food borne illness claims, perhaps as many as 95 percent, are settled confidentially out of court. Firms may settle because they believe they would lose in court, because the costs of defending themselves are greater than the cost of the settlement, or to avoid negative publicity. Such settlements limit the deterrence effect on other firms.

Incentives for firms to avoid large outbreaks of food borne illness are probably stronger than the incentives to avoid isolated, sporadic cases of illness, because outbreaks have greater potential to damage firms. Public health authorities are also more likely to become involved in outbreaks, and technological advances have improved the chances that widely scattered cases will be traced back to a source and linked to each other. According to one attorney experienced in food borne illness litigation, it is primarily the business disruption and negative publicity of the catastrophic food borne illness or outbreaks that cost firm's money, so it is these extraordinary, nonrecurring illnesses or outbreaks that have the potential to substantively shape corporate behaviour. In the rare instances where food borne disease outbreaks are linked to particular firms, the impact on those firms can be large.

In 1998, the Center for Food Safety, on behalf of a collection of scientists, religious leaders and consumer advocates, filed suit against the Food and Drug Administration, asserting that the FDA's permissive policy on genetically engineered foods violated several federal laws. The plaintiffs asked the FDA for compulsory labelling and safety testing of engineered foods. The suit was dismissed by the judge on Oct. 2, partially on the grounds that the FDA's 1992 statement on genetically engineered foods was not a binding policy at all. In other words, the United States Government has never had an official policy on transgenic foods. FDA is expected to announce new regulations soon-200.

RESTAURANTS AND ILLNESS LAWSUITS:

Nearly a third of food borne lawsuits tracked by ERS from 1988-97, targeted restaurants as the main source of the food contamination. The second largest category of defendants was "parent companies." The median award to winning plaintiffs was $25,560, while a few much higher awards raised the mean to $133,280 (1998). Plaintiffs were more likely to win if they could link the illness to a specific pathogen, and more severe illnesses tended to result in higher awards.

Both food firms and consumers make food-handling errors that lead to food borne illness, but the proportion of illnesses due to each is unknown due to data limitations.

1. Limited Incentives: Legal observers suspect that most food borne illness claims, perhaps as many as 95 percent, are settled confidentially out of court. Analogies with other types of product liability cases suggest that those settled out of court may have the strongest claims, while those that go to trial may have serious disputes about the causation of the illness or the amount of damages to be awarded. With confidential settlements, direct economic signals from the legal system about the costs of producing pathogen-contaminated food are usually restricted to the responsible firm and its insurer.

Because jury verdicts find firms responsible for microbial contamination in relatively few cases, the legal system provides only limited feedback to firms about the need for greater food safety. Nonetheless, such firms cannot ignore the potential legal consequences and catastrophic losses of making or distributing contaminated food products that might cause illness or death.

The small percentage of food borne illness lawsuits that are resolved in the public view may indirectly influence the behaviour of other firms. This is particularly true for lawsuits that attract adverse media attention. Other firms may decide to increase investments in food safety after observing the economic costs to defendant firm's accused of producing contaminated food products that caused illness.

For example, an effective, industry-generated, food safety reform occurred after the large 1993 outbreak from hamburgers contaminated with _E. coli_ O157:H7 and subsequent litigation. The restaurant chain revamped its food safety program and significantly altered the practices of the fast food industry with respect to meat products. As we are increasingly able to identify the source of a food borne illness, the power of litigation to shape industry behaviour about food safety will increase. Legal incentives probably work better in outbreak situations, less well for sporadic cases.

Incentives for firms to avoid large outbreaks of food borne illness are probably stronger than the incentives to avoid isolated, sporadic cases of illness because outbreaks have greater potential to damage firms. Public health authorities are also more likely to become involved in outbreaks, and technological advances have improved the chances that widely scattered cases will be traced back to a source and linked to each other.

2. Common Lawsuits: Food borne illness—and the reasons for litigation—may decrease if firms continue to improve quality control practices to ensure safer food. In contrast, improvements in pathogen detection and identification techniques (including DNA fingerprinting and more rapid microbial tests) may increase the chances that food borne illnesses (particularly outbreaks) will be detected and linked to specific food products and firms.

Food Safety Protection Conclusion:

In practice, it is difficult and expensive to test each food product, so food safety standards are often a mix of product outcome, process standards and regulatory requirements. It would enhance the long run efficiency of the meat industry if scientists can agree on appropriate performance standards for microbial pathogens in meat. This would encourage firms to find ways to reduce the incidence of these pathogens in the food supply.

The ongoing development is the mandated use of Hazard Analysis Critical Control Point (HACCP) systems of food safety management. HACCP requires that processors identify critical control points and develop procedures for monitoring controls and addressing any failures that occur. This reflects a growing recognition that it is important to prevent and control hazards before they reach the consumer. HACCP, in fact, signifies prevention than cure.

The preventive methodology entailed in HACCP not only provides safety to human health but also automatically reduces economic losses. Benefits from reducing food borne illnesses are potentially very large, ranging from $2 billion to $172 billion, reflecting the varying estimates of the extent of food borne illness and different methods for valuing life and health.

All factors point to the desirability of setting clear standards for microbial pathogens. Both consumers and ultimately industry would be better served by standards that are well understood. This may require changes in the dairy, bakery, meat and poultry inspection laws, as well as further research to determine the best sampling and testing methods. The government has concentrated the effort to consolidate the food safety and inspection functions of numerous agencies and offices into a single, independent food safety agency. It is to be hoped that the safety evaluation of GM foods takes an encouraging move as the public debate on genetically modified (GM) foods is showing depressing signs of following a similar path to that which occurred with irradiated foods.

A major difference is that irradiated foods were, and are, never likely to form a major part of the diet in any country, whereas the same may not be the case with some GM foods. However, every home in Canada and most of the United States enjoy microwave-cooked food. However, there is no solid evidence that microwaves cause any effect on food other than those due to rapid heating. Food cooked in a microwave oven does not present a radiation risk. Microwaves cease to exist as soon as the power to the magnetron of a microwave oven is switched off. They do not remain in the food and are incapable of making either it or the oven radioactive. However, difference in organoleptic evaluations and psychological barriers will continue to engage critics of microwave oven.

Similarly public awareness of Bioterrorism has gained momentum in public eye. Countering Bioterrorism is comprised of a number of essential elements one such element is the expeditious development and licensing of products to diagnose, treat, or prevent outbreaks from exposure to the pathogens that have been identified as Bioterrorism agents. Considering and identifying all threats to food safety, much action is required on prevention. Hazard Analysis Control Points stands on seven principles, which are the basis of prevention, and corrective actions, which eliminates recurrence. For the human welfareness, food safety protection is much needed today than ever before.

Qamrul A. Khanson

Chapter: 03
HACCP Costs to Industry

Overview:

The cost factor in any profit-oriented industry is an operational strategy for the success of the business. In all the businesses we conduct for the purpose of commerce we do business to make earnings and to keep happy the customer. In food industry we ought to satisfy food safety requirements by implementing government regulations and SOPs in order to keep customers coming back for continual purchases paving the way for a continual moneymaking. The cost of implementing a HACCP system varies from plant to plant depending on the requirements of the impending state regulation, current technology, current equipments, management's attitude, and available resources to the plants in the food industry-07.

Design and implementation of a food safety system do not come in the form of inexpensive financial deal but they are worth the cost. The biggest conclusion of HACCP food safety system is the spirit and fortitude of protection being created in the food industry. After HACCP became mandatory in 1997 in North America, industry has, since then, put in time, effort and money, on an equal basis, to comply with the law, producers pay the bulk of HACCP costs but have yet to balance the cost of incremental hazard reduction against risk.

With the induction of HACCP in North American food industry, all food manufacturers will be open to audits and inspections. Many small-scale producers should also change or could shut the business due to lack of resources. Until now, very little information was available about food safety practices by small food manufacturing businesses. If government regulations improve the safety of the food supply irrespective of the size of food business, consumers benefit by having fewer food borne illnesses. New regulations, however, may raise producer costs in the short term or long term and require purchases of new equipment, new worker training programs, or investment in new research and development. Whether society sees net benefits from a regulatory intervention depends on the size of the public health protection benefits compared to the costs. Benefit and cost analysis does not necessarily allow one to reduce the risk of all activities to zero, but it does allow one to balance the costs of a proposed undertaking against the benefits the undertaking may provide. With such information, one can then assess which food safety proposals are not only economically feasible, but also which reduce the most threatening kinds of risk to the largest number of people. The cost of improving seafood safety and quality at various levels of health risk reduction achieved by using different processes within different regulatory rapprochement regimes (ranging from harmonization to coordination) needs to be determined and compared over.

Sheila A. Martin and Donald W. Anderson (2000) conducted a survey on behalf of US-FDA to determine the current and projected status of plants with respect to HACCP and related food safety practices. Their findings reveal the degree to which different sectors of the food industry will have to change the way they do business to be compliant with a HACCP rule-[07].

Approach: The survey was part of a larger study to determine the cost of prospective HACCP regulations for plants regulated by US-FDA. Plants producing seafood were not included in the study. The first step of the analysis was to determine the baseline level of compliance with HACCP and food safety-related practices. The second step was to determine the per-plant cost of making the changes required to implement these practices. The survey was designed to meet the objectives of the first step of the analysis.

Because HACCP is difficult to define, especially for such a broad industry, they constructed a survey instrument that asked industry about current practices with respect to HACCP training and implementation, sanitation procedures, and other food safety-related practices. The survey was customized for each plant interviewed based on the nature and complexity of the plant's operations.

Survey Procedures: US-FDA's Official Establishment Inventory, a list of all the plants that are inspected by US-FDA, defined the survey universe. They stratified the sample by industry sector and company size, using the Small Business Administration's definitions of large and small companies. The total numbers of respondents were 595, for an overall response rate of 32 percent.

The survey was administered via telephone. In the recruitment phase, they identified a respondent in each plant and mailed the respondent information that would help him or her complete the telephone interview. In the interview phase, they collected the responses during a prearranged telephone interview.

HACCP Training and Implementation in the industry were analysed. Large companies and small companies had been included in the survey. The extent of written and implemented HACCP plan for the different products was studied. The study also analysed the implementation mode according to the type of food products and the size of food manufacturing companies.

HACCP diffusion in the existing workology can never be instant in adoption. An observation of its diffusion in the present food manufacturing atmosphere and its understood implications by the industry operators were also studied.

Sanitation system in the food industry is regarded as equal to processing system for a common purpose of food safety. It's importance as nucleus of food safety, regulatory pre-requisite adoption, standard operating procedures, record keeping of what is categorised as sanitation and the understanding of sensitivity to different products were observed in the study.

Related food safety processes like different stages of manufacturing and procurement of ingredients were also studied. The extent of HACCP implementation by large and small food businesses with reference to vendor guarantees of their raw materials and ingredients were studied.

COMPONENTS OF HACCP COSTS:

Cost of a HACCP regulation for most industries will depend not only on the requirements of the regulation, but also on the current status of food safety-related practices of the plants in these industries. This chapter will deal with the results of a survey that the Sheila Donald team conducted on behalf of the FDA to determine the current and projected status of plants with respect to HACCP and related food safety practices. Until now, very little information was available about food safety practices. The team's effort sheds light on the degree to which different sectors of the food industry will have to change the way they do business to be compliant with HACCP rule.

1. HACCP Training and Implementation: Sixty-three percent of plants surveyed have employees who have received some kind of HACCP training. Employees of large companies are more likely to have had HACCP training and are more likely to rate themselves "very familiar" with HACCP.

While seventy five percent of plants owned by large companies have conducted a hazard analysis for at least one product, only fifty one percent of plants owned by small companies have done so. Forty-four percent of all plants surveyed have written and implemented a HACCP plan for at least one product. Large companies lead small companies in HACCP plan implementation by 30 percentage points.

Among plants owned by small companies, the animal products industry is leading the implementation of HACCP. Among plants owned by large companies, cereals/ grains/baked goods lead HACCP implementation.

2. HACCP Diffusion: It was observed that HACCP diffusion has been relatively rapid since 1990 and had another surge of activity in 1994. It has slowed since 1996. While a significant number of plants plan to implement HACCP within the next year, about 30 percent of plants owned by small companies and 12 percent of plants owned by large companies say that they will never implement HACCP if FDA does not require it for their plant.

3. Sanitation: Despite current Good Management Practices (GMPs), only 71 percent of plants owned by small companies currently have a written sanitation program, and only about 73 percent of plants owned by small companies maintain records to verify sanitation inspections. The sensitive products, animal protein products, and cereals/grains/baked goods sectors lead in having sanitation programs.

4. Related Food Safety Processes: Plants owned by large companies, lead the plants owned by small companies in implementing most food safety processes. For example, 86 percent of the plants owned by large companies required written vendor guarantees of the specifications for raw materials and ingredients. However, only 67 percent of the plants owned by small companies required such vendor guarantees. The team of researchers collected information from approximately 105-food safety processes-07.

5. Concluding Observations:
- The baseline adoption of HACCP in many industries is almost certainly being influenced by the promulgation of HACCP rules for other industries.
- Consequently, some industry segments are adopting HACCP faster than others are.
- Large companies are adopting HACCP at a higher rate than smaller firms.
- In many cases, implementing HACCP will require more significant changes in plants owned by small companies.
- The process costs of HACCP are significant.

Cost factor cannot be ignored in a food manufacturing business but it is to be economised without compromise otherwise very purpose of business will be lost. The implementation cost of HACCP may sound excessive to those who count the numbers but comparative evaluation between the cost of consequential safety failures and HACCP, one would agree to adopt HACCP either by consent, understanding or by regulatory enforcements otherwise the food business shall cease to exist.

Economics of HACCP Application:

Quality concept can be applied to a product when it is innocuous, nutritive, and appetizing, and if it satisfies the expectations of the market. The additional consideration of the process technology and competitiveness of the product require the application of economic engineering techniques to the Total Quality Systems. The evaluation of the quality cost and its relationship to the level of product quality constitutes a useful tool for decision-making intended to implement systems of quality assurance. Their analysis permits the establishment of the basis to evaluate the effectiveness of the proposed system and to optimize the technological process.

The aims of economics of HACCP application are to analyse quality, financial and technological parameters. To study the relationships of these parameters to the quality costs, total production costs, final product quality and selling price.

The behaviour of the quality costs in installed plants of the fishing sector is analysed using the PAF model (Prevention - Appraisal-Failure) developed by Feigenbaum. Total quality control uses quality as a strategic business tool that requires awareness by everyone in the organization. Feigenbaum defines total quality control as excellence driven rather than defect driven, and suggests that quality costs are divided into controllable (prevention and evaluation) and resulting costs (external and internal failures). Feigenbaum defines that cost and quality are complementary rather than conflicting objectives. It is observed that the more representative controllable costs to reach a good level of product quality are inspection of raw material, training of labour and production control mechanism.

For food processing plants, the values found for low quality products, are 5, 25, and 70, expressed as a percentage of the CP, CA and CF, with respect to the total quality costs. If the actual relationship between the components of the costs of quality is the one exposed before, there are many failures, and no preventive actions. If the goal is to produce at a better quality level, these figures indicate the direction to follow: an increase in the preventive efforts that reduce the defects and simultaneously increase the quality.

Quality costs for the Argentine export fishing industry of the following manually elaborated products: frozen blocks of hake fillets (*Merluccius hubbsi*) and salted anchovy (*Engraulis anchoita*) were analysed. Data were collected in selected installed plants in Mar del Plata, the main Argentinean fish landing port.

Starting from the results obtained from previous work, a lineal correlation between initial raw material quality and final product quality were observed.

Parameters related to quality as raw material and final product quality, number of critical control points in the HACCP plan implementation, economic variables such as raw material and final product prices, investment, and production parameters as daily capacity, raw material yield and labour productivity were analysed.

In salting plants, the initial raw material quality was measured by the proportion of belly burst. An increase in yield for good input quality (average yield 85%) can be observed when compared with poor quality (average yield 70%). In terms of costs, the reduction in yield is extremely important, since raw material costs are on the average 74.7% of the total cost of the finished product (salted anchovy).

Processing optimum quality raw material reduces production costs (about 48%) and increases benefits through an increase in the quality of the product, even if a higher price is paid for the raw material. The same behaviour was also observed in freezing plants.

Results show that due to the poor quality of inputs, failure costs are over 95 percent of total quality cost. For a very good quality level, failure costs descend below 20 percent of total quality cost. Without the recognition of the existence of failure costs, the optimization of quality costs is impossible. In those cases, the usual actions of the companies are the reduction of prevention and appraisal costs that lead to lower quality levels. The company could decide an increase in the prevention and appraisal costs above the minimum point based on considerations such as volume of sales, safety, prestige (brand image) and company reputation.

Average total production cost per unit of product was analysed, showing that it continues reducing beyond the point of minimum quality cost per unit. This is due to the decrease of production costs by the increase in plant productivity associated with high levels of quality. Total quality costs descend from 40 to 21 percent of total production cost when the quality level is increased from bad to very good.

On the other hand, if the relationship between the final product quality and its selling price is considered, a maximum benefit point is obtained, not necessarily coincident with the previous minimum points. Consequently, an interval of quality level exists, within which the company will decide the optimum operation point according to the characteristics of demand function associated with the product.

Different minimum points for total quality cost and total production cost and a maximum benefit point are observed, indicating an advisable working zone within 80-90 percent of the optimum quality level.

In the United States, using the most conservative assumptions and new CDC cost estimates; Economic Research Service (ERS) found that HACCP provided net benefits of $7 billion or more over a 20-year time horizon. When the analysis assumed higher rates of pathogen control and lower interest rates, the present value of the net benefits provided by HACCP increased to a maximum of $42 billion [82].

HACCP Transformation Costs:

Preventive measures does not provide a quick fix for food safety and quality problems and it is a long-term business concept in which returns for doing things right may not be direct or immediate. The whole process of transformation from existing stage to HACCP implemented stage involves Cost of Transformation (COT). If things are done right the first time then the cost of transformation could have been minimal. If it is to be clearly understood, HACCP program involves use of a systematic approach for preventing problems or defects from occurring and for documenting the elements by which processes are controlled.

Any company involved in the transformation, production, packaging, handling, and transporting, warehousing, catering, distributing or serving food is liable to put in place proper procedures to comply with HACCP self-regulations. The HACCP guidelines do not impose a specific set of rules for all companies to follow.   Instead, they require every organization to analyze and identify all the critical points relating to their organization. The correct implementation of the regulations then demands that an appropriate plan is drawn up. The HACCP plan or checklist must catalogue all the critical points, instigate proper checks and controls and take preventative measures should a problem arise as well as how the controls effected should be documented.

Furthermore implementation and sustaining the HACCP system is not effortless and the transformation was difficult for some producers to grasp and to capture at the essence of the system and learning how to implement it efficiently. All this cost money! In a typical situation following sectors transformation cost may be involved for a satisfactory and viable Food Safety System (FSS).

1. Cost of Motivation for HACCP: To remain quality competitive in the present food safety conscious time, Canadian food industry and food processing organizations would have to adopt food safety management system - Hazard Analysis and Critical Control Points (HACCP). It is obligatory to comprehend; therefore, in what way the system helps the continuity of profit, earning the trust of safe quality food and improvement of business reputation, and, what are the costs of HACCP implementation. While food safety to consuming customers, a leadership role in the food business, export oriented food manufacturing, regulatory necessities and production related factors motivate firms to employ HACCP; food trade associations could play an important role and become instrumental in promoting the system.

HACCP transformation costs and maintenance or operating costs vary with the type of food sub-sector, status of the plant and the size of firm. The costs of implementing and operating HACCP vary between individual food manufacturers according to their own particular circumstances and the prevailing standards to which they operate. The motives for implementing HACCP may differ between individual businesses, even though the food sector is subject to a legal requirement to implement a HACCP-based food safety control system. It is evident that the food safety concerns, requirements of customers, pressure to conform with regulatory requirements, GMPs, GHPs and quality standards, as well as the need to improve internal efficiency have all played a part in motivating businesses to implement HACCP in the Canadian and US food industry.

The motivating factor for HACCP is also appears to be an increased ability to hold onto existing customers. The main impact of HACCP is to enable food-manufacturing organizations and businesses to meet the increasing demands of the marketplace as well as to obtain real competitive advantage over imported foodstuff from overseas.

The internal cost failures in manufacturing organizations are the major factor, which motivates food businesses to seek protection of their operations through a science, based system approved by CFIA and FSIS respectively guaranteeing the future of business. The elimination of internal and external cost failures help increase profit which will compensate the cost of maintaining HACCP in the long run of a food business. There is no business wisdom to continually sustain punitive fines, consumer's neglection, and acting on reactive measures. The loss of financial investments due to quality and safety failures would definitely prompt for a comprehensive solution. Thus the cost of motivation for HACCP in North American food industry will vary from the cost of product failures to the cost of punitive numeric. Abiding to good manufacturing should eliminate cost of motivation and enhance the science based safety system in the food industry.

In Canada, a safe, high-quality food production is influenced by financial stability along with consumer and market demand, rather than government enforcement. However, CFIA remains a motivating factor in the shadow of a regulatory body. By not inspecting their operations frequently and providing areas of improvement, the government may allow producers to continue with procedures that do not ensure complete safety of food produced. CFIA's initiatives would eliminate unhealthy business activities who have been commenting such as " We have been in business for 20 years with the same procedures and never had a problem so why should I change now?" such statements could only be made by traditional processors who have no glimpse of modern food technology and food safety understanding. Such businesses do not keep track of their safety failures and ignorantly boast of problem free. Such food manufacturers should realise the impact of food safety issue and strive to transform to HACCP in the interest of consumer safety and their business.

The larger food manufacturing companies have motivation in consumer and market demand and to gain market leverage. Therefore, in Canada if HACCP were made mandatory for all segment of the food industry, as it is being debated in the United States only those larger operations that are financially stable would survive. The Canadian government has been active in helping manufacturers produce a clean product that tastes good, that customers will accept, is economical to produce and will be competitive without high risk to consumers or the industry. Thus CFIA helps the Canadian food industry to minimise cost of motivation by providing technical, regulatory, and motivational assistance to the Canadian Food Industry.

2. Cost of Consultancy: In Canada many consultants of international fame are available to provide their assistance as well with complete package to train, document and implement HACCP and quality related systems. Registrar selection is critical, and with the number of accredited Registrars the task becomes more difficult.

Verify consultants and registrars, through either personal contact or phone conversation, the support given prior to and after registration is one of the criteria for a selection. Also verify for other criteria such as auditors meeting registrar requirements e.g. RVA (Dutch council for accreditation; Raad Voor Accreditatie), IRCA (International Register of Certificated Auditors), IEMA (Institute of Environmental Management and Assessment), RAB (Registrar Accreditation Board) and other internationally recognised auditors for adequacy or registration. The Registrars should be recognised and accredited by Internationally recognised accreditation bodies like RVA, IEMA, IRCA, RAB, SCC (Standards Council of Canada) or UKAS (United Kingdom Accreditation Service) or are in process (also, Registrars themselves may be an accredited body) and may have more than one accreditation. CFIA is the right agency to assist and advise food manufacturers in Canada. The Guelph Food Technology Centre (GFTC) is Canada's largest HACCP trainer and consulting group, they have worked with hundreds of companies who have implemented GMPs and HACCP in Canada.

Consultant will assist in developing HACCP program or review existing documentation for compliance with HACCP principles, verification of existing plans and monitoring of long-range performance etc. The total cost of package could be obtained directly from consultants and registrars in different locations of Canada. Most of the consultants are located in Toronto and Vancouver.

A food processor would require specialist help in the food safety and quality business but often do not want to recruit a senior manager with a high salary and benefits package. HACCP requires unbiased, professional, and balanced guidance in specific areas of food manufacturing stages on an ongoing basis. To appoint a well qualified Quality Director in Canada for a company employing 100 people will cost at least Can.$ 70,000. What a food manufacturer of that size may look in to is the equivalent of a Quality Director and confidant to assist the Quality Assurance Team and the management team push the business forward profitably and considerably cheaper than the Can.$70,000 a full-time specialist would cost. Expert advice on an ongoing basis in vital areas of food safety and quality assurance at considerably less cost, but with the same dedication as a full-time retained executive may be obtained from a competent consultant. However, bigger organizations prefer to appoint top experts in the field and pay the price considered worth than the risk faced to food safety system.

Individual independent consultants for HACCP and Quality Assurance Management could be paid on hourly basis and on contract basis. A HACCP consultant in North America may charge

Can.$ 100-150 per hour for his services that may exclude transport and lodging depending on the agreement.

With the increasing importance of Food Safety all over the world, ever-increasing horizon of food safety risk and fight against terrorism add to the cost of overall food manufacturing and safety. Food Businesses are often aware that they can save money but do not have the time and expertise to take best advantage of certain saving opportunities available in food manufacturing and food safety sector. There are consultants who offer a cost consultancy service through cost management and profit enhancement in safe food manufacturing. In hiring such consultants, please consider quality and reliability of services are as important as reduced costs. The food processors who are spending over Can.$100,000 per year on HACCP system need to consult such cost saving consultants who provide not only effective systems but assist in utility savings, by-product dispension and cycle time reduction with out compromising food safety.

In Agricultural food production, consumer resistance to the use of chemical pesticides, together with the growing problem of pest resistance, is encouraging farmers to adopt organic farming methods, or production systems, which make minimal use of chemicals. Japan and India are important producers of technical grade pesticides. Korea and Taiwan also produce technical grades. Most of these are generic pesticides (i.e. the patent has expired), which can be produced at a low cost. Most other countries in the region import technical grades and process them locally into required formulations. The need is expressed for safer formulations, such as WDG (Water Dispersible Granules) granules rather than wettable powder. This is another area where a short term advice could be obtained from relevant agencies and high cost of chemicals could be reduced by the use of generic but safe pesticides or other cheaper organic means. By any standard, the safety of food products and economics of it should be guaranteed.

Food Science engineers are also part of our food safety system. They help solve design, processing plants and packaging machinery, which critically measures food safety related HACCP issues. Food industry building, equipment design, equipment layout to address Occupational Health and Food Safety are the best examples. In the twenty-seven years of experience in food safety, the author has analyzed that the time of quality is in the forefront and safety issues should be critically analysed not only from raw materials and ingredients but the very design of the plant and machinery itself.

Let us take few examples; the meat industry slaughter, boning, processing, packaging design, to address plant layout, equipment selection, food and personnel safety parameters, electromechanical set up, hydro mechanical design, application and control of low and high speed production equipment in sterile, clean or dirty environments require professional consultancy. In the meat processing facilities paddocks, holding yards, lairage for beef and small stock, a slaughter floor and boning room, chilling and freezing facilities and fully equipped small goods plant, Automatic Carcass Splitter, Automatic Cattle Stunner, Boning room ergonomics, Beef Rib Deboning, Sheep & Beef Meat Safety concerns are to be looked by a proper equipment manufacturer as well by your consultant who would help install a zero defect concept in processing and packaging.

Similarly in Fruit Juice Production, one needs Automated fruit sorting system concepts using an imaging system to grade, sort and orient the fruit, Automated harvesting system concepts etc., are the critical points to be consulted to meet quality and food safety parameters. It goes in honey decanting, cheese processing equipment design modifications, including vats, cheddaring table, and a Mozzarella stretcher etc. The emphasis is on right consultancy, which pays in the long run in terms of hazard free manufacturing system enhanced by HACCP process. Such costs will not form the part of HACCP but will form the part of a right Plant and Machinery expenses. Only matter to be the concern of a cost consultant is to separate these costs and add to the machine procurement budget or charge to the profits of a machine supplier rather than adding as a modification costs due to HACCP implementation.

Food processors are also required to enlist legal consultants in case of food safety associated litigations though no one would ever think to reach such a crucial stage of food safety related issues. The consultant or adviser would have the knowledge of relevant legislation and offences, codes of practice, powers of inspection and obstruction, gathering evidence, notices and emergency provisions, the decision to prosecute, whom to prosecute, formal cautions, due diligence defences, examination-in-chief and cross-examination of local authority officer. The cost of such a consultancy may require Can. $ 200-300 per hour. The best saving will be to invest in prevention rather than cure, though cure should remain handy.

3. Cost of Training: Any course offered to learn HACCP should include a complete subject matter covering all aspects of its principles. The cost range for an individual may vary from Can$

3000-5000. Sometimes a specific portion of HACCP course may be required for an individual; in such circumstance cost will be much less. For example an auditor's training could cost Can. $1200-1800.

A HACCP workshop is an important aspect of training where the common sense approach to assuring food safety, embodied in the principles of HACCP, is explained with the use of a case study. Such a course may cost around Can. $1000. The importance of HACCP training supersedes the value of expense when it comes to the safety of food during manufacturing and until the purchaser consumes it safely. More than training is the outcome of training and its value imparted in the attitude of trainee when he/she implements the knowledge in the practical field of safe manufacturing and safe handling of food. The sensitivity of food involved and the criticality of the parameters for a particular food require a food technology background in a trainee. Otherwise, the value of training cannot be earned fully and could incur doubtful outcome endangering the process and the product out of it. Additional costs to retrain or expand the horizon of training could be burdensome and unnecessary.

To minimise the cost of training, a right candidate to train, specific requirement to impart, right schedule, right atmosphere, open discussion with out barriers, a just right trainer and established educational materials would utilise best of training and its implementation.

Another matter to be considered is to "Train the Trainer". An internal trainer would cease the need to invest extra money on external resources and it would encourage the need to invest that money in providing resources to internal recognition of talents, provisions, initiatives and training to the manufacturing staff. The external cost of transportation, production time, material expense, and external hiring could be minimized. The will and necessity of training expenditure cannot be compromised but it can be economised for better results wherever and whenever applicable.

4. Cost of Audit: Qualified auditors shall be availed to review the facilities for compliance with regulations and corporate standards. By using routine audit services, manufacturing staff will become more aware of food handling practices. A full report after each inspection will help identify where problems existed and how to correct the deficiencies. Follow-up visits will insure that corrective measures have been taken and will reinforce proper food safety practices. Cost for audits could range from Can. $90 an hour to Can. $650 per day. Additional "travel costs" are added if auditors travel from the long distances.

Beside HACCP Audits, the auditing services could include, Supplier's Audits, and Sanitation Audits. The value of external audits can be increased and its expenditures minimised if external audit is followed after internal audits. A self-assessment exercise rectifies many discrepancies and prepares the manufacturing units for a referral audit. If a spiritual internal audit leads to external audits then added values are expected rather than alternative solutions. That is a remarkable achievement of the factory indicating the thoughts and attitude of the management and commitment of the staff. This helps stabilize the cost and economize the operations in terms of reduced auditing hours, eliminated corrective actions, absence of verification hours, and renewed confidence in HACCP implementation process.

The cost of audits could be minimised when there is no need for repeated audits due to one failures or the other. The personal style one uses in working with others in a food-manufacturing atmosphere depends on many factors. One is the background and human perspective of the management teams themselves. The characteristics exhibited by employees towards food safety issues individually or as a group, may also impact how a manager will approach an issue. Management dealing quite differently when acting with one-on-one discussion with an employee about food safety issues, communicating to the entire organization about the opportunities for learning that will be imbedded in a new company initiative on food safety is the points to be considered. Last not the least is the management style one follows to achieve perfectness in proposed food safety plans. The overall success and near perfectness will require only formal one time audit to accredit the HACCP system in a well valued food manufacturing and handling organization.

5. <u>Cost of Layout</u>: The design and layout of food processes and plants shall be such that raw materials enter from one end and the final products exit from the other end. This is required to prevent cross contamination of processed food with that of raw ingredients. Unfortunately, few of the old manufacturers in Canada had laid their plant on first come first basis and with out any scientific reasoning for the installation of plant and machinery. That will cost significant amount of money to rearrange the utility work, product flow pipe work, CIP lines and replacing the existing equipments with the right and updated ones or the same unit at right place.

Most of the work in the layout involves drawings, food-processing equipment placements, and utility support for the equipment, pollution control equipment, monitoring devices and sanitary pumping. Normally a project manager designs and constructs food plants. Plant layouts are required in the dairy, beverage, confectionery, bottled water, and canning industries. The cost of doing such a job is highly variable and requires research to settle with most trusted, experienced and economical bet.

6. Cost of building renovation: Their can exist such a situation where the infrastructure was sufficient and the only thing was to clean up and stay clean, but that situation is very rare. When one intends to renovate older buildings instead of building new, significant quantities of materials and energy are saved, thus benefiting the environment. In addition to reducing project costs, there may also be significant savings in time and money associated with reduced regulatory review and approvals. Additional reduced costs can occur with sustainable aspects of site and construction debris management.

With sustainable renovation projects, just as with new building projects, integrated building design can often result in initial cost savings, particularly with energy savings. Savings can often be found by eliminating dropped ceilings. While some of these savings may be offset by needs for pendent light fixtures, additional painting, special fireproofing measures, and exposed ducts, other cost and energy savings may become available. Deeper day lighting penetration opportunities or reduced floor-to-floor height or access flooring potential may result. Access flooring offers opportunities for energy savings, improved indoor air quality, and easier continuing reconfiguration of space with particular value in public buildings. Construction costs are most likely to be reduced if integrated design with access floors enables savings elsewhere.

The most important but riskful aspect of a food processing building renovation is the concurrent production activities and the on sight renovation activities. It has to be shrudely and judiciously managed so that contaminants are restricted to construction zone only. The chances of microbial, physical, and chemical cross contaminations are to be eliminated and severe preventative methods enforced for food safety.

Flexibility is probably the biggest trend in new food plant construction. With new materials in construction of food plant floors proliferating and old ones discontinued, facilities need to accommodate multiple lines and allow quick changeovers. Flexible facility design is an emerging trend, but sanitary facility design just as important. Because food safety and quality issues are receiving more attention, facilities are looking for a higher quality of design and construction material to improve the overall quality of food plant building.

With the growing emphasis on doing more with less, it is infinitely more effective to renovate or expand rather than construct a new facility.

Irradiation is a new issue for most food plants, and construction projects need to address the material handling and safety questions associated with it. A plant's layout and ultimate construction would be specifically impacted by this technology; HACCP rules could impact the construction to meet inspection requirements. The food processors should look ahead with the food safety issues as this core issue will dictate the most radical changes in terms of site selection, site development, drainage and sewage construction, plant construction, ingredients and finished food products storage construction.

7. Cost of Extra Space: In older food manufacturing plants, expansion space to facilitate science based installation and growing business is a challenge. Such plants could manoeuvre for a very short period and will be forced to move out to new construction when enough is enough reaching its limit. However, the urge to merge may have hidden benefits for food companies looking for extra and existing facilities. At the same time opportunities exists to acquire new sites, as there are a lot of buildings available due to downsizing or consolidation.

Without a doubt, new food industry regulations have an enormous impact on plant construction projects. HACCP has sustained and invigorated a pre-existing trend toward more food sanitary facilities with deliberate design focus and with the highest priority given to food safety.

Flexibility, consolidation, automation, sanitation and food safety— the same issues that dominate daily food plant operations—are the same issues driving expenditures for new food plant construction, expansions and renovations. Urge for extra space my lead to acquisition of adjacent facility or economisation in existing facility. Any economisation must see increased automation and higher levels of plant hygiene required for a safe and quality food production.

The utilization of multi level production plant installations to economise on available space is another alternative. The design of the plant, type of installation, food products to be manufactured, machinery, local construction and safety regulations could impact such an endeavour. The construction of such a plant shall require specialist approach to building construction design, building load strength, building construction materials, comparative advantages, production monitoring and total comparative cost.

In the dairy industry, such a construction is more feasible as Milk Silo Towers (MSTs) are installed outside of the production hall but the remaining milk storage tanks can be installed on the first level of the production hall. The first level facilities could include raw milk storage, Pasteurizing unit, Laboratory facilities, Production Manager's office, Packaging conveyors, Crate cleaning and empty plastic crates storage etc. The ground floor is generally utilised for Milk receiving platform, Milk recombination unit, Homogenizing units, Pasteurizing units, and Packing machineries and stacking units. The moving machines like Homogenisers, heavy load milk pumps, packing machines, and shrink-wrap machines are installed on ground level because of Vibration force, which impact the construction's strength load. The utilities like air compressors, chilling plants and water purification systems could go for underground installations. The steam generation and diesel storage facilities shall be always on the ground level and away from the main production hall for safety reasons. With such considerations one could save a lot of valuable space and save cost.

8. Cost of Hygiene: The cost of hygiene in the food industry should be seen from two angles. The consequential cost of a poor hygiene and the cost of good hygiene, an achievement would indicate the importance of a compatible hygiene system. The balance between of cost of hygiene failures in terms of losses incurred and the cost of maintaining an effective hygiene system would influence the earnings and successful running of a business. Cost of hygiene is not directly related to HACCP implementation but associated with the GMPs of the manufacturing business. GMPs are essential for HACCP and the business.

The food hygiene elements should be in place to assure management, workers, and clients that potential health risks related to food safety in food production processes are minimized. The primary element to control workplace hazards to food and personnel safety is to use engineering controls. Emphasis should be placed on closed food transfer systems and process containment with no open handling of processed food. A thorough program of reviewing the recommended additions and potency of added food ingredients to be manufactured and new materials to be used should be in correct amounts and in correct place. Processes should be evaluated and characterized through complete and documented industrial hygiene monitoring surveys to confidently predict the exposure potential they present to the food processing system.

Local exhaust ventilation system testing and maintenance should be in place including at least annual face velocity measurements of all hood and duct velocities and fan speed measurements. Records should be kept of testing and maintenance and repairs made as required. Food testing laboratories in manufacturing units may require that a Chemical Hygiene Program conforming to OSHA regulations be in place. Effective cleaning and decontamination procedures should be established for equipment and operating suites. A food personal hygiene and uniform laundering program should be in place. Effective environmental controls and procedures to prevent contamination of wastewater and air with products should be in place and maintained especially where fermented food products are manufactured. These elements mentioned here are to protect manufactured food and workers health and may involve additional elements depending on food products, processing and packaging equipments. All such initiatives of hygiene costs are interrelated with HACCP and the food safety. Added cost on such preventive measures will become a part of transformational cost to HACCP.

Workplace hygiene procedures are strictly followed in accordance with prevalent science based standards and legal requirements with in Canada. The cost of dairy hygiene inspections should be included in maintenance cost of HACCP. Such inspections could cost Can. $250 – 300 per inspection. Today's dairy producer must think about efficient, quality milk production on the farm.

The Codex Committee on Food Hygiene (CCFH) has been drafting *The Code of Hygienic Practice for Milk and Milk Products* (Milk Code)—a set of harmonized hygiene standards for internationally traded dairy products. Milk Code will have an immediate affect on the industry: For the past 15 years, the Codex Committee on Food Hygiene (CCFH) has worked continuously to harmonize international dairy hygiene standards. Progress has stalled primarily due to differences between the United States and France regarding the acceptable level of public health risk associated with raw milk products, particularly cheese. In order to assist in the development of the Canadian position, comments by the industry are being submitted to the Codex Contact Point for Canada.

The cost of prevention is much economical than cost of correction. The cost of food plant hygiene should be based on preventive measures and any chance of reactive philosophy should be eliminated.

9. Cost of Sanitation: Without a doubt, new food industry regulations have an enormous impact on plant construction projects. New food industry regulations have influenced new food plant projects in terms of upgrading processes to achieve better and more automatic cleaning and sanitization. New regulations mean attention to Chemical material selection, Description of materials, Human safety data, Food safety data, Sewerage pollution data, Special drainage requirements, Anti-clogging drainage for fatty productions, Non stagnating drainage (no standing water), Clean air flow, Air filtration rates, Temperature control on fluctuations for the safe cleaning and sanitization of a plant.

Cleaning and Sanitization are like oxygen to living individual as it is to food safety. Without a satisfactory cleaning and sanitization process, a food-processing unit will become a breeding ground for microorganisms and a health risk to consumers. In the food plant installations, cleaning and sanitization is an integral part of the process. Every effort is devoted to facilitate the number one priority of cleaning and sanitization. The use of only stainless steel material, proper chemicals flow pipe work, turbulence pumps, right chemicals, right dosages, built in CIP in packaging machines and human safety measures add to the cost of cleaning and sanitation.

Specialist chemicals cost more than the classical chemicals like sodium hydroxide and nitric acid. It is up to the production manager what type of cost savings he foresees for his operations. There are advantages and disadvantages to use specialist's chemicals. The only disadvantage one could come across is the huge cost of these chemicals. In some situations these huge costs outweigh the benefits. However, in some situations like twenty-four hour pasteurization operations, high degree of sanitation requirements, nil microbial counts requirement benefits, outweighs the costs. One is to decide according to requirements, planned arrangements and to balance the costs.

We in Canada see more stringent clean designs and improved plant operating criteria as a continuing trend. Previously less stringent food processors are now adapting clean design protocol from other food markets that were long accustomed to higher levels of hygiene. With the introduction of HACCP and its implementation, increased cost of sanitation is worth sustaining. The suppliers of cleaning and sanitizing chemicals in Canada belong to internationally reputed companies who are continuously striving to maintain and improve the efficiency of their products with reduced costs to food manufacturer. Speciality chemicals have taken place of traditional chemicals increasing the cost in the name of safety and efficiency. These chemicals in turn do affect the cost of wastewater treatments in the food industry. Thus an interconnecting sequence exists between the costs of hygiene, sanitation, and sewage disposal systems. The range of cost for sanitation-specific equipment is estimated to range from $100,000 to $500,000 in Canadian Market.

10. Cost of Pest Control: The Pest control programme is a part of pre-requisite requirement of HACCP system, which is to be implemented to safeguard stored raw materials, plant, machinery, water system, processing system, packaging materials and finished products from pests. The establishments planning to a pest control system should look for a comprehensive established solution, which may involve renovation of doors, fixation of traps, adequate fencing, removal of vegetation from manufacturing and storage area. The estimated transformation cost from zero point in Canada is about Can. $20,000. The maintenance cost of a contractual pest control system in a milk plant of 150,000 Lts/day could cost Can. $10,000/year.

11. Cost of Sewage & Garbage Disposal: Illegal discharges of oily wastes, garbage, sewage, and noxious liquids from dairy industry and other food industries put unnecessarily burden on municipal ecosystems and result in punitive actions by regulatory agencies in Canada. More than 10% waste stream is comprised of food and organic material, it is important to educate food waste generators on food waste reduction, reuse, and composting. Always try to prevent the generation of food waste first, and then look towards donating or composting the leftover material. Disposal of solid waste and liquid waste from food processing plants need management so that municipal acceptance standards are met.

A liquid waste treatment plant in a food manufacturing establishment may be needed to an efficient settling system, reduced odours, with very low investment and rental option, which utilises low energy and homogeneous basin mixing. In sewage treatment plants, the energy consumed by aeration constitutes a significant portion of the overall operating budget. All treatment plant efficiencies are geared to the waste that they receive. Once a treatment plant has been built, the factors that will affect the biomass growth rate, such as flow and aeration rate, have already been established and therefore the only changing factor that remains that can affect the process is the incoming waste stream. An affordable treatment system for poultry processing, meat processing, milk processing, bakery processing, food oil processing waste water would diminish the temptation of illegally dumping potentially harmful waste water endangering the food safety with in the vicinity. A 100,000 gallon/day dairy effluent treatment plant could cost Can.$500,000, which is a direct investment cost and cannot be considered as a HACCP cost. HACCP system gets support from good waste management practices.

Wastewater disposal has become an acute problem for abattoirs, particularly for plants, which are not served by municipal sewers. Municipalities often charge a premium rate for industrial or commercial discharge into their sewers based on wastewater strength. Abattoirs served by municipal sewers may choose between paying the surcharge and retreating their effluent to reduce its strength prior to discharge. Rural abattoirs do not have this option. Slaughter plants located outside of the sewer network must either pay to have their effluent hauled off the premises or provide on-site disposal. Providing adequate wastewater treatment to meet the strict criteria for discharge into an open watercourse is cost prohibitive for all but the largest slaughter plants.

In Ontario, a hydro geological study is required before a certificate of approval to operate an industrial or commercial private sewer system is granted. Subsurface discharge is limited by hydro geological conditions: there is a maximum volume of water, which will infiltrate into the soil before it begins to break through to the surface. Furthermore, poorly designed subsurface discharge systems have the potential to contaminate the plant's water supply. Enlarging the subsurface disposal field is not necessarily the most economical or even a viable method of increasing the allowable discharge rate. Plants with existing approved subsurface discharge systems are certified to discharge at the designed rate. If the plant is to expand its production and produce more wastewater, a new certificate of approval is required. The site conditions may be deemed to be inadequate for handling the increased hydraulic loading.

It is possible to meet Agriculture Canada's requirements for a recycling system to be considered for approval. The costs and reliability of such a system would have to be determined in full-scale trials. In order to reduce and eliminate risk to food safety in a manufacturing plant, a properly managed wastewater treatment plant and a swift solid waste compacter and disposal management would be of great importance. The cost factors should be analysed according to the size, type, and location of the business. In some cases wastewater treatment requirement could be eliminated if waste in the liquid can be contained through proper drainage and solid containment system. That will definitely save money for other productive and safety uses.

12. <u>Cost of quantitative demand</u>: This refers to expanding market and the expansion expenses in plant, machinery and built in safety accessories with it. The increased volume production carries a cost of extra expenses on safety matters. This cost is only incremented when new acquisitions are sought.

In the manufacturing management, numerical quotas for the workforce and numerical goals for the people in management jeopardize the objective of food safety and quality-[127]. It has been observed in few of the developing countries where enforcement is not enough to control quality, quantitative importance supersedes the qualitative importance. It results in the deterioration of quality, increase in risk of food safety and loss in long term business. In such a situation the cost of food safety is more in terms of volume of risk, liability suits, health endangerment, reduced business and a bad name in the market.

Quantitative demands should never be allowed to supersede food safety during manufacturing and handling of the food products. The HACCP system should be made compatible to the factory's production capacities and operational schedules. Over stretching the plant and machinery will result in more wastage, increased cost, dwindling safety guarantees, and increased psychological pressure at the cost of food safety and quality. Late night extra shifts result in more stretching troubles than the daytime shift when the management has a vulture's eye on the deviating performances. The best way to deal with the quantitative demand is to re-assess the plant capacities and work on expansion plan, produce what is safe to produce, do not work on numerical figures and work on zero defect policy. Any expansion to accommodate HACCP based manufacturing system is a bright side of a food manufacturing business.

13. <u>Cost of upgrading processing equipment</u>: Presently, 95% of machine manufacturers lease some of their equipment and almost every business, sooner or later, must acquire equipment in order to reduce immediate cost. Tetra Pak, International Paper, and Elopak have evolved such type of deals to attract more customers and continued confidence in their products. To upgrade certain portion of the plant in order to meet HACCP and other quality requirements one must consider such possibilities.

The increase in demand for more products means more strains in available capacities. Instead of replacing equipment with borrowed money, upgrading of capacities is always a possibility. A heat exchanger to pasteurize liquid food could be upgraded to another 1000 – 1500 Lts. Packing machines could be upgraded to extra 15-20% capacities in some cases. Such possibilities should be explored. In doing so, product safety consideration must be measured and risk prevention steps should be taken. The cost in this case will be comparatively minimal and it should be HACCP oriented.

In most cases one need to change out some of the old equipment for new hygienically friendly equipment. In some processing industries, where one cooks the product in the processing (shrimp), the change to HACCP needs massive reorganization/renovation of the plant housing. That alone requires serious capital investments.

14. <u>Cost of replacing obsolete gadgets</u>: In the old plants, pH indicators, temperature monitors and in certain cases humidity detectors are never found to be functional and need replacements. The pH value ranks as one of the most important indicators of food quality and safety. The pH of raw ingredients such as milk and meat is measured to ensure that quality standards have been properly met. The pH is also monitored at different stages of food preparation and transformation to guarantee safety, improve production, and enhance quality.

Without a credible opportunity for year-over-year revenue growth, investors will not see capital gains and must be attracted to make their food manufacturing more functional in terms of risk detection and prevention. That is the strategic investment to secure the future of their business. Capital formation, return on investment, market share - these are hardly the natural instruments of management for food safety. To be sure, increasing margins generally result from reductions/elimination in product recalls, quality failures, and bad publicity. Since food safety is generally required by the mandate under the force of law so investment is automatic but manufacturers can still precise their cost.

15. <u>Cost of Required Instrumentation</u>: Up until recently, food hygiene and sanitary checks were carried out by governmental organizations responsible for public safety. Spot checks and random tests were usually made on site at production plants and distribution points. Such checks and controls however resulted in what amounts to an after-the-event investigation. Inspectors found themselves merely reporting on damaged goods due to substandard procedures and were rarely in a position to point out the exact reason for the presence of pathogens or toxic material.

HACCP regulation is an attempt in changing this procedure. HACCP is based on identifying and controlling all the critical points in different phases of production and distribution that can have a detrimental effect on the quality of food. Therefore, instruments to monitor temperature during milk pasteurization and milk chilling, detection of foreign body in bread, on the spot microbial count on the surface of meat and detection of spoilt egg require online detection of risk factors. Instruments are available for such monitoring and should be installed according to its importance. For example, sanitation measurement can be quick with ATP bioluminescence to determine sanitation effectiveness. It is faster (10 Min.), sensitive and effective method than the conventional technique-186. Built in thermographs in Pasteurizers are other examples of instrumentation where one may acquire the technology by following PMO guidelines.

16. Cost of Calibration: Calibration is a set of operations that establish, under specified conditions, the relationship between values of quantities indicated by a measuring instrument and the corresponding values realized by standards. In practice, Calibration is essential comparison with a higher standard. Higher standard means higher accuracy and better resolution. Calibration is a mandatory requirement in HACCP. Calibration has to be viewed as an essential element of reliable measurement. Inspection, measuring, and test equipment should be recalibrated periodically, as specified by the manufacturer.

The cost of a contracted calibration by external service shall be included in the HACCP cost. If it is internally done then it remains the overhead cost with in the company's finance. The testing and calibration of a chilled water unit to give an output of 6000 L chilled water per hour may require a calibration contract of $300/year. Thus, keeping all the equipments e.g. packing machine, feed pumps, pasteurizing units, steam generation, chilling units, cold stores, homogenizing units, air compression etc., would require contractual agreements or internal team to calibrate at a given interval.

17. Cost of upgrading equipment: All the food manufacturers have to package their products. The best way to keep packaging machinery updated and operating efficiently without replacing it and sinking countless dollars into the effort is to upgrade with little additional cost to accommodate safety requirement. For example a cup-filling machine can be added with complete sanitary hard plastic hood cover to avoid foreign body falling in the cups during packing.

Take conveyors for another example. Up until 3-5 years ago (in some places still today) conveyors where not built for cleaning. They were almost impossible to clean and it was virtually impossible to get them free of bacteria. With more advanced designed in terms of accessibility for cleaning, the risk of bacteria in conveyors were decreased dramatically. Such costs could be minimised and spent somewhere else where another critical control is needed.

A recent trend in the packaging machinery industry has been to integrate bottling lines, utilizing new machinery whenever necessary while rebuilding and upgrading existing or previously owned machinery. This type of arrangement offers the manufacturer significant cost savings. Incorporating pre-owned machinery, even if completely rebuilt, is a fraction of the cost of a new machine. Rebuilt machinery often comes with warranties that include parts and service. By performing a simple cost comparison of replacing a machine completely, vs. rebuilding and upgrading, a clear basis for investment decision-making will become evident.

Another advantage is the flexibility. Why replace a complete bottling line if it is not really necessary? If each component piece of machinery in that line is evaluated, some machines will perform to growing production demands by upgrading controls and/or completely rebuilding the piece. Thus, the existing line remains functional and grows with production needs. There may also be surplus equipment that could be upgraded and integrated with other machinery to form a bottling line that operates like new.

18. Cost of Schematic Diagram: These diagrams are needed by the HACCP plan and could be obtained from food engineering services available by all food machine manufacturers. The schematic diagram shows, by means of graphic symbols, the electrical connections, and functions of a specific circuit arrangement. The schematic diagram is used to trace the circuit and its functions without regard to the actual physical size, shape, or location of the component devices or parts. The schematic diagram is the most useful of all the diagrams in learning overall system operation. The cost of such diagram could ranges from Can.$3000 – 5000. The diagram helps in the analysis of food safety, operation, monitoring and tracing back the link.

19. Cost of Documentation: Food Safety requires a systems approach. HACCP must be implemented in day-to-day operations. Procedures must be developed, records must be maintained, and management must continually review how effectively the system is working. Often, Food Safety must be integrated into existing Quality Management systems. All manufacturers including primary producers, main manufacturers, foodservice companies, and healthcare organisations that take food safety seriously must maintain all procedures and day-to-day records. The complete solution to Food Safety Management is available from innovative services all over North America. HACCP modules allow the coordinator to rapidly create whole HACCP plans and documents.

The HACCP software guides the user through a HACCP study in a logical and systematic way, prompting the HACCP team on points that need to be considered at each stage. The program allows a comprehensive range of established and custom-made process flow diagrams to be generated. It also applies a decision tree to each hazard at each process step to determine the critical control points. The program available are designed for PCs running Windows 95 or above or Windows NT. The cost of such programs may range from Can.$1200-1500 per copy. The mean wage of employees involved with writing the plan is approximately $20.00 per hour.

20. <u>Cost of Assessment</u>: An internal assessment of HACCP process is the first step in the systematic operation. Then State Enforcement Audits, Corrective Actions & Follow-up activities take place. Audit frequency is decided as per the intensity of operation and corrective actions resulting in increased costs. A minimum period or interval for audits is fixed. First Year initial audit may be followed by next 30 to 45 days; 4 month follow ups and subsequent audits every 6 months & compliance follow up - listing evaluations every 2 years.

HACCP audits are conducted to verify that HACCP Plans comply with the seven Codex Principles. HACCP plan and operation will be assessed to determine that significant hazards have been identified, that critical control points (CCPs) are appropriate and are correctly identified, that CCP monitoring procedures are implemented and are effective, that appropriate corrective action is being taken and that the system is supported by comprehensive record keeping. Verification procedures will be evaluated to determine whether the HACCP Plan is subject to necessary review processes.

Food safety audits encompass prerequisite HACCP programs that are essential to the successful development and implementation of HACCP plans. These support programs play an important role in controlling potential food safety hazards and can include Good Manufacturing Practice (GMP), cleaning and sanitation, pest control, Supplier's Quality Assurance (SQA), staff training, calibration, incident management, food safety maintenance, Good Laboratory Practice (GLP), Good Distribution Practice (GDP) etc. Support programs will be evaluated and assessed to determine if they are appropriate and effective. Suppliers play a crucial role in maintaining manufacturer's brand image. Independent supplier audits provide you with the confidence you need to protect your brand name and to ensure that quality and food safety specifications are continually being met. Suppliers of assessment services can design and implement a supplier-auditing program that is customized to requirements. Audits can be scheduled in any country including the Middle East and Asia-Pacific region.

HACCP is an internationally recognized means of assuring food safety from harvest to consumption. HACCP Accreditation Contract is normally signed in advance. The cost for an on-site audit is approximately Can.$1,500 per day; plus expenses, per auditor. Typically two auditors conduct a two-days audit. The cost of a manual review is approximately Can. $1200. Having discussed different costs of transformation, one may envisage a huge task of transformation. Regulatory authorities are very understanding in providing time to transform gradually. A deadline is always provided to accommodate manufactures convenience. However more and more plant owners and manager are realizing that despite the increased cost of capital and higher operating cost the end result is positive. From HACCP comes a consistent and safe product that can give better price. The new installations could include the HACCP cost in a Turnkey Project.

21. <u>Cost of Hiring Extra Employee</u>: An estimated 20% of the companies hire extra personnel to run day to day HACCP operations, to handle HACCP requirements such as record-keeping or to manage sanitation in a factory. The average salary for a new employee, based on reports from Canadian companies, is at least $30,000. The transformation cost will include only the cost of hiring which is estimated to be Can. 2000. The yearly salary or yearly personnel cost for HACCP will add to HACCP maintenance cost.

The total transformation costs could vary from Can. $172000 to 265,000 for a milk and milk processing factory with a handling capacity of at least 150,000 Lts/day. These costs are estimated and should not be considered statutory. The costs keep on varying due to economic variables in North America. The constant costs are one-time costs, which are necessary to meet HACCP system's demand. The utilization of internal resources from the inventory and labour could further minimize the cost of transformation. The variable costs are never fixed as they vary according to individual plant's requirements and the business demands of the organization. Table 3(1) – HACCP Transformation Cost to a 150,000 Lt/day Milk Plant; is indicative of the total cost involved in a HACCP operation. The figure of Can.$265,000 could still go up according to the transformations required by the stakeholders to meet the market demands. The transformation costs would be paid back with in less than of a year from the day of HACCP certification due to increased reputation, product confidence, employees' motivation and management's positive attitude towards food safety, productivity, minimal wastages and quality assurance.

Table 3(1) – HACCP Transformation Cost to a 150,000 Lt/day Milk Plant

No.	Elements of Cost	Constant Cost*	Variable cost*
1	Cost of Motivation	Can.$2,000	Can.$10,000
2	Cost of Consultancy	30,000	50,000
3	Cost of Training	5000	10,000
4	Cost of Audit	2000	10,000
5	Cost of Layout:	10,000	-
6	Cost of building renovation	10,000	10,000
7	Cost of Extra Space	-	10,000+
8	Cost of Hygiene	5000	10,000
9	Cost of Sanitation	20,000	-
10	Cost of Pest Control	20,000	-
11	Cost of Sewage Disposal	56,000	100,000
12	Cost of quantitative demand	-	Variable+
13	Cost of upgrading equipments	-	10,000 +
14	Cost of replacing obsolete gadgets	-	10,000
15	Cost of Required Instrumentation	-	10,000
16	Cost of Calibration	1500	-
17	Cost of upgrading packaging equipment	-	25,000+
18	Cost of Schematic Diagram	5000	-
19	Cost of Documentation	1500	-
20	Cost of Assessment	2000	-
21	Cost of Hiring Extra Employee	2000	-
	Total Constant Cost	**172,000**	**265000+**

* Variable costs differ from plant to plant as per the individual needs of the plant manufacturing operations.
* Constant costs are normal to all plants; its variation is due to different quotations and resources.
+The cost could go further high as per the demand and expansion budget of the company.

Table 3(2) – HACCP Transformation Costs to Food Industry; indicates the expected costs to different segments of the food industry in Canada. The cost variables are dependent on the food safety changes required due to sensitivity of the product, types of processing, packaging, preservation, and storage requirements.

HACCP Maintenance Cost:

Once the initial investments are sustained to upgrade a food manufacturing factory in a food handling company to a level when it is accredited as a HACCP certified organization, the maintenance of HACCP based operations become much economical. Since HACCP establishments involves for all the product processes and includes the one which is used to create new products, the hassle of non-conformity becomes a secondary issue while zero defect preventive process becomes the first priority. By the establishment of HACCP many myths surrounding HACCP with in a factory erodes to reality, like most other Canadians, few farmers have more than a fuzzy notion what the acronym HACCP stands for.

The implementation of HACCP by Government, food industry, and even marketing boards are touting HACCP as the key to prosperity for Ontario farmers, even though they are acting more on faith than hard fact. The one who has already implemented, put efforts to observe the process, realises the mental satisfaction, sees the profit numeric increase and failure costs disappearing, he does not go unguarded on HACCP issues but maintains continually the HACCP momentum. It becomes a continual risk preventive and food safety process. The maintenance cost of HACCP will involve the following elements to function as per the laid arrangements and procedures.

Cost of Continual Documentation: In any organization, same personnel with extra financial incentives could do the job without extra hiring. The actual financial cost could be calculated against the number of hours utilized to document the records, procedures, or printing of formats for the HACCP process.

Cost of materials: Like stationery, chemicals and laboratory expenses which are utilised to perform the task of observing and maintaining critical control limits in a manufacturing atmosphere.

Table 3(2) – HACCP Transformation Costs to Food Industry

No.	Different Food Segments	Size Of Operation	Total Estimated Cost
1	Bakery	150 metric tons/day	$90,000
2	Beverage	150,000 Lts/day	$ 120,000
3	Dairy	150,000 Lts Raw Milk Handling/ day	$130,000
4	Meat	150 Metric tons of Red Meat/day	$110,000
5	Sea Food	150 Metric Tons/day	$112,000

The cost of material will also include specific equipments used to manage HACCP in the plant and the surroundings.

HACCP Coordinator: An extra employee for the manufacturing team will be hired to work as a permanent HACCP Coordinator of the company and could cost at the rate of Can. $40,000 – 55,000 per year.

Preventive Maintenance Cost: The maintenance department/engineering department also performs this without any extra cost to the Quality Assurance and food safety Department. Most of the maintenance cost is never added to HACCP budget but to the Maintenance cost of plant and machinery. The timely and preventative maintenance costs are added in to the cost of transformational costs.

Internal Audit Cost: Such a cost is not much as regular staff members are trained to become internal auditors to impart cross-departmental audits coming under HACCP jurisdiction. Such an audit may not cost much as resources are still available from the establishment. However, an allocation of Can. $600 per anum is a positive step to facilitate recreational and obligatory internal requirements.

External Audits: If annual audits are mandated, the cost of its execution is to be sustained which may vary from Can. $2000 – 6000 per year. However, the size of the company, food safety violations, and process change may increase the costs dramatically.

Regulatory Audits: These audits do not involve extra expenses unless violations have occurred due to food safety lapses. In such a situation, cost of punitive actions, reimbursement, litigation fee, criminal suit, civil suit and defamation of reputation will find depleting finance at elevated loss.

A. <u>HACCP cost to Bakery:</u>

Food legislation, regulation, and inspection are the areas of shared jurisdiction in Canada. A federal-provincial initiative has been undertaken by the Canadian Food Inspection System Implementation Group (CFISIG) to develop a Common Legislative Base for food law in Canada. Bakery or any other food industry has the Common Legislative Base aimed at food safety and quality, thereby facilitating the adoption of any future harmonized regulations and standards.

The baking industry is part of a mature market segment kept dynamic by both rapidly changing consumer needs and acquisition. It is clear that the leaders in the baking industry are going to be faced with a variety of choices regarding the technologies they select to maintain profitability in this safety conscious environment. Muffins, Cakes, Sweet Dough, Cookies, Breads, Buns, Rolls, Biscuits, Hot Cereals, Puddings, Cream Pies, Pancakes, Dry Mixes, and more are very much needed by the consumers, but of good quality, which are safe and nutritious to their health.

Safe and quality products achieved through applied technology, superior products, excellent productivity, quality ingredients, cost, and differentiated end product benefits show a bright future for any baker. Small bakers of the time fear the need to incorporate safety costs, which are a bit extra of their budgeted finance. Beside the fixed asset costs, bakers are faced with cost management: Formula Cost Management, Production Cost Management, Process Cost Management, and now it is the HACCP Cost Management. Is there any extra cost to implement HACCP process in the bakery? It is a bad news for the small operators who are still primitive in their operations, unable to afford investment and closing the doors would be a better idea than producing bakery products with health risks. The modern bakeries with state of the art technology would only need to incorporate the HACCP at the negligible cost as they already apply GMPs, SOPs, SLPs, and food safety principles.

HACCP cost management would not add any extra financial burden but a proper training to all so that they convert their skills to produce safe bakery products. All the bakeries in Canada produce excellent tasting goods; added value in terms of safety would develop confidence among customers and consumers. HACCP cost could be balanced by incorporating Formula Cost Management; by reducing milk and egg use to simplify formulas, increased acceptability by different consumer groups, creative ingredients combinations for better economics and by allergen management and indications on labels. Production Cost Management; concentrates on rheology such as improved crumb structure, strength and resiliency, improve moisture retention, migration control, improve glaze stability, gloss retention, reduce breakage and many other parameters to release cost burden by improving mentioned qualities. Process Cost Management; improves dough handling/tolerance, improve fat absorption control, improve fermentation tolerance, improve safety by improving thermal treatments, safe packaging mechanism, proper packaging materials, metal detection and proper storage conditions. Incorporation of safety measures in all these processes does not need extra cost but a sensible utilization of available resources. HACCP offers indirectly competitive prices by being cost conscious, minimizing waste and vigorously pursuing continuous improvements, resulting in lower prices and greater values to bakery industry.

Let us take the sceneric example of a cigarette butt, which could be found in a loaf if the food employees are not following dress codes and standard hygiene in a manufacturing atmosphere. Food Safety Act (FSA) in Australia encompasses the necessity that the food manufacturers harmonize their operations with the seven principles of HACCP. The failures by the traditional bakers to adopt GMPs, SOPs, and proper hygiene have lead to the contamination of products by contaminants like cigarette butts, ashes, pocket pens, and coins falling in to the products. In Australia, a cigarette butt found in a loaf in the month of January 2003 cost a bakery owner $6000-27. To add up all, it will be many times more expensive than implementing the HACCP process in full.

The trained bakery staff members do understand that HACCP is an important cost factor. The competent baking technologists should understand the functionalities of all ingredients used in the production of breads, cakes and sweet goods including but not limited to: flour, yeast, mineral yeast food, salt, water, fats and oils, sweeteners, milk and milk replacers, malts, oxidizing and reducing agents, dough strengtheners and crumb softeners, enzymes, mold inhibitors, leaveners, egg products, soy products, gums, starches, enrichment, wheat gluten, spices and flavours, etc. He/she is to learn and get trained in HACCP system and process, which is an easy task with the given technologist's baking background. The three levels: Superintendent level, Supervisor level and Operator level in bakery function must have good bakery techniques and practical knowledge of food safety.

The superintendents must be fully knowledgeable of the food product safety principles in producing, handling, storing, distribution of bakery products and ingredients. The superintendents must be competent and knowledgeable in all aspects of sanitation, safety procedures, government regulations, personnel practices, statistical process control, purchasing, management, labour laws, contracts, skills in working with unions, interpersonal skills, the ability to communicate both orally and in writing and have an understanding of costs, marketing and the profitability of their company. These skills must be passed on to those they supervise through example. They must have the ability to motivate people to produce top quality products in a safe and sanitary environment. By hiring a superintendent of that calibre, one could save cost failures in a bakery set up.

The supervisors must have complete knowledge of the food safety principles in producing and handling products that are produced in the area for which they are responsible. In order to control quality and safety factors, the supervisors must have good problem solving skills, pay attention to detail, have the ability to coordinate and supervise the activities of their subordinates, be able to communicate both orally and in writing to their subordinates, co-workers and supervisor. This individual must also be a leader, a teacher, a counsellor, and a coach. In order for those with ambition to advance and grow in their organization, they must be aware of all management skills necessary to be successful. By hiring a supervisor of that skill and qualifications, one could help eliminate cost failures in a bakery set up.

The process and machine operators must understand the food safety principles in their area of responsibility. They are the ones whose activities directly impact the safety and quality issues. The operators must have a good attendance record, follow directions explicitly, have a good attitude, and be responsible for their actions both at work and in their personal lives-34.

By hiring operators with proper communication skills and imparting training to develop these skills, one could eliminate safety cost failures in a bakery-manufacturing unit.

A competent baking technologist who could be a quality assurance operator understands the food product safety principles in producing, handling, storing, and distribution of bakery products and ingredients. Coordination between him and rest of the staff would lead to the process of defect elimination and increased productivity. At the same time, baking technologist develops new products with its safety to human consumption in mind. This authority recommends ingredients and its procurement source, processing, packaging, storage, and distribution conditions. By hiring skilled baking technologists with a food technology background and specialization in bakery production, one could eliminate safety cost failures in a bakery-manufacturing unit.

The bakery safety cost and the process will have to incorporate improved capacity to respond to opportunities for growth, improved competitiveness of baker's commodity, products and services, increased amount of added value, increased diversity of commodities, increased capability to manage risk, improved environmental stewardship, continued excellence in bakery food safety and improved management of the regulatory requirements.

By implementing a food safety and food quality program, bakery industry can eliminate costs that result from poor quality and unsafe food products. Poor quality in a bakery, for example, can be spotted as defective product, wastage, and product returns. In addition to the cost above, there are other costs associated with poor quality control such as a reduction in shelf life, loss of customers, reduction in repeat sales, production line downtime, excess inventory, and product liability. In the United States and

Canada, major customers demand that bakery suppliers implement GMP's and HACCP programs. Further, if bakery suppliers intend to export then HACCP becomes a prerequisite. By implementing HACCP, bakery industry could eliminate costs that result from poor quality and unsafe food products.

Administering the legislative, regulatory and policy environment enhances competitiveness and saves cost of operation in the long run of any business. Encouraging investment in value added items, partnering with CFIA and FSIS to enhance food safety will develop opportunities and reduce constraints. Time, efforts, and intent in food safety cost much less, and pro-active food safety approach attracts appreciation from the industry, enhancing chances of new and expanded market. HACCP is a value-added investment in the bakery industry, which enhances public awareness of your efforts to serve the community and understanding of the value-added bakery products. It is prescribed to encourage increased knowledge and skills among employees that encourage independence, self-reliance and minimize risk from adverse events. The relationships with CFIA/FSIS and/or other HACCP regulatory agencies should be developed as of a partnership to produce quality and safe bakery products rather than as an intimidating and punitive adversary.

In North America, general bakery growth has been relatively stagnant; the specialty bakery area has experienced 6% to 8% growth. Snack Food sector continues to experience 6-7% growth each year, usually fuelled by new products. Specific opportunities in private label or healthy lines of snacks exist for the Canadian manufacturer. It is estimated that the Confectionery market in United States is almost $8.5 billion[76].

It's important to note that, imported items from Canada are capturing more of this market each year. Consumer perception of these items appears to be improving because of quality and trustworthy Canadian name in safety. Definite opportunities exist for Canadian marketer as their Canadian manufacturers are positioned as the producer of "imported and safe" products in the United States.

In summary, the cost incurred in improvements would pay back many times the incurred expenditure. The unit cost of bakery products would give dividend in the form of market value and the increased sales. The six HACCP prerequisite programs focus on premises, transportation, & storage, equipment, personnel, sanitation & pest control, and recalls. An effective prerequisite program will actually decrease the number of critical control points during the hazard analysis of the product/process. In contrast, HACCP looks at the actual manufacturing process of the product. It is a systematic and scientific approach of controlling food safety during the bakery manufacturing process, though procurement of right raw material is a quality issue more closely related to safe ingredients. All points in the bakery production interrelate in such a manner as to prevent situations that are outside standards and specifications, therefore those points could cause a major hazard without the information being picked up through the monitoring system. HACCP cost to bakery is an investment, which will multiply business many times than ignoring it to the safety cost failures.

B. HACCP cost to Beverage:

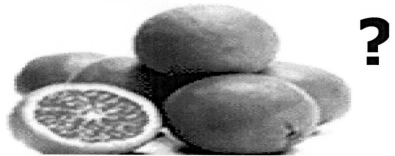

Fig: 3(1) – <u>Juice from Orange fruits is rated Top</u>

Thanks to hunger for excellence, HACCP and food safety drive, consumers in North America have never before been offered such a vast array of goods, safe, convenient fruit juices and fruit drinks, at competitive prices as it is now. A healthy and competitive food chain has always been considered vital for Canadian economy. Opportunities to capitalize on the public's perception of Canada exist across both the food and beverage services and retail facets of the food business. It is clear that the first decade of the new millennium is the most important ever for public health and safety. Food safety regulatory directives and its implementation costs can no longer be considered "Nothing inflates costs like government red tape".

The urgency to safeguard public from drinking unpasteurized juice may add little cost in terms of declaration on labels and education. That is worth than losing the dear ones to <u>E. coli</u> O157:H7 and other pathogens. For the labels "pasteurized" and "unpasteurized" to be effective, the consumer would need to know more about the term pasteurization, which eliminates pathogens from beverages. One may argue that the consuming public does not fully understand the safety ramifications of pasteurization; therefore, using the term "pasteurized" or "unpasteurized" alone is insufficient. Although they know that pasteurization does something to apple juice, which make it safer for human

168

consumption. The consumers strongly support CFIA and US-FDA efforts to place warning labels on raw juices.

Members of the raw juice industry, including juice bars, continue to promote the benefits of raw juice as a "health" related product. Parents, and consumers seeking to improve their health such as people with weakened immune systems, seniors and pregnant women, can thus be led to believe that raw juice is superior to pasteurized juices. In contrast, the American Academy of Paediatrics comments that, with respect to children, "Juice offers little of nutritional value." Raw juices, if contaminated with pathogens, can be life threatening, particularly to the at-risk groups. Small businesses can create juice that is just as lethal as that of larger businesses. Therefore, small businesses should not be treated differently. Certain guidelines recommended by CFIA and FSIS should be followed voluntarily instead of facing the cost of business closures and health risks. To protect consumers from pathogens in juices, the US-FDA announced a rule on January 18, 2001, requiring juice processors to use Hazard Analysis and Critical Control Point (HACCP) programs for juice processing. Similarly in Canada, the Recommendations for the Production and Distribution of Juice has been developed as a co-operative effort of the juice industry and government to provide general guidelines for the production of safe juice-175.

In the United States, One of the most rapidly developing sectors of the soft-drink industry is the bottled water business. Bottled water isn't necessarily safer than tap water. Bottled water is expected to plateau its growth rate with only a 4-8% increase in the next 5 years. Per capita consumption of soft drinks is estimated to be around 50 gallons. Much of this increase can be accounted for by the overall growth in demand for bottled waters by American consumers-76. How are we going to safeguard our water supply with minimum cost, is a question to ponder about.

According to industry estimates, about one-quarter of bottled water is tap water that has been processed and repackaged. US-FDA and EPA standards on water are not identical. For example, the EPA requires that tap water be monitored for asbestos, while the FDA imposes no such requirement on bottled-water manufacturers, maintaining that the sources aren't likely to contain asbestos. The bottled water industry must limit fluoride and lead. At the same time Bottled-water companies aren't required to disinfect or test for parasites such as *Cryptosporidium sp.*, or *Giardia sp.*, - a requirement for city tap water. The US-FDA says that the sources of bottled water are unlikely to harbour these parasites. As far as safety of human health is concerned, the drinking water should have a unified standard for bottled, tap and manufacturing water. Cost of unified regulation and changes in the industry accordingly will benefit health of public in general and reputation of water industry in particular.

Such a change in regulatory unity had furthered the bottled water business flourish in the year 2003. Industry analysts had predicted that bottled water sales will reach more than $8 billion by the year 2004 and the noted shipment value of bottled and canned soft drinks is increasing by 2.5 percent annually. In the United States, bottled water isn't cheap; prices average about 89 cents for a 1-gallon jug, the kind supermarkets sell. At that rate, a typical household would spend $214 a year for drinking water. In addition, if they wanted it delivered at home, add about $325 or more per year. So slicing out a negligible portion of huge profit margin should absorb change in safety issues-76.

Unsafe Beverages should be considered as an item of quality cost failures in the beverage industry. The intended human consumption of beverages should not come in the form of water from hotel sinks, restaurants and public restrooms, unprocessed or chemically untreated water, beverages from glasses with moisture on them, carbonated drinks that are served with ice, bottled water without a manufacturer's seal and raw milk. Under normal understanding of beverage safety, boiled or otherwise purified water, internationally known brands of bottled water, carbonated drinks without ice, pasteurized juices and pasteurized fruit drinks are considered as safe beverages. Here we have identified a clear line of safety.

When contaminated beverages come from manufacturing companies, formal kitchens, licensed vendors making consumers sick because of the consumption of these beverages, a product safety issue may arise. A contaminated beverage from a manufacturing company or any formal beverage selling company recognises a quality failure at some stage of their manufacturing to distribution. The manufacturer of such a contaminated beverage has just incurred extra cost in terms of damage claims, litigation expenses, regulatory fines, and bad name in quality, brand failure, and probable suspension of business.

Add the total cost in terms of finance and compare the cost of a unit of that contaminated beverage. The cost of failures would be thousand times more than the cost of a can of beverage. While in preventing this failure, the added cost per unit would have been negligible.

Demonstrate an understanding of beverage safety practices and procedures in the beverage-manufacturing environment by training and creating understanding among employees. Fig.3 (1) highlights the importance of safe juice for consumers and its affect on business.

The safety Zealots could change to aseptic packing ensuring complete microbial safety. Aseptic packaging is the packaging of a product in germ free atmosphere. The product to be packed should be aseptically processed. Aseptic processing involves, heating the product rapidly to a temperature of 137-140 degrees centigrade, holding it at that temperature for a few seconds and quickly cooling down to room temperature. This kills spoilage causing bacteria without affecting the taste or nutrients in the product. The entire process takes place in a closed, pre-sterilized system to prevent re-infection.

To safe guard the high microbiological quality imparted by the process, the aseptically processed milk is conveyed to the packaging machine in a closed, pre-sterilized system and metered aseptically to packs, which are sterilized and formed inside the machine.

If safety is the whole issue then a complete transformation of plant and machinery and additional training is required. These days a plant producing 3000 Lt juice per hour may cost 3 – 5 million US dollars only in terms of plant and machinery. Such investments are advantageous when safety of products is required for distance transportation and long-term shelf life.

In pasteurized beverages, safety through preventive measures could save 95-97 % of the consumers in North America. While unpasteurized beverages with CFIA recommended GMPs and recommended labelling may satisfy pro-natural minority at the cost of risks involved. No matter what preventive measures are taken, unpasteurized beverage would still be posing possibilities of health risks. Is there any point in trying to protect a product from external contamination if it is already vulnerable to possible contamination? Is it worth to drink an unpasteurized beverage where one is not sure of its safety? It remains a matter of personal choice and readiness to pay the cost.

No doubt that the food and beverage processing sector is Canada's third largest manufacturing sector. A sound HACCP program can lead to enhanced product quality & safety, increased productivity, consumer confidence and access to markets.

Results oriented technical outsourcing for HACCP based line extensions, start-up operations, recipe & Formulation development, contract packer sourcing if needed, manuals, implementation, monitoring, development and execution of HACCP programs, nutritional-CFIA-FDA label preparation, regulatory liaison, proper writing of company policies, procedures, specifications, management of raw materials & packaging materials, complete manufacturing quality assurance; aged stock and distressed product retribution; product retrieval; competitive cuttings, audits (Systems, Procedures, Plant & Product), spot & contract purchase inspections, proper project management and other additions would help minimize the HACCP cost of implementation.

C. <u>HACCP Cost to Dairy Industry</u>:

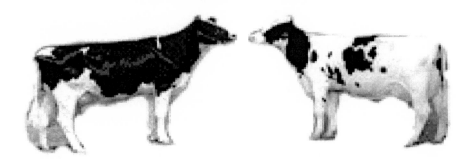

Fig: 03(3) - <u>Beginning of Dairy HACCP right from Milk Cows</u>?

If one in a modern dairy plant with an up-to-date Plant, Machinery and Building Design trying to manage a clean dairy operation, already maintaining SOPs to turn out good quality products, and working according to GMPs even though the plant staff may not know that there is a name for clean and preventive work, the cost of implementing HACCP should be the lowest. If, on the other hand, one is addressing a slovenly draughty plant with cobwebs, processing million germs per ml of milk, it may be quite costly exercise for the implementation of HACCP. Such plants may not survive to see next financial year of operation and profit. One would have to start by changing the faces and figures.

Basically, it is useful to recruit (at least temporarily) someone who knows the jargon, how to do the initial paperwork, and who is good at leading HACCP management meetings. It is essential that the management really want HACCP. The rest is all about changing the mindset of the whole staff, top to bottom. A decade ago, we in Canada were less enthusiastic about HACCP, but now Canadian dairy has an ongoing HACCP conversion, and most operators find it extremely interesting, useful, and enlightening.

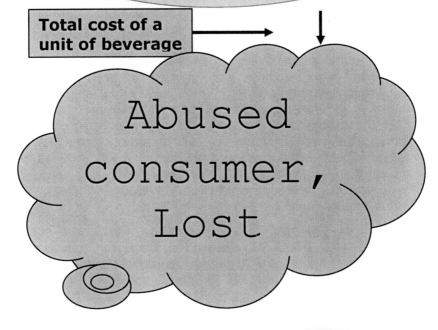

Added cost of quality failure

Total cost of a unit of beverage

Abused consumer, Lost

Fig: 03(2)-Importance of HACCP

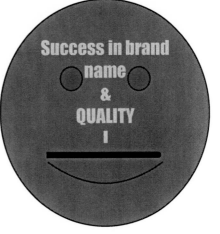

A guaranteed quality and safe can of beverage based on HACCP Principles

Success in brand name & QUALITY !

Canada is a best food planner and strategist. Through the Agricultural Policy Framework, the Government of Canada is committed to ensuring that food produced in Canada continues to be among the safest and highest quality in the world. Canada is putting in place national, seamless food safety systems on the farm and throughout the Agri-food chain - from the field to the fork. The dairy industry is an important sector for HACCP implementation. Since dairy industry is very versatile due to various food produced from milk, its safety parameters and planned safety arrangements with fluid milk, flavoured milks, table cream, coffee cream, whipping cream, single cream, double cream will be different than fermented dairy products like plain set yoghurt, plain stirred yoghurt, fruit yoghurt, cultured buttermilk, white cheeses and Labneh etc. Same is for the frozen dairy products like ice creams, dairy desserts, dairy puddings and milk ice drinks etc. The hard cheeses would require different food safety parameters. The HACCP cost to different segments of milk and milk products would vary after the pasteurization process. The common cost of HACCP from farm to the pasteurization unit will be almost same. Its cost application to post pasteurization manufacturing will differ due to different control parameters, regulatory standards, and sensitivity of the products, storage conditions, microbial factors, and distribution requirements.

By any means, the HACCP Transformation Costs and HACCP maintenance costs would be almost the same as in any other sector of the food industry. The general expected variations in cost would be in equipments, size of the plant, volume of production and stringent parameters to meet. The fermented dairy products would tilt the balance of the cost slightly in their favour. Most of the pathogens causing disease find milk constituents like lactose a suitable medium for the growth under certain conditions. The milk food products carry the crucial and specific critical points in different segments of the milk and milk products food chain.

The Government of Canada is working with farmers and the industry to build on existing food safety measures while undertaking new measures to enable the tracing of dairy food products back to the dairy farms, improve milk food quality and share critical information. These measures will improve the sector's ability to identify and respond to food safety issues and concerns, while improving market access and opportunities for the different segments of the dairy industry and different food sectors. The most variables concerning food safety issues in Canadian and US situations are communication among lower ranked employees and the management, training criteria, employee hygiene, human rights issues, personnel safety issues, sanitizers and general hygiene.

Communication within the large dairy food factories may be complicating effectiveness of improvements efforts on food safety. Complicating the challenges in this sensitive industry are high turnover rates in many segments of the industry and the increasing likelihood that the language spoken by supervisors is not the first language of many line operators and dairy workers. Spanish is more likely to be spoken than English in the break rooms of many plants, and many other languages like Arabic can be part of the mix.

Training in Canadian dairy sector requires a multilingual approach as sizable number of East Europeans, Pakistanis, Punjabis, Spanish, Caribbean, and East Asians form the bulk of workforce often lacking fluent English. Bilingual signage and instructional manuals fall short of what is needed in most of the instances. In a multicultural society like Canada, a picture - and symbol-based approach to employee training and instruction is badly needed for an understandable communication. If language is a barrier, visual instructions can be an affordable, valuable, and effective solution. Imagine if quality-assurance personnel in white laboratory coats come into the plant to discuss food safety and hygiene issues with machine operators and a common worker. It looks like a classical American movie conversation with ethnic Indians of the old times. The food code, bacterial contaminants, viral threats and food poisoning become more scary notions rather than preventive drive, no one fully understand technicality and severity of the safety drive. Though workforce is intelligent, it's the communication, which bars a direct understanding. Such individuals should be imparted with communicable language training and then the HACCP awareness training.

A digital camera and a $300 colour inkjet printer are all that is needed to produce signs that convey expected behaviour. The modem is to show it, don't explain it. Learning by visual aids and seeing the learned work may very well prove learning by doing and seeing believes.

Most training materials stick to English and Spanish, but the quality of the Spanish versions are uneven at best, according to Jeff Tenut, vice president of product development at the National Restaurant Association Educational Foundation (NRAEF), in Chicago. NRAEF is a not-for-profit organization dedicated to fulfilling the educational mission of the National Restaurant Association.

Dialectical differences can wreak havoc on translations. Entomologist Frank Meek of Orkin Pest Control recalls a Spanish instructional poster used in South Florida that, when used in southern California, became, "Put a bomb in the bucket."

Training the dairy personnel is one of the keys to the accomplishments in dairy food plants. Training by food-safety experts can be expensive, of course, and content can be generic. When executives at John Morrell and Co. in Cincinnati decided to institute a company-wide sanitation program as a fundamental step for improved HACCP-based food safety, they opted for internal training programs. Gene W. Bartholomew, corporate manager of HACCP and regulatory affairs, outlined that initiative at Food Engineering magazine's Plant Tech 2001 conference.

The Smithfield Foods subsidiary operates seven plants, including units operating under the Iowa Quality Meats, Mohawk Packaging, Saratoga Specialties, and Curly's Foods names. A wide of the mark recall would cost the firm $4.5 million, Bartholomew estimated. A HACCP plan could minimize any such losses, and a comprehensive approach to sanitation; pest control and personal hygiene underpin and bolster HACCP.

Service companies are addressing the affordability issue with do-it-yourself training options. Ecolab-Minneapolis, for instance, offers in-house training kits on food safety, including student and leader workbooks and support materials.

The package is geared toward sanitation workers and includes English and Spanish language videos detailing safe chemical handling, how to interpret a Material Safety Data Sheet and what to do in the event of an accident.

The normal food safety kit contains information for general staffers and supervisors alike. Materials range from sample GMP policies and HACCP decision trees to background on U.S. public health policy as it relates to food handling. The section on hand care suggests that 10%-20% of food borne illnesses may be attributable to poor personal hygiene—a figure some sanitation experts view as conservative. In author's point of view, poor personal hygiene contributes to 50% of food borne illnesses when such hygiene is applied to soft cheese manufacturing.

There are few things more critical to a dairy operation than sanitation. In addition, dairy processors, like other food manufacturers, must develop the right strategies to ensure that sanitation standards are not only met but produce better results in terms of quality excellence, guaranteed shelf-life and safety to human health.

Table 3(3) – <u>Yearly HACCP Maintenance Cost to 150,000 Lts/day Milk Handling Plant</u>

No.	Elements	Can.$	Remark
1	Cost of Training	3000	Continual
2	Cost of Building renovation	12000	Continual
3	Cost of Hygiene	12000	Continual
4	Cost of Sanitation	5000	Continual
5	Cost of Sewage & Waste Disposal	24,000	Continual
6	Cost of Calibration	1200	Interval
7	Cost of Documentation	1200	Continual
8	Cost of External Audit	2000	Interval
9	Cost of Preventive Maintenance	4200	Timely
9	Cost of Internal Audit	600	Interval
10	Cost of Internal review	1200	Interval
11	Personnel Expenses	60,000	Continual
12	Cost of Communication	1200	Continual
13	Cost of Pest Control	10,000	Continual
14	Contingency Expenses	2400	Optional
	Total	**140,000**	

Table 3(4) – <u>Yearly HACCP Management Cost to 150,000 Lts/day Milk Handling Plant</u>

No.	Elements	Can.$	Remark
1	**Cost of Training**	3000	Continual
2	**Cost of Documentation**	1200	Continual
3	**Cost of External Audit**	2000	Interval
4	**Cost of Internal Audit**	600	Interval
5	**Cost of internal review**	1200	Interval
6	**Personnel Expenses**	60,000*	Continual
7	**Cost of communication**	1200	Continual
8	**Contingency expenses**	2400	Optional
	Total	**71600**	

*Many organizations do not hire extra personnel for HACCP management but give incentive to incumbent food technologists, supervisors, and managers to take extra responsibility of HACCP coordination. That saves 70-80% HACCP management cost. Under such a situation, the HACCP management cost could range from Can.$ 14000 – 25000. The remark column represents the elevation of costs as per individual requirements.

Whether the mission is disinfecting against a virus or ensuring that soil and microbial contamination have been removed from floors and surfaces, processors invest significant time and effort in teaching and reinforcing the sanitation message to employees.

Employee hygiene could be the leading cause of food contamination, thus enforcing a standard on personal hygiene would add value to food safety in the dairy industry. All those bilingual posters and chemical cleaners are good, but hand washing is the number one food safety intervention. A lot has to be done on personal hygiene as experience with workers indicate that 25% of female and 42% of male food industry workers still do not wash their hands after using the rest room. Some processors are going to extraordinary lengths to win employee compliance with this fundamental sanitation step. Atlanta's Buckhead Beef Co., a supplier of prime cuts to restaurants throughout the eastern United States, installed keypad controls on hand sanitizers throughout the plant. Workers key in part of their Social Security number to activate the dispenser and activation data is fed back to the payroll system, and employees found deficient in dispenser use are subject to financial reprisals.

Wiping in dairy plants is an intruding source of contamination. Elkhorn, Wisconsin based San Jamar recently introduced sensor equipped paper towel dispensers to replace hand cranks that can be a source of cross contamination. The units also count the number of towels dispensed and correlate the data for supervisor retrieval via a palm pilot or other remote device. GoJo Industries Inc. of Akron, Ohio, offers the Signal dispenser. The unit beeps once, then twice 20 seconds later to signal users that they have washed their hands sufficiently.

Personnel safety parameters during lifting, milking, factory operations and exposure to hazards are common all over north America and do not require any extra cost to HACCP. Human rights are well covered and protected and it does not add to the food safety concerns unless individual sabotage is in the offing with out the knowledge of the management. Crises management teams pre-empt such events amicably.

Sanitizers play a decisive role in dairy plant terminal sanitation and general hygiene. In most of the cases, it is used for terminal disinfection followed by product processing and packing. Rather than asking plant managers and supervisors to train and motivate employees in sanitation procedures, many stakeholders of the processing industry turn to experts such as the American Institute of Baking, Silliker, Ecolab, Steritech, and others. Helping expand the specialists' role in recent years is the U.S. Department of Labour's Hazard Communications Standard, also known as the Right-to-Know Law. The liability should be put squarely on employers' shoulders to make sure employees receive periodic training on safe handling of chemicals, including the wide range of food-plant sanitizers.

Chlorine dioxide, acidic peroxygen, iodophors, and quaternary disinfectants are part of the sanitizing arsenal for many food processors and the food-plant options on sanitizers are expanding. Chlorine's days may be numbered as a sanitizing agent, with an outright psychological ban looming among the processors. Chlorine has been found to be misused by employees of the food industry, chlorine does a lot of damage to the food contact parts of stainless steel unless non-corrosive agents are included and chlorine sometimes causes incidents of grave consequences when admixed with other chemical agents.

The standard sanitizer used to be bleach, but it's probably not the best to use. Bleach at $1 a gallon is hard to beat on an economic basis, but it disintegrates if it is stored for any length of time, and the by-products it produces are bad for the environment. Chlorine dioxide, Para-acetic acid, and peroxide are some of the chlorine alternatives, and a switch to any or all necessitates training in handling.

Presenting information on chemicals and cleaning procedures to a group of workers does formally accomplish a formal session but little in itself. Sometimes, the author had the experience of giving the training to supervisors and they said yes to everything explained. To the authors surprise when it came to practical application, they did follow the procedures but they did not realise the dangers out of it. If we tell them, they'll do it, but that's not always the case. One has to move people from awareness to actually doing something with the knowledge right in front of the provider (educationist).

Pest control is a part of HACCP system. Some food clients to quickly identify and address any infestation hot spots in their plants are using contour mapping and spatial analysis. Service technicians use hand-held computers and bar-code charts to track activity levels at various locations, and then use the data to identify trends and problem areas. However, labour intensive and expensive to set up, spatial analysis enables processors to proactively manage pest control, and it complements the movement away from sprays, poisons, and other active ingredients and toward more strategic placement of materials.

Technology alone can't control pests anymore than chemicals alone can sanitize a plant. They require active support and understanding of both managers and workers, and the kind of buy-in made possible by effective training-74.

Table 3(3) – Yearly HACCP Maintenance Cost to a 150,000 Lts/day Milk Handling Plant indicates budgetary expenses of Can. 130,000, which includes the cost of sewage water and solid waste disposal. One may resort to contractual disposal of sewage water or may install a plant to treat sewage water to meet municipal requirements so that it can enter the municipal streams without any hindrance. However, the choice and mode of treatment and disposal of industrial affluent will reflect the cost of liquid and solid waste disposal.

Table 3(4) – Yearly HACCP Management Cost to 150,000 Lts/day Milk Handling Plant indicates a yearly cost of managing HACCP, which only includes the material and salary expenses. Many may like to budget out non-management expenses to Factory Operation budgets. A HACCP budget may well be confined to the management expenses of HACCP as indicated in Table 3(4). Under such a decision, HACCP yearly expenses will be confined to five digits, which will help HACCP management team to ward off financial burden and pressures of the budgetary control. However, the HACCP system cannot exclude the transformational costs, which are necessary parts of the HACCP pre-requisite program.

D. HACCP Cost to Meat Industry:

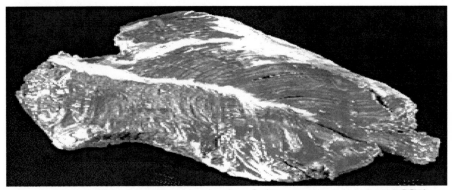

Fig 03(04): Canadian Tender Beef. (Courtesy: CANADA-BEEF)

HACCP Regulation implications and increasing cost of operations in meat industry are worth discussing. Most of the pathogens causing disease find meat a suitable medium. The food animals are the crucial critical point in the meat food chain.

The Food animals related safety issues to meat industry become devastative when diseases like Bovine Spongiform Encephalopathy (BSE) is diagnosed or identified in beef. During nineties, over the possible link between BSE and the human disease Creutzfeldt - Jakob disease (CJD) led to a significant loss of consumer confidence in beef throughout much of Europe. On May 20-2003, the single beef cow with the first confirmed case of BSE in Canada during the last decade apparently spent time at two cattle ranches before it joined a herd of 150 cows near the community of Wenham in north-western Alberta. The CFIA announced on the day that tests confirmed that a cow slaughtered on Jan. 31 had BSE. The news had devastated the Canadian beef industry. Agriculture officials in the U.S. — Canada's biggest market — moved immediately to temporarily ban beef imports from Canada. Australia, South Korea, Japan, Taiwan, New Zealand, and Mexico quickly followed suit. The result was an economic loss to almost five billion dollar beef industry in Canada. The cost of recovery from this incident when compared with the cost of HACCP implementation as preventive measure would be many fold higher. It is the beauty of already existing HACCP system that only one cow was found with BSE and it was never allowed to reach for human consumption.

Cost Study can be conducted by developing a framework for measuring the plant-level cost of quality regulations, based on models of the production of quality-differentiated meat products. This framework may emphasize the potential importance of the impacts of regulations on both variable and fixed costs of meat production. Evidence on the potential impacts of food safety regulation on variable costs of production should be studied.

The structure of cost functions for meat plants producing quality-differentiated products, focusing on the jointness properties of conventional inputs and quality control inputs can be undertaken. This structure could be used to explore how the plant-level costs of performance standards and design standards can be measured, including difficulties in ex ante assessment when only parameters of the pre-regulation technologies are known. A topic has been identified for future research is to compare the accuracy of ex ante estimates of the costs of regulation with the observed ex post costs of regulation.

The results from the research could be used to investigate implications for the costs of the HACCP regulations being implemented by USDA. In its regulatory impact assessment, the Food Safety Inspection Service of USDA assumed the HACCP regulations would not affect the productivity of meat plants or their variable cost of production. Estimates of variable cost functions for beef in the United States show that variable costs of production are an increasing function of product quality, and variable costs of production are a large share of total cost. Once again, the HACCP Transformation Costs and HACCP maintenance costs would be almost the same as in any other sector of the food industry, only variables pertaining to meat industry would add up to the HACCP cost.

It is always expected that safety regulations that significantly affect the efficiency of the production process can significantly raise the cost of production. These costs were not included in the FSIS' regulatory impact assessment of the HACCP regulations. When it is assumed that the cost of production will increase with the effectiveness of the regulations, the expectation remains that the costs of the regulations will likely to equal or exceed the benefits estimated by FSIS. Small beef plants are likely to experience a greater cost increase than the larger plants, and that beef plants' costs are likely to be increased more than pork or poultry plants[128].

According to FSIS regulatory impact analysis, the final rule on HACCP-based regulatory program has potential annual public health benefits of $990 million to $3.7 billion because of reduced food borne illness costs such as medical care and lost work time. It has been estimated that the cost of implementing HACCP would be one-tenth of a cent per pound of meat. Over a four-year period, the estimated cost to the meat and poultry industry for developing, implementing and operating the proposed pathogen reduction and HACCP systems is estimated at $305 to $357 million, averaging $76 to $89 million per year This is significantly lower than the annual estimated cost of implementing the proposed rule, which was about $244.5 million per year, or slightly more than 2/10 of a cent per pound of meat. The recurring cost after full implementation of the pathogen reduction and HACCP systems is estimated at $99.6 to $119.8 million per year[134].

The cost of HACCP to meat industry starts with the Cattle feed, Pre-handling of Cattle, Cattle Management, Factory Hygiene Management System, Stunning & Bleeding, Slaughtering, Dressing & Hide Removal, Evisceration, Carcass Storage, Cutting, Inspection, Cleaning, By-products Management, Differentiated Product Manufacturing, Packaging, and Storage. The Feed and Animal Nutrition Association of Canada has developed a HACCP program for feed mills. Mills will be expected to implement a full HACCP program not a HACCP-based program. In Canada, there are 3 mills that have been certified under the HACCP program and seven more should be ready this year for certification.

The cost of Factory Hygiene Management System (FHMS) is an essential element of HACCP. It is estimated that FHMS cost may be with in the range of two cents per pound of processed and packed meat, which is a necessity. The FHMS should cover the whole process of slaughtering and meat processing, from when the animals enter the slaughterhouse to shipment of the final products. It should include all the equipment and how it is set up, and how that equipment is cleaned and maintained. It should cover water management. All the water being used on-site must be clean, and all the wastewater must meet government regulations with regard to BOD and other limits. Finally, the hygiene management system must include training for employees in plant operations.

By-product management may open a channel in cost saving by processing and packing organ meats such as liver and kidney fetching a higher price in many Asian countries than steak.

However, traditional markets for organ meats and other edible meat by-products are gradually disappearing. Often, it is the use of these by-products, which determine whether a meat processing plant is profitable. They make up a large part of the carcass. For example, by-products such as organs, fat, skin, feet and bones make up around 66% of a cattle carcass. It has been suggested that 7-12% of the income from slaughter comes from the sale of animal by-products. Since the cost of live animals often exceeds the selling price of the meat, it is the value of the by-products, which must cover the cost of HACCP implementation and generate a many fold profit.

HACCP cost estimates will be relatively higher for smaller firms as compared to their larger counterparts. Small firms may incur an estimated average of 25 cents per pound of processed and packed products. Meat processing firms would enjoy lower marginal costs with HACCP systems as opposed to their marginal cost prior to HACCP implementation and firms without HACCP systems are expected to be less cost efficient than firms with HACCP systems.

HACCP can improve the overall efficiency of the meat industry by training and efficient reallocation of labour use and quality carcass purchases. Small firms that may not have output price incentives or economies of scale incentives can enjoy cost cutting incentives with HACCP systems. HACCP will be economically beneficial to small and large firms. HACCP has the potential as a quality management tool to reduce production cost and improve the efficiency of the industry. Meat industry would gain by implementing food safety system and the benefits would outweigh the cost of implementing HACCP in the short and long runs.

E. HACCP Cost to Pork Industry:

New regulations and greater public awareness are leading to increased demand for food safety in meats. Pork is a potential source of several microbial pathogens that pose relatively high costs to society, including _Campylobacter jejuni_, _clostridium perfringens_, and _Listeria monocytogenes_, _Salmonella sp._, and _Staphylococcus aureus_. The pork processing industry faces strong incentives, especially in export markets, to improve food safety, extend product shelf life, and achieve greater consumer acceptance of product. Both industry and regulators need better information about how to reduce pathogens with most effective cost saving.

Swine is considered as a scavenger to serve as a living, breathing, and garbage disposal. It was fashioned to serve as nature's way of eliminating filth and disposing of waste. Numerous physical illnesses can be directly attributed to the pork industry. There are many diseases carried from swine to man, particularly parasite infestations It also carries a wide host of parasites and worms, namely: Faciolopsis buski, Paragonimus, and the sucking worm _Clonorchis sinesis_. In addition, of course there is also the danger of infestation by the extremely dangerous trichina worms which live and breed in swine flesh and which are known to infect one out of every four humans who ingest its poisonous meat. Dr. Glen Shepherd wrote on the dangers of eating pork in Washington Post (31 May 1952)."One in six people in USA and Canada have germs in their muscles - trichinosis 8 from eating pork infected with trichina worms. Many people so infected have no symptoms. Most of those, who do have, recover slowly. Some die; some are reduced to permanent invalids. That is why Old Testament forbids the consumption of pork.

".... The pig also because it is a splitter of the hoof but there is no cud. It is unclean for you. None of their flesh must you eat and carcass you must not touch. " (Deuteronomy 14:8)

Humans are free to exert their choice of food and west are a worldly heaven when it comes to the freedom of choice. HACCP approach in the pork industry is more important with the sense that it is beyond the risks of beef, mutton, fish and milk products. Pork is not poisonous as to kill people right on the spot but latent. A HACCP system approach would help safeguard human health and could help eliminate the risks. However, every food consumed in safe conditions does exert its influence in the long run. One can make a choice of consumption accordingly.

HACCP is one approach to improving food safety with pork that helps firms decide where to intervene during processing for control of pathogens. Control of existing processes through monitoring and verification may be inadequate to reduce pathogens to desired levels, and therefore firms may consider additional interventions. Let us examine four pathogen reduction technologies in pork processing: carcass rinses, sanitizing sprays, steam vacuums, and hot water Pasteurizers. Many large plants have already adopted three of these four; the Pasteurizers is the newest technology. These technologies would most often be used in post-evisceration, before chilling and fabrication. As plants adopt and add to existing processes, they may want to identify the least cost combinations to achieve pathogen reduction. Choosing such combinations must take into account that interventions may affect different pathogens to varying degrees.

It is estimated that the cost of individual technologies based on data from input supply firms and estimates of pathogen reduction from selected meat science studies will constitute the HACCP cost elements in the pork industry. The cost of individual interventions varies from 3 cents/carcass for a cold-water wash to 20 cents per carcass for hot water pasteurization. Higher cost interventions achieve greater pathogen reduction. It is better to use a simple optimization model to find the least cost combinations to achieve multiple pathogen reduction targets. The highest cost combination of rinses and sprays costs 47 cents per carcass, would reduce pathogens to very low levels, and is comparable to combinations of technologies currently employed in some plants. Use of a hot water carcass Pasteurizers might reduce costs to 29 cents per carcass to the total costs of comparable levels of control, and may be particularly cost-effective in improving shelf life.

It is clear that the cost function is upward sloping for microbial pathogen reduction in the pork industry, and that some interventions or combinations of interventions are more cost-effective than others. The costs of specific interventions are less than 2 % of total pork processing costs, so improvements in food safety can be achieved through relatively modest investments by large plants. Of course, the highly competitive nature of the industry means that firms need to find the most cost-effective interventions. We caution that these results are preliminary in several senses- more studies of pathogen reduction under plant conditions are needed; new technologies are emerging to control pathogens; and the technologies represent only part of the costs of a full HACCP system that includes monitoring and verification-115.

F. HACCP Cost to Seafood Industry: Governments across the world are increasingly mandating the use of Hazard Analysis and Critical Control Points (HACCP) approaches to assuring food safety in the seafood industry. In the United States, HACCP was first mandated in 1995 for the seafood industry, with full implementation by December 1997. The adoption of HACCP as a regulatory approach in the United States is based in part on an estimation of the approach's benefits and costs. However, accurately estimating benefits and costs prior to implementation was considered difficult. As implementation has commenced, better estimates will be coming in due course of time based on actual experience. Cost estimates should distinguish between several different measures of the costs of HACCP adoption. Such costs are not transformational discussed earlier. Except the cost of HACCP adoption, which is the part of HACCP transformational cost, the cost of minimum FDA requirements and incremental cost of FDA regulations will be additional and these costs will be amalgamated with ongoing process of the HACCP system.

1.Total Cost of HACCP Adoption: Cost of HACCP plans as adopted by the companies may include more critical control points

(CCPs) than required by the FDA regulation. The cost is counted regardless of whether the plan was adopted in response to the FDA regulation. It therefore includes voluntary and mandatory adoption. The Food and Drug Administration (FDA) estimated benefits of implementing the HACCP programme for seafood range from US$1.435 to US$2.561 billion. The cost of implementing the programme was estimated to range from US$677 million to US$1.488 billion. Cost estimates were based on several models of seafood processing plants and included such costs as training, HACCP plan refinement, sanitation audits, costs of implementing CCPs, equipment cleaning, record review, eliminating pests, and administration. Costs also were assigned to those activities that would be borne by domestic manufacturers and exporters, major plant repair and renovation, Sea Grant expertise, repackers and warehouses, rejected product at the harvesting level, shellfish vessels and foreign processors-[122].

Cost per plant for domestic manufacturers was estimated to be an average of US$23000 the first year and US$13000 per year in subsequent years. This will exclude the salary of HACCP Coordinator who could be paid at least US$30,000 per anum. Prices for seafood were also estimated to increase by less than one percent in the first year and less that one-half of one percent in subsequent years with the larger increase expected to decrease consumption by less than one-half of one percent. It was recognized that small plants would suffer a greater impact than larger ones, but the entire reduction because of HACCP would be borne by the small plants that would exit the industry for other economic reasons-[122]. Cost of HACCP to fish industry can be manipulated by cutting edges and absorbing the change with in the old set up, the estimates provided in Table 3(2) – HACCP Transformation Costs to Food Industry are just guidelines for an extreme practical approach.

2. Cost of Minimum FDA Requirements: This is the cost for the companies of adopting a HACCP plan that met FDA minimum requirements (i.e., had the minimum number of CCPs to meet mandated requirements). The cost is counted regardless of whether the plan was adopted in response to the FDA regulation and, therefore, includes voluntary and mandatory adoptions.

On December 18, 1997 the long anticipated regulation for a new method of inspection for food safety in the seafood and aquaculture industry became effective and enforceable by the U. S. Food & Drug Administration (US-FDA). Each system has specific costs related to its development and implementation.

Every processor shall conduct, or have conducted for it, a hazard analysis to determine whether there are food safety hazards that are reasonably likely to occur for each kind of fish and fishery product processed by that processor and to identify the preventive measures that the processor can apply to control those hazards. Such food safety hazards can be introduced both within and outside the processing plant environment, including food safety hazards that can occur before, during, and after harvest. A food safety hazard that is reasonably likely to occur is one for which a prudent processor would establish controls because experience, illness data, scientific reports, or other information provide a basis to conclude that there is a reasonable possibility that it will occur in the particular type of fish or fishery product being processed in the absence of those controls. Every processor shall have and implement a written HACCP plan whenever a hazard analysis reveals one or more food safety hazards that are reasonably likely to occur. HACCP plan shall be specific to each location where fish and fishery products are processed by that processor.

The HACCP plan shall, at a minimum; list the food safety hazards that are reasonably likely to occur, list the critical control points for each of the identified food safety hazards, including as appropriate, list the critical limits that must be met at each of the critical control points, list the procedures, and frequency thereof, that will be used to monitor each of the critical control points to ensure compliance with the critical limits, include any corrective action plans that have been developed in accordance with Sec. 123.7(b) of seafood HACCP regulation, to be followed in response to deviations from critical limits at critical control points, list the verification procedures, and frequency thereof, that the processor will use in accordance with Sec. 123.8(a) of seafood HACCP regulation; and provide for a record keeping system that documents the monitoring of the critical control points. The records shall contain the actual values and observations obtained during monitoring-189.

The estimated cost to achieve such requirements could be calculated and budgeted from HACCP Transformation Costs and HACCP Maintenance Costs. There is expectation that generic costs will not vary much but varying HACCP understanding for the seafood could fluctuate the cost of transformation and maintenance from plant to plant.

3. Incremental Cost to the FDA Regulation: Cost for the companies of adopting HACCP plans that meet the minimum FDA requirements net of voluntary HACCP adoption that did or would have occurred without the regulation.

In this study, a sample of eight companies processing breaded fish in Massachusetts were interviewed on their costs of implementing a HACCP plan based on the costs of complying with the FDA's requirements, and views of the HACCP regulation itself. The cost data were collected in personal interviews with quality control personnel using detailed interview protocols and survey instruments. The results show that cost estimates vary greatly depending on how the cost of HACCP is defined.

The average first-year total cost of transforming and implementing HACCP in a seafood manufacturing set up is estimated with the figure of US$112,000. The average first-year cost for implementing only the US-FDA minimum requirements could be estimated as US$35,000. This gives the impression that companies had implemented much tougher and more expensive HACCP plans than required and often included non-safety related CCPs within their plans. The cost of implementing only the minimum FDA requirements was 30% of the actual costs companies incurred. It is a psychological and imperative impression that force minority of the seafood companies to implement HACCP because of the FDA regulation. The trend shows that US-FDA generally underestimated the first-year costs of HACCP adoption, such as the costs of writing a HACCP plan and taking corrective actions, but accurately estimated the costs of monitoring and record keeping.

Conclusion:

As we have studied and reviewed the different aspects of costs in food industry, we can conclude that the baseline adoption of HACCP in many industries is almost certainly being influenced by the promulgation of HACCP rules for other industries. Consequently, some industry segments are adopting HACCP faster than the others. Large companies are adopting HACCP at a higher rate than smaller firms. In many cases, implementing HACCP will require more significant changes in plants owned by small companies. The process costs of HACCP are significant.

Smaller companies with their old age technology have many challenges. First of all, the management of such companies should understand the importance of food safety for their business. Once they are convinced, application of regulatory requirements will need substantial finance to fulfil the prerequisites. After the prerequisite investments, an improvement in Plant, Machinery, Laboratory facilities, and Monitoring system would require added investment. Sometimes, installation design of small companies is found as per the "first come first installed basis in available space", which is the bottleneck constraint in food safety improvements. Under such circumstances, an auditor may not press for complete overhaul of the system as long as it satisfies the minimum food safety obligations. However, future expansion may require complete face-lift. Therefore, the cost of HACCP for small and old companies are enormous and the changes have to be budgeted in such a way that safety is maintained and business remains viable.

The small plants are certainly facing a different situation because of the structure of their costs. While some costs are certainly likely to be higher for small plants, the fact that they have fewer people to train and that they might have less turnover may mean that some of the costs are lower. Some small plants process more than one kind of animal, thus posing the potential for cross-species contamination. They may need to move to single-species processing and meet the more restrictive food safety controls.

Larger companies already have better quality management system in place. Better equipments, right installations, process monitoring, standard procedures, and an urge to improve continually. Such companies with the state of the art equipments need fewer improvements which include training of their staff in HACCP, documentation of their arranged plans, decisions, reviews, records, eliminating recurrence of a defect or contamination and motivating employees with imparted knowledge of food safety. The added cost of each segment of HACCP in modern plant will be of consultancy, training, and documentation and of a coordinator of the HACCP process. However, size and volume of operation will influence the cost HACCP at incremental rate. Large plants have some inherent advantages of their own in absorbing costs. In larger plants the costs can be spread over more of the product. Irradiation, an intervention-step technology that was recently approved for commercial use in certain meat products, is not in wide use yet. Its cost for ground beef is estimated at 2 to 5 cents per pound at the retail level, a relatively high amount. Because of that cost, irradiation would likely be used in combination with other technologies. Technically, the ideal place to irradiate product is after it has been packaged as maximum insurance against potential cross-contamination.

Much needed experimentation will be necessary before the products could be put for human consumption. Some technologies like pasteurization dominate the industry and some will prove to be more cost effective like UHT where preservation at ambient temperature and long shelf life is guaranteed.

Chapter: 04
<u>HACCP EVOLUTION</u>

Overview:

In previous chapters we have acquired knowledge of HACCP, which stands for Hazard Analysis Critical control Point. A system to help guarantee the safety of food products by controlling raw materials, manufacturing process, plant environment, plant machinery, manufacturing procedures, evaluation procedures and food manufacturing employees.

Deming concepts, which formed the foundation of HACCP, were taken from the teachings of world-renowned quality guru, Dr. W.E. Deming. Dr. Deming developed the Total Quality Management (TQM) approach that emphasised a "total systems" strategy in manufacturing. The total systems approach involves the integrated effort of everyone in an organization to improve the quality and performance of the company at every level. The premise is that if one improves quality, then costs will be lowered and resources better utilised. Deming's best-known contribution to food safety has been his emphasis on education, training, and self-improvement for everyone. The drive to improve constantly and forever the system of production and services is today's theme, which is one of the fourteen points Deming contributed to transform western management.

We can gain and add up to the HACCP system in the appreciation of the Total Quality System; quality operational organization is a system of interrelated components with a common purpose of food safety and quality. In food safety and quality, first thing to understand is changing one part of the system affects the other parts. Second is the Knowledge of Variation; Every thing in the process is variable, but understanding whether the variation is due to chance cause or random cause will change what action should be taken e.g. upper and lower control limits. Third component is Theory of Knowledge; No learning has occurred if there is no theory that allows prediction. In theory what can go wrong it could well go wrong. Operational definitions are necessary in order to allow theories to be useful in preventing measures. The fourth component is Psychology; it should be properly guided with objectivity of the purpose. We should not forget that we all want to be appreciated.

Philip B. Crosby is another important quality guru who has impacted HACCP from a different angle. He defined quality as conformance to requirements. Fulfilment of requirements from internal and external customers would satisfy the purpose of a business. He meant by quality management as prevention. If a product is manufactured with all preventive defect measures with conformity to requirements then the end product will be free from defect. Thus prevention is the first criteria of his philosophy and HACCP is a prevention based food safety process. However, Audit, inspection, testing, checking, corrective action, and verification are the part of HACCP process only to eliminate recurrence. Prevention reduces reliance on end product analysis and immediate reaction to resultant defects in the product. Crosby believed in conformance not elegance, it is always economical to do the job right the first time, only performance measurement is cost of quality, there is no such thing as quality problem and the only performance standard is zero defect.

HACCP being a preventive process aiming at zero defects but does not ignore the possibilities of defects. That is why a corrective action and verification is purposeful in eliminating recurrence of those defects. Holding a Zero-defect day in a manufacturing plant will impact employees to rely that there is a change in the air.

The current trends in the approach to obtain food innocuity show a favourable scenario for an extensive use of the HACCP System in the future, as a cost-effective and versatile tool that allows its application in the different links of the food chain. Voluntary adherence to its use, especially by the private initiative, is visible in some countries, and this can be proof that, today, many Canadian companies have understood the system as a tool that contributes to improve the efficiency of the food productive process rather than an obligation imposed by regulatory authorities.

The HACCP evolution process must be considered irreversible, notwithstanding the natural resistance that, in cases such as this, generates the necessary change of attitude. As to the scientific aspects of the HACCP development, contributions are expected that can add quantitative approaches in the definition and estimation of risks, especially the microbial type, which relates to the use of such tools as the predictive models and the epidemiological surveillance systems of food-transmitted illnesses. Likewise, the development of quick microbiological analysis tests will allow its use as a support of monitoring and verification activities within HACCP Plan, as long as they show their capacity to produce rapid and reliable results.

The trend in the different segments of the food industry indicated long back that the HACCP would be essential in food manufacturing processes as the development of new products; new design of facilities and long preservation of food became a necessity of world food trade. If these aspects are analyzed before materializing their development, evaluating inherent risks to the process or product, resulting in the adoption of structural and functional designs excluding to the maximum extent the likelihood of hazards, and that will also lead to elimination where hazards cannot be eliminated or reduced to acceptable levels.

Another aspect in HACCP process is the greater importance given to control of suppliers. Because food producing industries find that greater demands as to their suppliers' innocuity give them a big advantage in preventing risks in their processes. Therefore, the HACCP application trend is to be extended as time goes by, up to the production link in order to control food's primary contamination at that stage, a crucial point in controlling pathogens. Possibly, that is the strategy allowing to hugely advancing in the intent to consolidate innocuity control from the farm to the table. The evolution of HACCP took a long course of development and adoption, it would not have been realized if geniuses in technological advancement did not take a lead in human development. The necessity is the mother of invention and our vision in food safety shall travel to the outer periphery of this planet.

HACCP Takes A Start:

The Pillsbury Company pioneered the HACCP concept with the U.S. Army and NASA in the 1960s. The challenge was to perfect a "zero defect" program to guarantee safety of foods for astronauts while in space. HACCP emphasised control of the food process as far upstream in the processing system as possible.

The HACCP System for foods was originally developed in response to a request by NASA to insure that space foods used on manned space flights were safe. Thus HACCP got its start in the 1960s. NASA's food safety concerns were; how would food particles behave in zero gravity and could they detrimentally affect intricate electrical equipment? How to guarantee absolute assurance that the space foods were not contaminated with microbial pathogens, toxins, chemicals, or physical hazards? Developing bite-sized foods coated with a specially formulated coating, which held the product together solved first concern. However, the second concern was much more difficult. At that time, the current technology to assure 100% safety relied solely on end product testing. With this method of quality control it was statistically impractical to assure a 100 % safe food product.

In 1959, Dr. Howard Bauman with Pillsbury Company was the first contacted person by NASA to reconcile the problem. Dr. Howard Bauman concluded after extensive evaluation and brainstorming that by using standard methods of quality control, there was absolutely no way one could be assured that there wouldn't be a problem. Thus the only way, they could succeed, would be to establish control over the entire process, the raw materials, the processing environment and the people involved.

The joint effort of NASA and Dr Howard Bauman led to a zero defect policy in food production. It was with good intent but did not find appropriate for food products. This again was an end product testing, what they needed was a preventative system besides end testing. Next, they got the U.S. Army Natick Research Laboratories involved and evaluated one of their engineering systems Failure, Mode, and Effect Analysis (FEMA). This system, used for medical supplies, looked at what can go wrong at every step, stages of a process, operation along with possible causes and likely effects, before invoking effective control mechanisms. After close evaluation, Pillsbury and NASA adopted this technique as their model and began to make modifications to specifically apply this to food manufacturing. This technique allowed them to evaluate each step of a process for what might go wrong as a hazard, then select critical points in this process where it could be determined if the process was in control. Thus, Hazard Analysis Critical Control Point (HACCP) system for food products was born.

Thus Howard Baumar, Pillsbury's Vice President of science and regulatory affairs made a commitment to improve on already good quality programs by using same techniques they developed to supply food to NASA's astronauts. He was the key figure in the development work for the space program and its later application throughout the company.

This original system; unlike current HACCP system, which has seven principles; consisted of only three principles:

Identification and assessment of hazards associated with growing/harvesting to marketing/ preparation.

Determination of the critical control points to control any identifiable hazard.

Establishment of system to monitor critical control points in the production of food.

Along with these principles, critical control points were identified as points where loss of control would result in an unacceptable food safety risk. Before the HACCP acronym was identified Pillsbury had taken the food safety system outside the research-and-development and pilot-plan mode and put it in to the East Greenville, pre-refrigerated dough plant in 1970. The original objective was to use expanded computer capabilities developed in Minneapolis, MN, to focus on product controls, specifications, and automated recall capabilities[219].

In 1970, a Pillsbury drink powder called Funny face was withdrawn from the market because it contained cyclamate sugar substitute, which had been suddenly declared a possible carcinogen. This led to the establishment of the Product Control and Identification System (PCIS) task force. The task force, under consultant John Haaland, developed what was referred to as the Product Safety Documentation Instructions by 1972. This manual covered the workings of the Corporate Food Safety Committee and its relationship to the freestanding business or profit centres in regard to food safety. This manual had some significant resemblance to the concepts and format of what are now the ISO 9000 standards and the U.S. military standards.

The similarity is not surprising since the original HACCP work was done with what became Natick Laboratories of the Army, the Air Force Space Lab group, and NASA. Thus even at its first commercialisation, HACCP is the cornerstone of the building blocks used to design and produce a safe food product. The overall program as implemented at Pillsbury elevated food safety to a corporate culture. It changed a reactive system into a proactive, preventive system from design to documented conformance.

Started in 1959 and used in Pillsbury plants for several years, the HACCP system wasn't publicly recognized until 1971. At the 1971 National Conference of Food Protection, Pillsbury presented their program and soon afterwards received a contract by FDA to train FDA personnel on the HACCP system. There were several conferences and papers conducted and written in the 70's and early 80's concerning this "new" preventative system. During this time FDA issued the low-acid and acidified canned food regulations, which were based on HACCP principles but did not recognize HACCP specifically. In fact, few companies really took the ball and ran with it until the mid 80's.

In 1985, the National Academy of Science published a report entitled "An Evaluation of the Microbiological Criteria for Foods and Food Ingredients." The NAS committee--actually the Sub-committee on Microbiological Criteria for Foods and Food Ingredients--stated that a preventative system (HACCP) was essential for controlling microbial hazards in food products[95].

From this committee recommendation sprang a flurry of interest in HACCP, not only in the United States but also internationally with Codex Alimentarius Commission. NASA recommended that a National Advisory Committee on Microbiological Criteria for Foods be established. This committee has since embraced HACCP and more importantly further refined it to what we know it as today.

HACCP, as part of a food company policy and management system, is not even economically justified today but even more applicable for consumer protection in today's environment. Previously botulism incidents led to the Low Acid Canned Foods Regulations of 1973 that formally utilised the HACCP principles. Now the challenge to other segments of the food industry is to become more scientific and technologically capable to meet a common objective: to supply unadulterated food to the consuming public in an efficient cost effective way.

Not stated in that objective is a whole world of quality and nutrition, relative to various markets or consumers. Unadulterated food does not necessarily mean uncontaminated which plays a defiant role in litigations. All areas are dealt with in a comprehensive quality programme for safe food, which matches consumer needs with product attributes and spending price. Additional management systems, including ISO 9000 requirements, can deal with these areas in a formatted and effective manner. Further on there is a distinction between scientific food safety compliance through HACCP and other regulatory requirements such as adulteration, mislabelling, net weight, and so on.

What to include in a working HACCP plan has been an area of debate for the 25 plus years since HACCP was introduced publicly in 1971 at the National Conference of Food Protection. Pillsbury incorporated some regulatory compliance issues into many original HACCP plans. For many years, the HACCP system helped train personnel to prevent problems but did so through considerable, possibly excessive, documentation.

The HACCP systems of today correctly put many of the important but not critical control points (CCPs) in to prerequisite programs. The National Advisory Committee on Microbiological Criteria defines prerequisite programs for Foods as "procedures including good manufacturing practices that address operational conditions providing the foundation for the HACCP system." This approach puts the emphasis on doing the job with a reasonable amount of documentation to train, instruct, monitor, or try to measure such things as sanitation effectiveness or employee hygiene in supporting systems. It leaves the few critical points in the process to be dealt with in the HACCP program through measurable, documented data incarcerate.

Food Safety Realization:

Not long time ago, food managers often thought of food safety as passing inspections. Government regulation and inspection have given us this attitude as a reaction to complex and inconsistent regulations. The basic approach to food safety has changed the climate not only in North America but most of Europe and Asia. Government agencies are beginning to talk to each other, clarifying regulatory responsibilities and shifting the responsibility for food safety management to the manufacturer, distributor and retail grocer or restaurant.

The reliance on science based food safety programs is gaining momentum. Scientific understanding of the pathogens causing food borne illnesses is increasing and the focus is on prevention. HACCP engulfs the points of concern into point of prevention through Supplier Controls, Good Manufacturing Practices (GMPs), Sanitation Standard Operating Procedures (SSOPs) Standard Manufacturing Procedures (SMPs), Standard Analytical Procedures (SAPs), Standard Operating Procedures (SOPs) and all these are meant to prevent pathogen growth rather than discover it in finished products-when it may be too late. Though final testing of products in factory premise remains an integral part of the system, an extension of monitoring products until a purchaser consumes it remains the essential part of the whole food safety drive. The approach is preventive than reactional and intends a zero defect in food products based on regulatory stature.

Many would develop confidence with this change in approach in the food supply chain. It means that the responsibility and liability for executing food safety programs will rest squarely with the company processing, distributing or selling food. It is if one takes food safety management seriously and creates a business culture that promotes safe food handling practices. Solid food safety programs can then turn in to positive marketing tools to customers and the end user consumer. The consumer also is responsible how the food is handled under his jurisdiction. Though any illness caused by food consumption immediately targets the manufacturer, the mishandling; storage temperatures etc., of products by consumer could also increase the microorganisms from permitted limits to un-permitted and illness causing counts.

Food safety, product recalls or food poisoning risks are well reported by Canadian and other North American media. Will the increased emphasis on food safety eliminate fear and develop confidence in our food system. People in food business or who are already involved in food processing know the answer. Sanitation Standard Operating Procedure (SSOP) has been required for those under USDA inspection for some time. In addition, Good Manufacturing Practice (GMP) is the basis for safe and sound food production. Large and medium size meat processors are now both required to have a HACCP (Hazard Analysis and Critical Control Points) plan. HACCP has already been extended to small meat processors in January 2000 and eventually it is the food safety standard for other segments of food production and distribution.

Food safety realization underlines the new threats to global food supply posed by the rapid increase and deep market penetration of new and exotic foods from a variety of trading partners. That may constitute a safety or disease hazard; by environmental contaminants, especially in traditional food sources in Canada's Far North, which are also a threat to safety; and emergencies or disasters, which can cause problems such as contamination from hazardous chemicals or disease-causing microorganisms.

The lack of knowledge about preparation and storage of foods is identified as a threat, mainly at the household level. Actions to ensure safe supplies and safe handling include enhanced public education, better product labelling, enhanced biotechnology assessment, improved monitoring methods and stronger multisectoral partnerships.

Consumers are increasingly aware of the relationship between nutrition and health, and there is no doubt that they place a high priority on food safety and quality. The nutrition and metabolism component of the Food for Health program is recognized as an area of research excellence in Canada.

There are scientific groups in North America who have been working with food safety because of its importance and realization of complex food safety requirements. One component of that scientific group is the scientists in University of Alberta. The internationally recognized group of scientists had discipline focused research areas of strength and the group is currently at a stage of expanding its research capacity. The academic staffs with expertise in Food Science and Technology was brought together with the merger of the Departments of Food Science, Foods, and Nutrition to form the Department of Food Science and Nutrition in 1993. A subsequent merger with Departments of Plant Science and Animal Science followed this merger in 1994 to establish the current Department of Agricultural, Food, and Nutritional Science (AFNS). Compared to other similar groups across North America, the Food Science and Technology Group are in a unique position to take an integrated approach to food research from the "farm gate to the consumer plate-90.

Members of the Food Science and Technology Group collaborate extensively with researchers both within the University of Alberta and within other agencies, such as Alberta Agriculture, Food and Rural Development and Agriculture and Agri-Food Canada that together bring an unparalleled level of expertise contributing to value-added research in food safety and production.

Innovations in production efficiencies and new value-added technologies and products are expected to significantly diversify the Canadian economy and create new food sales opportunities in foreign markets. The Food Science and Technology Group are working closely with the Agri-food industry and other research partners. Ongoing research activities of the Group already have a substantial impact on the Agri-food industry in Alberta. Realization of the research potential of the Group through expansion of the intellectual capacity and establishment of the infrastructure needed to facilitate research in value-added product and process development and food safety will enhance contributions to the growth of Alberta and Canada's Agri-food sector. These contributions are based on internationally recognized sound science-90.

Similarly in Ontario, there is a constant need for Ontario's food safety system to keep up with new technology, scientific advances, new and evolving food hazards, and changing trade requirements. Within the last few years, there has been a realization that some of the known risks could be introduced at the farm and therefore makes more sense to address them at the farm level. In Ontario, The food safety program's goal is to eliminate or minimize to a suitable level any chemical, physical, or biological hazard that poses a threat to human health. Overall purpose of the on-farm food safety program is to identify and address hazards before they happen, rather than further along the food chain when more time, money, and effort are required to control the hazard. The on-farm programs developed to date are based on three simple principles: Say what you are going to do to maximize food safety. Do it and Document it-170.

Health Canada estimates that each year in Canada there are about one million cases of food-borne illness. Today, food safety is one of the highest priority food issues for consumers, producers, federal, provincial, and territorial governments alike.

In 2002, Agricultural ministers of the European Union (EU) finalized the creation of the European Food Safety Authority

(EFSA), a new EU food safety body. EFSA's role is to provide scientific advice to EU policymakers and to provide general public information on food safety. The authority will also operate a consumer alert system for possible food risks and recalls. EFSA will be similar to the U.S. Food and Drug Administration (FDA) in some functions, but the organization will not have FDA's broad enforcement authority. EFSA will cover issues from the farm to the fork, including animal feed safety, animal disease prevention, animal welfare, food labelling, food safety, and inspections-[63].

In the United States, the years of 1992-93, and subsequent _E. coli_ O157:H7 outbreak, food safety efforts evolved with great progress, with improvements in a number of key areas. Mandatory safe handling labels were first on the list implemented in 1994. The Pathogen Reduction and HACCP rule went in place in 1996, and was implemented in phases beginning in 1997. In addition, in 1997, the President's Food Safety Initiative set in motion a number of activities that have contributed greatly to reducing food borne illness. Although NASA and a large food processing company invented HACCP, it had not been widely embraced by the meat and poultry industry. However, evolution of HACCP in USA can be boasted back to year 1960.

The cost of medical treatment and productivity losses associated with only four food borne pathogens is estimated at $9.2 billion to 11.2 billion annually. The latest estimates on the incidence of food borne disease in the United States from the Centers for Disease Control and Prevention are that 76 million people get sick, 325,000 are hospitalized, and 5,000 die each year. These statistics indicate that food borne disease is still a very serious problem and a threat to the public health. In addition, all of us are paying for the costs of treating these illnesses through our insurance bills and taxes that support Medicare and Medicaid. This factor further evolved the adoption of HACCP by USDA-[83].

HACCP System and Future Food Safety -[100]

The current trends in the approach to obtain food innocuity show a favourable scenario for an extensive use of the HACCP System in the future, as a cost-effective and versatile tool that allows its application in the different links of the food chain. Voluntary adherence to its use, especially by the private initiative, is visible in some countries, and this can be proof that, today, many companies have understood the system as a tool that contributes to improve the efficiency of the food productive process rather than an obligation imposed by regulatory authorities.

In a world markedly influenced by the globalization, competitiveness plays an important role in keeping positioning in the markets. This will determine, in the next century, an important transition as to what to do with industries and governments in relation to food innocuity. Therefore, regulatory mechanisms based on HACCP principles will become essential. Governmental authorities, on their part, will have to reconsider their control strategies, turning to a role that will highlight their capacity to verify the industry's control programmes, which will imply, also the necessary review of its regulatory framework to adapt it to the new reality.

Although it is imperative to acknowledge the importance acquired by HACCP in the light of the agreements related to the World Trade Organization (WTO) and the regulatory demands for food trade, countries should also take into account the importance that food control for internal consumption is starting to have, since it is more and more reasonable to think that, if a country has succeeded in developing efficient control programmes for the food consumed by its population, this is a good indicator that the innocuity philosophy and culture have pervaded its population, and this is the best scenario to deploy successful approaches such as HACCP.

In this respect, it may be necessary to make a joint government-industry effort to support the mechanisms facilitating the adoption of HACCP in the small and medium enterprises. In home-made production, that entails the greatest proportion of the food industry in any country confronts serious limitations of different nature that demand assistance to facilitate their incorporation to this new approach. The HACCP evolution process must be considered irreversible, notwithstanding the natural resistance that, in cases such as this, generates the necessary change of attitude.

As to the scientific aspects of the HACCP development, contributions are expected that can add quantitative approaches in the definition and estimation of risks, especially the microbial type, which relates to the use of such tools as the predictive models and the epidemiological surveillance systems of food-transmitted illnesses. Likewise, the development of quick microbiological analysis tests will allow its use as a support of monitoring and verification activities within an HACCP Plan, as long as they show their capacity to produce rapid and reliable results.

Other trends, which indicate that HACCP will be essential in such processes as the development of new products and in the design of facilities for food production, these two aspects, are analyzed before materializing their development. In the light of the risks inherent to the process or product, which will lead to the adoption of structural and functional designs would give an opportunity to exclude to the maximum extent the likelihood of hazards. Analysis before materializing the development will also lead to the elimination of any product development where hazards cannot be eliminated or reduced to acceptable levels.

Another aspect that will markedly influence HACCP usage is the greater and greater importance given to control of suppliers, because food producing industries find that greater demands as to their suppliers' innocuity give them a big advantage in preventing risks in their processes. Therefore, the HACCP application trend is to be extended as time goes by, up to the production link in order to control food primary contamination at that stage, a crucial point in controlling pathogens-100. Possibly, that is the strategy allowing to hugely advancing in the intent to consolidate innocuity control from the farm to the dish.

RISK ANALYSIS AND HACCP
Covello and Merkhofer (1994) define risk as a combination of something that is undesirable and uncertain. More specifically "the possibility of an adverse outcome and uncertainty over the occurrence, its timing or magnitude of that adverse outcome" is risk. Risk analysis was first formalized by the U.S. National Academy of Sciences—through its U.S. National Research Council—in 1983, in a publication commonly referred to as, The Red Book-39.

With the emergence of new food borne diseases, sporadic poisoning outbreaks, and bio-terrorism, international concerns over food safety have accelerated the evolution and implementation of HACCP and risk assessment. Risk assessment and HACCP are indispensable to each other and are constituents of the overall risk analysis process.

Risk analysis includes risk management, risk communication and risk assessment. The 1983 NAS-NRC model (National Academy of Sciences)/(National Research Council's) explicitly distinguished between three stages of risk analysis: Risk Assessment, Risk Management, and Risk Communication.

Risk Assessment:
Risk assessment is a scientific assessment of the true risk. It is an integral constituent of the series of activities that starts with Good Manufacturing Practices (GMPs) and culminates in microbiological criteria used for the management of microbial hazards for food in national and international trades. The essence of microbial risk assessment is describing a system in which a microbial hazard reaches its host and causes harm. The knowledge in each system and steps is combined to represent a cause-and-effect chain from

the prevalence and concentration of the pathogen to the probability and magnitude of health effects. In risk assessment, risk consists of both the probability and impact of disease. In this way, risk reduction can be achieved in either dimension—by reducing the probability of disease or by reducing its severity. Risk assessment consists of four steps: hazard identification, exposure assessment, dose-response assessment, and risk characterization.

Risk assessment procedures include several conservative assumptions about uncertainty. The NAS-NRC (National Academy of Sciences)/(National Research Council's) model of risk assessment consists of four steps:

Hazard identification—the determination of whether a particular chemical is or is not causally linked to particular health effects.

Dose-response assessment—the determination of the relation between the magnitude of exposure and the probability of occurrence of the health effects in question.

Exposure assessment—the determination of the extent of human exposure before or after application of regulatory controls is critical.

Risk characterization—the description of the nature and often the magnitude of human risk, including attendant uncertainty.

These components of risk assessment have been endorsed and incorporated into the principles of risk assessment adopted by the U.S. National Advisory Committee on Microbiological Criteria for Foods (NACMCF-1998). Despite such endorsements, the NAS-NRC (National Academy of Sciences/National Research Council's) paradigm had been criticized as unworkable and unrealistic. Covello and Merkhofer (1994) argue that "The state of the art of risk assessment does not permit questions of science to be clearly separated from questions of policy. In practice, assumptions that have potential policy implications enter into risk assessment at virtually every stage of the process. The ideal of a risk assessment that is free, or nearly free, of policy considerations is beyond the realm of possibility".

Even the use of conservatism—the risk assessor errs on the side of safety—is a value judgment deliberately introduced into risk assessments to account for uncertainty, which can produce highly distorted risk assessments, which affect the pattern of regulation, preventing limited resources for health and safety from being efficiently allocated.

Soby et al. (1993), in a review of risk communication research and its applicability for managing food-related risks, developed the concept of the risk management cycle. In this model, public and other stakeholder concerns are actively sought at each stage of the management process—including assessment. "The risk assessment procedure should involve an element of interactive public participation and mutual questioning, otherwise the decisions and conclusions reached are more likely to be challenged" -195, 191.

The U.S. National Academy of Sciences' National Research Council Committee on Risk Characterization (US-NAS-NRCCRC 1996), urges risk assessors to expand risk characterization beyond the practice of translating the results of a risk analysis into non-technical terms. The stakeholders are an integral part of any food safety issues and an analytical-deliberative approach shall involve stakeholders from the very inception of a risk assessment-207.

Of particular importance is that the Framework is conducted in collaboration with stakeholders and using iterations if new information is developed that changes the need for, or nature of, risk management. As Pollak (1996) has argued, due to the inadequacy of scientific knowledge and the lack of public trust in government and in experts, risk regulators should be concerned both with creating institutional arrangements likely to foster trust and mechanisms for providing concerned individuals with credible reassurance.

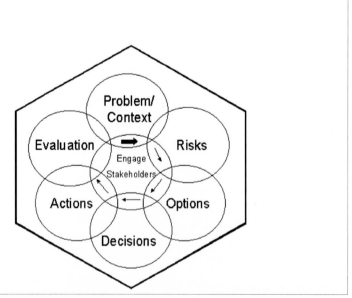

Fig: 04(1) - The risk management cycle. U.S. Presidential/ Congressional Commission on Risk Assessment and Risk Management (1997) -51A

Quantitative risk assessment of food-related hazards provides a focus for discussions among workers from diverse disciplines: farmers, veterinarians, professional agrologists, food-processing experts, microbiologists, and consumer behaviour experts. The model also allows for consideration and comparison of control strategies in a simulated environment (Lammerding and Paoli, 1998). Nevertheless, the large amount of scientific uncertainty inherent in a quantitative risk assessment means that an integrative approach incorporating management and communication considerations must be included in any policy about a particular food source, as well as a full and transparent accounting of the factors and uncertainties included in a specific risk assessment.

Risk assessment is the first of several key steps in managing hazards for foods. Initially the parameters and scope of the problem must be defined. Risk assessment next addresses hazard identification, including not only identification of the hazard, but also assessment of its impact on human health, and the determination of when, where, and how it has an impact on human health. Hazard identification can use LD50, ID50 and LC 50 techniques.

LD50 (Lethal Dose Test): LD50 is the amount of a material, given all at once, which causes the death of 50% (one half) of a group of test animals. The LD50 is one way to measure the short-term poisoning potential (acute toxicity) of a material.

ID50 (Infective Dosage): ID50 is used for the dose of an infectious organism required to produce infection in 50 percent of the experimental subjects.

LC50 (Lethal Concentration): LC stands for "Lethal Concentration". LC values usually refer to the concentration of a chemical in air but in environmental studies it can also mean the concentration of a chemical in water. For inhalation experiments, the concentration of the chemical in air that kills 50% of the test animals in a given time (usually four hours) is the LC50 value.

Hazard identification can also use laboratory, challenge studies, epidemiological studies, or observation of related products in similar environments. Risk assessment is only one integral component in a series of steps leading to the management of hazards for foods in international trade.

Full benefits of an effective HACCP program cannot be realized without a comprehensive risk assessment to customize the program to a specific situation. HACCP does not mandate or suggest any particular methodology for hazard analysis for risk assessment. Zurich Risk Engineering works with food companies using its proprietary Zurich Hazard Analysis (ZHA) is a team-based gross hazard analysis method that systematically identifies hazards and their trigger mechanisms, and assesses their associated effects in terms of likelihood and severity. Each hazard can then be assessed qualitatively for its relative risk, including comparative probability of occurrence and severity of effects, with due consideration for effectiveness of downstream controls.

Hazard Identification: In hazard identification, an association between disease and the presence of a pathogen in a food is documented. The information may describe conditions under which the pathogen survives, grows, causes infection, and dies. Epidemiological and surveillance data, challenge testing, and scientific studies of pathogenicity also contribute information. Data collected during hazard identification are later used in exposure assessment, where the impact of processing, distribution, preparation, and consumption of the food are incorporated.

Exposure Assessment: Exposure assessment describes the pathways through which a pathogen population is introduced, distributed, and challenged in the production, distribution, and consumption of food. This step differs from hazard identification in that it describes a particular food-processing pathway. Depending on the scope of the risk assessment, exposure assessment can begin with pathogen prevalence in raw materials or it can begin with the description of the pathogen population at subsequent steps (e.g., as input to a food-processing step). In any case, the intent of risk assessment is to track the pathogen population and estimate the likelihood of its being ingested by the consumer. By completing the pathway to the consumer, we incorporate the important issues of dose-response assessment.

Dose-Response Assessment: Dose-response assessment is used to translate the final exposure to a pathogen population into a health response in the population of consumers. This step is very difficult because of the shortage of data on pathogen-specific responses and because those responses depend on the immune status of the host (consumer). However, even limited knowledge of the shape and boundaries of a dose-response function can be informative in comparing the efficacy of alternate controls. The differences in response among various susceptible populations are important features in this step.

Risk Characterization:
Risk characterization involves integrating the information gathered

in the previous steps to estimate the risk to a population, or in some cases, to a particular type of consumer. In this step, by modifying the assumptions in the parameters of previous steps, we can study the effects of these alternate assumptions on ultimate health risk. Assumptions can be changed to study the impact due to lack of knowledge and the potential gains through further research or to suggest the impact of a suspected trend.

Risk characterization from an activity happens at the end of the risk assessment process, as many people understand it, to a continuous, back-and-forth dialogue between risk assessors and stakeholders that allows the problem to be formulated properly, and depends on an iterative, analytic-deliberative process.

Risk characterization takes place after defining the purpose for the activity, identifying the hazard, assessing the exposure, and predicting the dose response. Risk characterization integrates the sequential process to estimate the adverse effects likely to occur in the target population-94.

For this type of analysis, risk assessments are typically done in a computer environment to ease the computational burden and provide rapid responses to "what-if" questions using alternate assumptions and situations. Current spreadsheet applications and available "add-ins" allow generation of complicated probabilistic models that had previously only been available through expensive custom software.

Probable cost to the operator per year of customers getting sick or dying from a hazard is a part of risk characterization. The process of determining the qualitative and/or quantitative estimation, including attendant uncertainties, of the probability of occurrence and severity of known or potential adverse health effects in a given population based on hazard identification and exposure assessment characterises the risk.

As the interface between risk assessment and risk management, risk characterizations should be clearly presented, and separate from any risk management considerations. Risk management options should be developed using the risk characterization and should be based on consideration of all relevant factors, scientific and non-scientific. Risk characterizations should include a statement of confidence in the assessment that identifies all major uncertainties along with comment on their influence on the assessment, consistent with the Guidance on Risk Characterization. The degree to which confidence and uncertainty are addressed in a risk characterization depends largely on the scope of the assessment. In general, the scope of the risk characterization should reflect the information presented in the risk assessment and program-specific guidance.

Risk assessment is based on a series of questions that the assessor asks about scientific information that is relevant to human and/or environmental risk. Each question calls for analysis and interpretation of the available studies, selection of the concepts and data that are most scientifically reliable and most relevant to the problem at hand, and scientific conclusions regarding the question presented. For example, health risk assessments involve the following questions:

Hazard Identification: What is known about the capacity of an environmental agent for causing disease or other adverse health effects in humans, laboratory animals, or wildlife species? What are the related uncertainties and science policy choices?

Dose Response Assessment: What is known about the biological mechanisms and dose response relationships underlying any effects observed in the laboratory or Epidemiology studies providing data for the assessment? What are the related uncertainties and science policy choices?

Exposure Assessment: What is known about the principal paths, patterns, and magnitudes of human or wildlife exposure and numbers of persons or wildlife species likely to be exposed? What are the related uncertainties and science policy choices?

Corresponding principles and questions for ecological risk assessment are being discussed as part of the effort to develop ecological risk guidelines.

Risk characterization is the summarizing step of risk assessment. The risk characterization integrates information from the preceding components of the risk assessment and synthesizes an overall conclusion about risk that is complete, informative, and useful for decision makers.

Risk characterizations should clearly highlight both the confidence and the uncertainty associated with the risk assessment. For example, numerical risk estimates should always be accompanied by descriptive information carefully selected to ensure an objective and balanced characterization of risk in risk assessment reports and regulatory documents. In essence, a risk characterization conveys the assessor's judgment as to the nature and existence of (or lack of) human health or ecological risks. Even though a risk characterization describes limitations in an assessment, a balanced discussion of reasonable conclusions and related uncertainties enhances, rather than detracts, from the overall credibility of each assessment.

"Risk characterization" is not synonymous with "risk communication." This risk characterization policy addresses the interface between risk assessment and risk management. Risk communication, in contrast, emphasizes the process of exchanging information and opinion with the public – including individuals, groups, and other institutions. The development of a risk assessment may involve risk communication. For example, in the case of site-specific assessments for hazardous waste sites, discussions with the public may influence the exposure pathways included in the risk assessment. While the final risk assessment document (including the risk characterization) is available to the public, the risk communication process may be better served by separate risk information documents designed for particular audiences-220.

Risk Profile:

To determine the desired risk tolerance level and to compare this level to the potential frequency and severity of the catalogued hazards to determine unacceptable risks is called a risk profile. The 2nd HACCP principle, the identification of critical control points, becomes much clearer once the risk profile has been generated because it helps to identify CCPs with unacceptable risks. This helps to prioritize the hazards and simplify the completion of the HACCP program.

The production of food has numerous risks involved in the processes. A risk flow diagram of the particular food production processes consists of stages in food production, which should be listed to the left, and the associated risks involved with the stage to the right. When appropriate, the associated risks will be activated links leading to more information about the subject. Thus each stage of the process with identified associated risk could pave the way to eliminate it from the process. Risk profile for each product processing and packing would result in comprehensive safety provided all risks are identified, eliminated, limits controlled and performance monitored.

Food spoilage and food-borne illness are not random or chance events. All foods contain microorganisms and that is the way food is handled during processing and storage that determines if the food will become spoiled or will become a source of illness. All possible sources of microbial contamination should be profiled with respective food items, with needed processing, suitable packaging, and calculated shelf life. Microbial risk profiling has two main goals to eliminate: to prevent microorganisms from contaminating the product and to prevent microbial growth during the shelf life. Dairy products, fresh or processed meats, bakery products, and fruits and vegetables all have different handling and processing requirements. To handle, process, store and distribute safe food products, processors need to understand the special requirements of both their raw and finished products. All raw materials including packaging should be inspected upon arrival to ensure that they meet your product specifications as well as ensuring that the containers have not been opened or damaged and that perishable items arrive at the proper temperature.

Personnel risk profiling should be the part of safety drive. Bacteria may be found in the nose, mouth, throat, hair, face, skin, and hands, including under fingernails. Microorganisms can be easily transferred from non-food items to food by simply touching non-food items before handling the food. One example could be given of _Streptococcus aureus_, which produces a variety of diseases including food poisoning, impetigo, boils, carbuncles, osteomyelitis (infections of the bone), toxic shock syndrome, and fatal septicaemia (blood infections). Approximately 10% of the general public carry this organism. They are normal inhabitants of the skin and the nasal membranes of healthy food workers. Precautions must be taken to control the spread of such microorganisms from food handlers onto the food product. Processing facilities require proper hand washing stations, hand sanitizers, and footbaths that are conveniently placed at appropriate locations throughout the plant. All food handlers require training to understand how their work habits impact upon food safety.

Risk profiling during the cleaning process is another important factor. Let us take the example of milking cow, when cows are housed or graze in heavily stocked paddocks, external udder surfaces are usually grossly contaminated with bacteria even when they appear visibly clean, therefore routine udder preparation procedures should be followed. Whenever udders are washed they should be dried. The milk contact surfaces of milking and cooling equipment are a main source of milk contamination and frequently the principal cause of consistently high bacterial counts cleaning is the process where food, residue, dirt, and dust are physically removed from food equipment surfaces and the surrounding processing environment. Sanitizing is a later step in the clean-up process, which acts to reduce the number of microorganisms on surfaces to an acceptable level and kills all pathogens. All product contact parts in the food manufacturing chain shall be cleaned and sanitized in an efficient way, at the same time chemical from such process shall not pose threat of cross contamination and spill over to food.

Risk Management:

Risk management is the factor, which allows for the incorporation of non-scientific factors to reach a policy decision. The U.S. Presidential and Congressional Commission on Risk Assessment and Risk Management (1997) developed an integrative framework to help all types of risk managers—government officials, private sector businesses, individual members of the public—make good risk management decisions. The framework has six stages:

• Define the problem and put it in context
• Analyze the risks associated with the problem in context
• Examine options for addressing the risks
• Make decisions about which options to implement
• Take actions to implement the decisions
• Conduct an evaluation of the action's results

Risk management is a term borrowed from industries such as insurance, health care, and even the military. It recognizes that most activities have associated risk and once that premise has been accepted, actions can be implemented that help minimize the risk. Typically, zero risk is unattainable, but reducing it to a minimum, which does not impact negativity in the process and product, should be the objective.

For example, dairymen everywhere has to deal with the fact that cows develop mastitis and the consequences are always negative. Minimizing problems requires an appreciation of the causes, a risk management program aimed at identifying and eliminating problems plus an education effort for all people involved. Dairymen are faced with the fact that mastitis is an ever-present risk despite all the effort that has gone into determining ways of reducing or preventing it. The facts are that if you are a dairyman, there is likelihood that you face mastitis problems. The key is to minimize the risks by preventive measures and a proper Risk management Program.

Each risk nominally goes through different functions sequentially, but the activity occurs continuously, concurrently (e.g., risks are tracked in parallel while new risks are identified and analyzed), and iteratively e.g., the mitigation plan for one risk may yield another risk throughout the project life cycle on day-to-day basis. First step in risk management is to search for and locate risks before they become problems. Then Identify and analyze the risk; transform risk data into decision-making information. Evaluate impact, probability, and timeframe, classify risks, and prioritize risks. Plan and translate risk information into decisions and mitigating actions (both present and future) and implement those actions. Track the risks by monitoring risk indicators and mitigation actions. Control and corrective actions are required for deviation from the risk mitigation plans. The last is communication, which provides information and feedback of internal and external factors to the project on the risk activities, current risks, and emerging risks. However, verification is indispensable in all aspects of HACCP system.

Risk management steps should result in safe handling procedures and practices, food processing quality and safety assurance controls, appropriate food quality, safety standards, and safety criteria, which follow risk assessment. Risk management is a responsibility of food manufacturers, government regulatory agencies, catering industry, and the consumer. Implementation of an effective HACCP program provides a systematic approach to food safety. With dramatic increases in the variety of prepared foods, an effective food safety program is an important element of public health protection.

HACCP is a risk management technique, and the cornerstone to risk management is the proper definition of the nature and degree of the risks pertaining to a process. Without this first, fundamental understanding, risk managers' later decisions regarding intervention and monitoring techniques will be subject to question, and the HACCP system may fail in its purposes entirely. Risk managers in the food industry must plan and act with the knowledge that the reduction of the potential hazards inherent in food production crucially relies on a rational assessment of those hazards.

Food Safety Risks:

Improper cooking, processing, and storage of foods, poor hygiene, poor health of food handlers or an unsafe food source causes food poisoning and illness. By cooking food well, using good hygiene, and watching what you eat, reading the label on packaging, one will avoid consuming harmful bacteria, allergen, unwanted chemicals and other harmful contaminants. Reading label would only help safety from food allergens. Hazards and risk to human health can come from many sources; a food technologist must consider the possible risk factor in food operations. Following are the risk groups encountered in food safety system.

Chemical Risks:

Chemical risk causes Food Poisoning, which are usually caused by the consumption of contaminated food or water containing contaminants of chemical nature. There is a long list of chemicals, which pose risk to food safety during cultivation, procurement, factory processing, and packing. Some of the group examples are:

- DAIRY DETERGENT
- DAIRY SANITIZERS
- GENERAL CLEANERS
- HEAVY METALS
- HERBICIDES
- INSECTICIDES
- PESTICIDES
- REFRIGERANTS
- RODENTICIDES
- SOLVENTS
- INORGANIC SALTS

In the farm production, the proper use, storage, and application of Agricultural chemicals are regulated through the Pesticide Management Regulatory Agency (PMRA) of Health Canada and enforced through the Canadian Food Inspection Agency (CFIA). The use of antimicrobials are regulated and enforced by the CFIA. Chemical and heavy metal residues can also be introduced through the use of contaminated irrigation or dilution water, residues inherent in soil due to previous uses, or spill over from neighbouring operations.

Chemical hazards generally fall into two categories: naturally occurring poisons, chemicals, or deleterious substances that are natural constituents of foods, such as Aflatoxins or Mycotoxins, and are not the result of environmental, Agricultural, industrial, or other contamination; and, added chemicals or deleterious substances which are intentionally or unintentionally added to foods at some point in growing, harvesting, storage, processing, packing, or distribution, including pesticides, fungicides, insecticides, fertilizers, drug residues, and antibiotics, as well as direct and indirect food additives. This group can also include chemicals such as lubricants, cleaners, paints, and coatings.

A further impetus to the development of strict chemical-use guidelines was the passage of the U.S. Food Quality Protection Act of 1996 which established a health-based standard for all pesticide residues in food, and mandated that the U.S. Environmental Protection Agency (EPA) determine that there is reasonable certainty of no harm from aggregate exposure to pesticides from various sources, including the diet, drinking water, and residential use. Under the law, all existing pesticide tolerances will be reassessed in a process that is scheduled to be completed by

August 2006 (Coble, et al., 1998). The Act encompasses the broad principles of greater protection for the most risk-susceptible members of society, especially children, consideration of whether groups of pesticides have a common mode of action, and consideration of the aggregate exposure of pesticides in diet, drinking water, and non-occupational exposure throughout the process of pesticide registration and re-registration processes (Council for Agricultural Science and Technology, 1998). The outcome of the process could result in the cancellation of some pesticide registrations important to production of several crops.

There is already evidence that the European Union is gradually moving toward a Food Quality Protection Act approach to pesticide residues (Anon, 1998) and American producers are significantly concerned. Under the auspices of the Council for Agricultural Science and Technology, American producers produced a report calling for the prescription use of certain high-risk chemicals to retain their use while ensuring public safety. Regardless of the permutations, there will be an increased scrutiny of Agricultural chemicals in all foods, including processing vegetables. A prerequisite program for chemical inputs can provide both producers and processors with the data to support claims of product safety and to retain the confidence of international markets-52.

The chemical contaminants in food are defined as a specific combination of a chemical constituent or combination of contaminants and food, considered to pose potential threats to human health. Foodstuffs are an important source of exposure to a wide range of chemical hazards, which occur either as a natural constituent of the food or are introduced during production, storage, processing, or distribution. Routine monitoring and analysis of foodstuffs provides one way of detecting these hazards, and of directing action to reduce health risks.

Risk Phrases are available in many countries, which contain codes for certain notions of risk shown as R23, R45 etc. These risk phrase codes have the meanings: like R23 - Toxic by inhalation and R45 - may cause cancer.

The agencies involved in monitoring and providing information regarding chemicals related to food poisoning are FAO, Local authority, environmental health officers, National food agencies, National ministries of health, environment, Agriculture, UNEP and WHO - Food Safety Unit. The chemical monitoring of food products involves the routine sampling and analysis of food commodities, including drinking water, with the aim of assessing dietary exposure of the population to hazardous chemical contaminants or constituents. Hazardous concentrations are usually defined in relation to nationally or internationally agreed standards or tolerable/acceptable levels.

In Canada, Canadian Food Inspection Agency (CFIA) and Health Canada share the responsibility to enforce regulations and provide assistance to produce a safe food manufacturing system and safe food products for Canadian as well as export markets. Pest Management Regulatory Agency (PMRA), which works under Health Canada, registers and regulates pest control products under the Pest Control Products Act (PCPA) and regulates the use of chemicals on food products under the Canadian Food and Drug Regulations. Maximum Residue Limits (MRL) have been established for all chemicals used in the manufacturing of food products in Canada and National Chemical Residue Monitoring Program (NCRMP) of CFIA has the authority to monitor the compliance by the industry. In the monitoring phase, an unbiased selection of samples are taken from the normal food supply and tested for chemical residue. This testing allows for the detection of residue problems.

CFIA tested during the four-year period from April 1, 1994 to March 31, 1998; 44,379 shipments of fresh and processed fruit & vegetable products available in Canada for pesticide residues. Both domestic and imported shipments were sampled. An enhanced multi-residue method, capable of detecting more than 260 pesticides and their metabolites, was employed. Testing indicated that the violation rate was 1.2 % for domestic samples and 1.94 % for imported samples. An unexpected finding was that the difference between the violation rate for domestic and imports, which was traditionally 2.2 %, had decreased substantially to only 0.7 %. The diminution was due in equal parts to a reduced violation rate for imports and an increased violation rate for domestic samples. This may be, in part, due to the efforts at international harmonization of the maximum residue limits[86].

Hardness in food manufacturing water is a factor of long-term illness effect and should be considered by health conscious people. However, a hard water supply may not result in good quality manufactured food but the quality conscious food processors would also acknowledge that it is in their economical benefit to use soft water to safeguard their equipments, processed food and human health in the long run. A hard water supply of >100 ppm poses a risk of kidney stones, artery calcification, and skin diseases which most of us ignore. A serious thought is needed on the issue. Most of the people interviewed by the author in Mississauga responded by answering "I drink distilled water". The author does not recommend any particular water or brand for the purpose of drinking but does caution the public over the usage of high Total Dissolved Solids in water. The safe level of TDS should not be more than 35 ppm and should be the best maximum target.

Microbiological Risks:

In the food manufacturing system, risk to food comes from the contamination of food product from the farm, insufficient processing, improper storage, and poor hygiene. Microbial risk means occurrence of a microorganism that has the potential to cause illness or injury. Consequently, the food products provide growth medium at ambient temperatures and these organisms multiply manifold to cause illness.

Any HACCP-like on-farm food safety program must encompass the basic goals of HACCP -- to reduce or eliminate microbial risks associated with food products. Microorganisms are ubiquitous -- in birds, soil, and water. Because of the control on farms and proper processing, vegetables under the purview of the Ontario Vegetable Growers' Marketing Board (OVGMB) are subjected to a heat treatment, either through canning or blanching for freezing, microbes are of little concern, especially given the pre-processing environment.

There are many different types of microbial agents who enjoy the very same food as the humans. Microorganisms include yeasts, molds, bacteria, protozoa, helminths (worms), and viruses. Occasionally, the term "microbe" or "microbial" is used instead of the term "microorganism." Some of the known agents have been further classified as follows:

Bacterial Agents: Bacteria are very small. Yet despite their size they show a surprising degree of structural complexity. Bacteria vary widely in size and shape, but tend to be at least 10 times larger than viruses, or at least 1 micrometer (1 millionth of a meter) long. They are single-cell organisms that reproduce independently.

Disease causing bacteria (pathogens) have various structures that enhance their ability to cause illness. Movement is the character of many bacteria and is capable of movement in their environment either by flagella or by gliding motility. Growth is a natural process of multiplication by which bacterium grows. Mating is also with in the capability of microbes for exchanging genetic information. Dormancy stage in bacteria provides a resting period. Bacteria will take steps to insure their survival. The examples of some pathogenic bacteria are _E. coli_ 0157:H7, _Salmonella enteritidis,_ _Listeria monocytogenes_ etc.

Fungal Agents: Many fungi cause human diseases, some are controllable some are being investigated upon. They include yeast and mould. Fungi are more chemically and genetically similar to animals than other organisms this makes fungal diseases very difficult to treat. Some of the examples of fungus are *Aspergillus flavus, Candida albicans, Wangiella dermatitidis* etc.

Viral Agents: Viruses are the smallest of all infectious agents, averaging about 100 nanometres (100 billionths of a meter) in length. They have so few genes and proteins of their own that in order to reproduce they need to commandeer the machinery of the cells they invade. The common examples of viral agents causing disease to humans are Hepatitis Virus (HV), Coxsackievirus, and Poxviruses etc.

Protozoan Agents: Protozoans are the unicellular organisms with characteristics like an animal –like organism ranging in size from 0.005 to 5 mm. These minute organisms mostly live in water and their living process accomplishes with their one cell body. The common examples of protozoan inflicting illness to human are *Entamoeba histolytica, Giardia lamblia, Cyclospora cayetanensis* etc.

Parasitic Roundworm: A parasite is a living being or organism that exists by depending on another organism. Parasites that infect humans are much more widespread than many people realize. These diseases affect not only poverty-stricken peoples in remote areas of the world, but they also can be important health problems for rich and poor throughout. The examples are *Enterobius vermicularis, Ascaris lumbricoides, Trichinella spiralis* etc.

Bio-Chemical risks: The release of genetically engineered foods from the confines of the laboratory to farmers in the orchards, barns, and farms is often perceived as presenting new environmental and food risks endangering consumers. The possible transfer of introduced genes to other meat animals where they may take on a role from recessive to dominant negative role as in BSE etc. it could become a nightmare for health agencies all over the world. Health risks from eating food derived from genetically engineered animals, plants, birds, and modified food could be dangerous and catastrophic to human generations. The unforeseen effects of the genetically engineered plants on other species and ecosystems are a cause of concern where investigation and the outcome may take years to conclude. However, risks from normal breeding, natural plantation, and food processing have always existed with a perfect possibility to apply control measures. However, by genetically modifications and its effect on human health are not yet known and any adverse effect could take years of research to find a cure, as is the case with AIDS. That is where the risk is more alarming and in one sense more speculative and prevention is the only remedy unless scientifically approved measures guarantee its safety.

So far most genetically engineered crop plants currently under development involve the transfer of genes conferring resistance to pests, diseases, herbicides, and environmental stress, as well as quality traits such as improved post harvest storage, flavour, nutrition, and colour. The stability of gene performance in terms of where, when and to what magnitude a transferred gene is expressed in the plant can be accurately determined after the gene is transferred.

Potential hazards from genetically engineered food fall into three groups; inserted genes and the biochemical products directly resulting from their expression; secondary effects from the expression of the inserted gene; and genetic changes resulting from the random insertion of genes into the plant chromosomes. The belief they are safe to eat rests on an unfounded assumption -- the assumption that producing new varieties of food-yielding organisms through recombinant DNA technology ("genetic engineering") is inherently no more hazardous than doing so through traditional breeding.

Bioengineers isolate a gene from one type of organism and splice it haphazardly into the DNA of a dissimilar species, disrupting its natural sequence. Because the transplanted gene is foreign to its new surroundings, it cannot adequately function without a big artificial boost. Biotechnicians achieve this unnatural boosting by taking the section of DNA that promotes gene expression in a pathogenic virus and fusing it to the gene prior to insertion. The viral booster (called a "promoter") radically alters the behaviour of the transplanted gene and causes it to function in important respects like an invading virus -- deeply different from the way it behaves within its native organism and from the way the engineered organisms own genes behave. Each of these types of disruption can cause the generation of new substances that have never before been in the species, and these substances can be toxic or otherwise harmful. Such harmful by-products are unpredictable and difficult to detect.

Our bodies expend vital energy and nutrients in protecting itself from foreign substances. Reducing your exposure to certain substances will help your immune system fight other disorders that cause further degeneration. Hydrogenated oils not only contribute to heart problems but also to a higher risk of cancer, diabetes, decrease our immunity and they accelerate tissue decay. The result of hydrogenation is a poisonous molecular distortion of the fatty acids that turn them into harmful TFAs. Research shows that the warped fatty acids raise bad cholesterol and lower good cholesterol levels. The long-term dangers of using these bad oils far outweigh the savings.

Pharmaceuticals are daily health risks, which are toxic and foreign to our bodies that only trade immediate or temporary relief for more suffering. They interfere with our biochemical pathways and metabolism. Some can cover-up and temporarily alleviate the symptoms, but the cause is merely masked as further degeneration is taking place in our bodies. Some can bind minerals, destroy vitamin C, and cause bowel problems.

Pharmaceuticals to lower blood pressure (calcium channel blockers) increase your risk to heart disease. Others can cause confusion, disorientation, inflame the pancreas, liver failure and memory loss. The bad effect of these is never ending as new ones are developed.

There are other dangers when you take prescriptions by mixing them with certain beverages, foods, or vitamins. Repercussions can range from minor to lethal. Options include abstaining from drugs, do not eat, or find out more information. Your doctor or pharmacist should be able to warn you of any possible reaction and what to avoid. The right information can either save your life or take it for the lack of it. You cannot become a victim from the choices of others if you have the right information.

The more powerful painkillers attack the brain and spinal column that shuts down your support functions. The brain loses contact with the rest of itself. The pain and source of the problem still exist but are only being ignored. Prescriptions for pain cause constipation.

The older we are, the more reactions we will experience from them. Drugs will build to higher levels in the elderly because the liver and kidneys are less efficient in eliminating them from the blood. Those over 65 are three times more likely to the adverse effects than those younger.

All synthetics have consequences that can lead to one problem after another. Others are then prescribed to counteract the problem caused by the previous one used. The Downhill Roller Coaster Effect Into The Pit Of Dependency. Meanwhile, the doctors and pharmaceuticals get richer while the sick get sicker and different kinds of food may also become a source of discomfort when certain drugs are taken under prescription.

The raising of livestock for meat, milk, and eggs has been an integral component of the our food production system in Canada. Veterinary drugs are a critical and riskful component of food-animal production. Actual human health risks associated with food-producing animals may involve negative effects of antibiotics, Bovine Growth Hormones (BGH) and Genetically Modified Animal (GMA). Health of food-producing animals is intrinsically linked to human health. That affect food-animal health will, in turn, affect human health. The use of animal drugs, antibiotics in particular, is considered by some to pose an increased health risk to the people who consume the products from those animals. The use of all drugs (in humans as well as animals) creates both benefits and risks. What is required is a proper control limits in administration and control limits in residual contents in final food. With proper controls, the benefits should exceed the risks, and "new" risks will replace the "old" risks at a lower level of threat. Drug residues in animal-derived food products are an important consideration for consumers. Residues of drugs used in the food-animal industry threaten human health by being acutely or cumulatively allergenic, toxic, mutagenic, teratogenic, or carcinogenic. There is inconclusive evidence that antibiotic residues transferred to humans through food might set up a biological milieu that favours the emergence of microbial strains within a host.

The dominant issue in the use of drugs in food animals is the microbial acquisition of resistance to antibiotics. This issue dominates both the drug approval process and the risk—benefit aspect of drug use in food animals, and therefore it is central to our food safety system.

Capitalizing on opportunities and solving problems pertaining to food-animal production systems now and in the future will be best accomplished through an integrated process that continuously assesses the strengths and weaknesses of the total system, rather than the various components separately, and uses the expertise of all stakeholders. This will be successful only if the various stakeholders define the best long-term solutions instead of short-term wins and losses and have access to information that is relevant, comprehensive, and accurate.

Radiological Risks: The principal hazard is the release from safe containment of materials emitting ionizing radiation and contaminating crops, meat animals, milk animals, and their feed. The amount, type, and form of the material would depend on its source and the nature of the incident. Radioactive material released in an incident is likely to be carried by the wind, behaving like a plume of smoke, dispersing into the air and depositing activity on the ground. This will expose and contaminate virtually all-living cell, humans and food of humans are the main concern in this context. People and their source of food may thus incur: exposure to direct radiation from a radioactive plume or from radio nuclides deposited on the crops, animals, buildings etc., exposure to radiation from radio nuclides contaminating the body surface, clothing or possessions cannot be ruled out, internal exposure to radiation following inhalation or ingestion of radioactive substances as a result of direct atmospheric or environmental contamination or, subsequently, by radioactive material in water or food. Where the casualty's condition permits, the infected person should be taken to a hospital designated to receive contaminated casualties.

Irradiation of food destroys some of the essential nutrients, and may alter the taste and appearance of some products. No studies have been done to show what the long term effect of food irradiation will be, which makes one wonder how this was approved without this data. However, iridologists of the pro-irradiation lobby always argue that Irradiation is a physical treatment of food with high-energy, ionizing radiation. It can be used to prolong the shelf life of food products and/or to reduce health hazards associated with certain products due to the presence of pathogenic microorganisms. Extensive research has shown that macronutrients, such as protein, carbohydrates, and fat, are relatively stable to radiation doses of up to 10 kilogray.

Everything in our environment, including food, contains trace amounts of radioactivity. This means that this trace amount (about 150 to 200 Becquerel) of natural radioactivity (from elements such as potassium) is unavoidably in our daily diets. The food itself never comes into direct contact with the radiation source during the irradiation process. Some of the changes produce "radiolytic" products. The concern is from the changes it makes in food composition and its long-term affect on our health.

On November 23, 2002, Health Canada posted proposed new regulations to extend the use of food irradiation in Canada to include ground beef, poultry, shrimp and prawns, and mangoes. The proposed new regulations are amendments to the Food and Drug Regulations (1094 - Food Irradiation), under the Food and Drugs Act. Food irradiation is a method of food preservation in which foods are exposed to gamma radiation from Cobalt 60, Caesium 137, or an electron accelerator. The gamma radiation can sterilize or kill insects, and kill fungi and some bacteria that live in foods. Smaller doses can prevent sprouting of potatoes and onions, and delay the ripening of certain fruits. Irradiation can increase the storage life of some foods, allowing importers and distributors to ship foods further and store them longer. These foods do not become radioactive, but contrary to the conclusions of Health Canada, we believe that there are serious risks and drawbacks to the use of this technology.

The Sierra Club of Canada in cooperation with other organizations has been in the campaign to scrutiny the irradiation of food and they provide information to support their claim-48.

- Chemical by-products called "unique radiolytic products" (URPs) are created in foods by irradiation. Some scientific studies carried out on URPs link serious health risks with the consumption of irradiated foods.

- Irradiated foods are less nutritious than fresh foods because radiation damages some vitamins, amino acids, and fatty acids. Normal cooking methods and storage of foods will also cause nutritional losses, but irradiation plus cooking and storage decreases the nutritional value even more. Many vitamins are obtained from fresh fruits and vegetables.

- Irradiation has been hailed as an alternative to pesticides. However, at best irradiation might replace some post-harvest uses since pesticides will still be used in the field. Studies have not been done to determine the consequences of irradiating the pesticide residues commonly found in foods.

- Irradiation will not replace many additives commonly used in processed foods. In fact, some additives need to be used in combination with irradiation to control undesirable side effects.

- Irradiation of poultry is under consideration as a means for preventing salmonella food poisoning. In fact, less than 20% of salmonella poisoning cases can be traced back to poultry. A more effective solution is education about proper storage, handling and cooking of all foods in domestic and commercial sectors, which will be effective, safe, educational, and better than irradiation.

- Irradiation can actually cause food poisoning since treated foods may be contaminated but appear fresh. Microorganisms, which normally cause meat to look or smell spoiled, may be killed by irradiation, yet hardier bacteria, such as the one causing botulism food poisoning, may survive. Some organisms may even mutate when irradiated, forming new, more radiation-resistant strains.

- o Aflatoxins are toxic and carcinogenic (cancer-causing) substance produced by microorganism, which inhabits damp grains, beans and nuts. Aflatoxin poisoning is a major cause of death in Asia and Africa. Irradiation of this microorganism actually causes it to produce more Aflatoxin. Building dry storage facilities is a more practical way to control this organism.

- o Increased use of food irradiation will increase occupational and environmental hazards. The level of gamma radiation inside an operating irradiation facility is anywhere from ten to hundreds of times the level that would kill a human in a single short exposure. The gamma source for irradiation must be replaced regularly, so the risk of transportation accidents increases with time. Spent gamma sources also become radioactive waste, and there is still no acceptable method of long-term radioactive waste management-48.

Physical Risks: The physical contaminants are common in farm products. Before forwarding the products for marketing, the physical contaminants are removed. In food processing factories, all ingredients are assured contaminants free from the supplier though few companies still screen the incoming ingredients as part of preventive measure.

Physical hazards in finished products can arise from several sources, such as contaminated raw materials, poorly designed or maintained facilities and equipment, faulty procedures during processing, poor building and roofing, and improper employee training and practices. For example, glass can arise from bottles, jars, light fixtures, utensils, gauge covers; metal can arise from nuts, bolts, screws, steel wool, wire; plastics can arise from improper disposal of packaging materials; paint chips can arise from poorly designed or poorly maintained facilities and equipment; and extraneous objects such as pens, pencils, buttons can arise from careless employee practices. Some other examples of physical contaminants are Human hairs, foreign bodies, machine grease, stone, wood piece and jewellery etc. Real danger of physical contaminants is during the processing and packing of food in a manufacturing plant. GMPs are the best solution.

In farm-produced products, Physical hazards include a variety of materials referred to as extraneous materials or foreign particles or objects. A physical hazard can be defined as any physical material not normally found in a farm food that can cause illness or injury to a person consuming the product. Physical hazards such as glass or metal can be introduced during harvesting, sorting, and transportation of processing vegetables. Prerequisite programs provide the basic environmental and operating conditions that are necessary for the production of safe, wholesome food. All HACCP prerequisite programs should be documented and regularly audited. A well-written prerequisite program clearly communicates what is expected to be performed and at what frequency and who has responsibility.

Terrorist Risks: The World Health Organization (WHO) has warned that terrorist groups could try to contaminate food supplies and has urged countries to strengthen their surveillance. In a special report, the leading UN health agency, said an attack using chemical or biological agents in food could lead to people dying or contracting serious illnesses like cancer. Such a threat may not attract much attention in food manufacturing factories but vigilance for such a threat remains a critical point. Miscreants among employed people may also lead to such a risk.

Allergen Risks: Food allergy refers to the adverse reaction to food for some consumers. Such reactions bring nausea, vomiting, stomach disorders, headache and body fatigue. It is estimated that in Canada two percent of adults and up to eight percent of children experience true food allergies caused by certain protein allergens. Symptoms of food allergies appear throughout the body. The most common sites are the mouth (swelling of the lips), digestive tract (stomach cramps, vomiting, diarrhoea), skin (hives, rashes or eczema), and the airways (wheezing or breathing problems). There is no cure for food allergies; the only course is strict avoidance of an offending food.

In North America, the United States Food and Drug Administration has identified eight foods or food ingredients that are responsible for 90 percent of the food allergic reactions. Those foods are milk and milk products, eggs, legumes like peanuts and soy, tree nuts, wheat, crustaceans, fish, and molluscs. Thus it necessitates that food manufacturers evaluate for allergen hazards (a chemical hazard) and it should be a part of HACCP plan. It is important for the food manufacturers to label the products with allergens and continually enforce ongoing monitoring system to verify that all control points are being consistently met and allergen free. The risk factors become more exposed when allergen ingredients form the formulation of products being manufactured in the same plant with non-allergen ingredients food products.

Food Safety Objectives (FSO):
FSO is the next step after risk assessment and food safety management. A statement of the maximum level of a microbiological hazard in a food considered acceptable for

consumer protection is one way of expressing the objective. Though complete elimination is an ideal situation but far lower than the acceptable maximum limit is a much safer criteria. The FSO is a risk management tool linking risk assessment and effective measures to control identified risks. The FSO should be achieved through the application of general principles of food hygiene and HACCP program. The FSO requires a performance criterion defined as the mandatory outcome of an action that assures that the FSO is met. The process criterion is subsequently established by defining the control parameters of actions that can be applied to achieve the performance criterion. It is imperative that adequate GMP's are in place and that a HACCP program be developed by industry to assure that the FSO has been achieved with the use of performance and process criteria. Finally, experts with experience in the food industry can establish microbiological criteria where appropriate.

The concept of FSO has been under discussion within a number of countries domestically, and it is being discussed internationally as well--particularly within Codex. The Codex Committee on General Principles considered the FSO concept when it met in April-2000 and decided that its application was of a technical nature, and it was premature to generalize the concept with a specific definition. Further, the Committee agreed that the FSO concept could be further developed by other relevant Codex Committees in order to identify how it could be applied to specific food safety issues. Such activity, in fact, is already underway by the Codex Committee on Food Hygiene, which at its last meeting in October discussed the FSO concept in relation to proposed draft principles and guidelines for making microbial risk management decisions.

Over the next few years FSO concept is going to be an important discussion internationally. Countries do have latitude to set their own level of protection for their countries. The FSO concept should provide greater clarity to industry in understanding the tolerable level of a hazard that it is expected to meet. Health Canada recognizes that a safe and nutritious food supply is a major contributory factor to the health of Canadians and that there is a need to maintain reputation nationally and internationally as a supplier of safe food products.

Risk communication:

Risk communication involves the communication of a policy decision. Risk communication, the science of understanding scientific and technological risk and how it is communicated within a socio-political structure, is a relatively new scientific endeavour, dating back to Starr's 1969 paper-197, which attempted to offer a scientific basis for thresholds of risk, which would be accepted by the public. As public concerns regarding nuclear power gained prominence in the 1970s, investigators tried to establish general principles of public risk acceptability, usually based on mortality statistics and to minimise risk principle, which argued that if a risk can be effectively lowered to less than one additional fatality per million citizens, the risk is effectively zero (U.S. National Research Council. 1989)-209. Such an approach was uniformly unsuccessful.

In the 1980s, several groups developed models that incorporated the value systems of individuals, peer groups and societies into risk communication theory resulting in broad agreement that risks are viewed according to their perceived threat to familiar social relationships and practices, and not simply by numbers alone. The psychometric paradigm (Slovic, 1987)-192 described risk from a psychological perspective, drawing on various characteristics or dimensions, which may be important in influencing risk perceptions.

Douglas and Wildavsky (1982) first described the cultural theory of risk in which individuals can be allocated into cultural groups based on shared values and beliefs. Whereas the psychometric paradigm holds that risk itself is deterministic in generating perceptions, the cultural theory holds that the characteristics of the perceiver—rather than the risk itself—are central to an understanding of risk perception. Kasperson et al. (1988) developed the social amplification of risk theory, which suggested a way to integrate the aforementioned frameworks into a comprehensive accounting of the social, cultural and individual characteristics, which tend to magnify or amplify one risk over another.

According to a U.S. National Research Council committee on risk perception and communication (1989)-209, risk communication is now defined as, "An interactive process of exchange of information and opinion among individuals, groups and institutions. It involves multiple messages about the nature of risk and other messages, not strictly about risk, that express concerns, opinions, or reactions to risk messages or to legal and institutional arrangements for risk management." In essence, risk communication must be treated as a reciprocal process—not simply those with a vested interest in a message developing more effective techniques to sell their side of the story.

A body of knowledge has been created over the past decade, which can assist in the understanding of public perceptions of microbial food safety risk, how the media translates this information, and how government, industry and other organizations can better relate risk information over a wide range of disciplines. This approach to communicating technological risk has been successfully applied in a number of sectors, especially in the chemical industry-123.

The growth of interest in risk communication is driven by four motivations:

❏ **A** requirement for—or desire by—government to inform in the participatory democracies of Western politics, from informal consultation to legislated accountability (such as the U.S. Administrative Procedures Act of 1946 and the Community Right to Know provisions of Title III of the Superfund Amendments and Reauthorization Act of 1986);

❏ **D**esires to overcome opposition to decisions;

❏ **A** desire to share power between government and public groups;

❏ **A** desire to develop effective alternatives to direct regulatory control (U.S. National Research Council, 1989).

Underlying these motivations is a general recognition that decision-making in democratic societies is becoming more public and is increasingly driven by non-experts. Thus, the need for a paradigm or system such as the risk communication frame work which acknowledges this transition.

Sandman (1987)-188 notes that the public generally pays too little attention to the hazardous nature of risks, and experts usually completely ignore those factors, which fuel consumer unrest or outrage. These are two very different starting points and not surprisingly, experts and consumers often rank the relative importance of various risks very differently (Sandman, 1987; -188 Slovic, 1987-192). Scientists, in general, define risks in the language and procedures of science itself. They consider the nature of the harm that may occur, the probability that it will occur, and the number of people who may be affected. Most citizens, in contrast, seem less aware of the quantitative or probabilistic nature of a risk, and much more concerned with broader, qualitative attributes, such as whether the risk is voluntarily assumed, whether the risks and benefits are fairly distributed, whether the risk can be controlled by the individual, whether a risk is necessary and unavoidable or whether there are safer alternatives, whether the risk is familiar or exotic, whether the risk is natural or technological in origin, and so forth-188.

Problems in communicating about risks originate primarily in the marked differences that exist between the two languages used to describe risk: the scientific and statistical language of experts, and the intuitively grounded language of the public (Fig: 04 (2).

The expert assessment of risk is essential to the making of informed choices in everyday life: To ignore the results of scientific risk assessments; ever changing as they are, it is merely substitute of an informal deliberative process for a formal one (Powell and Leiss, 1997)-163. At the same time, citizens in a democratic society cannot allow experts to dictate lessons in risk management to them; on the contrary, their informed consent must form the basis for the collective allocation of resources for risk control and risk reduction. In general, therefore, society must manage the tension between these two profoundly different ways of representing risk, rather than try to eliminate the difference itself.

Therefore, both languages for describing risk are necessary, because the daily business about managing risks – both the personal business of individuals and the social allocation of risk reduction resources — cannot be conducted in either language alone.

At the same time, the strong differences between the two languages constitute barriers to dialogue and co-operative understanding. Good risk communication practice seeks to break down those barriers and facilitate the productive exchanges between the two spheres Information skills and participatory opportunities.

Powell and Leiss (1998) have located the work of risk communication in the gap that separates the evolving scientific description of risks and the public understanding of those same risks [Fig: 04 (3)]. Further, they suggest that the competing "expert" and "public" understandings of the same risks are equally legitimate and necessary.

In many cases regarding publicly debated risks, the gap cannot be closed appreciably because the scientific and public apprehensions of a risk are framed by fundamentally different assumptions or values.

However, in all risk situations where some public policy response is called for – to ban a substance, to control emissions, to warn consumers about food safety hazards — what occurs in that gap can have significant consequences for institutions and the public alike. One of the most serious manifestations of these "gap dynamics" is the emergence of a risk information vacuum.

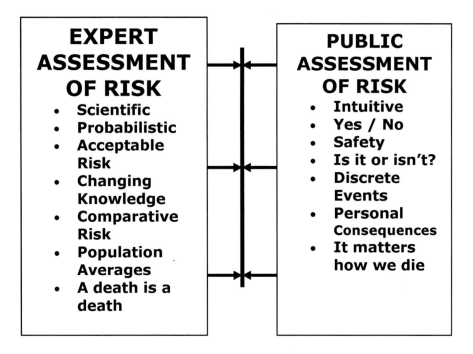

Fig: 04(2) - <u>Some characteristics of the two languages of Risk communication (Powell and Leiss, 1998)</u>-51C

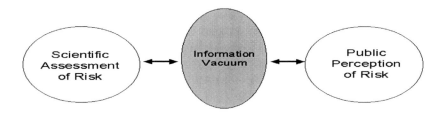

Fig: 04(3) - <u>The risk communication vacuum (Powell and Leiss, 1997)</u> -51C

The risk information vacuum arises where, over a long period of time, those who are conducting scientific research and assessments for high-profile risks make no special effort to communicate the results, regularly and effectively, to the public. Instead, partial scientific information dribbles out here and there and interpreted in apparently conflicting ways, all of which are mixed with people's fear. The failure to implement good risk communication practices gives rise to a risk information vacuum.

Society as well as nature abhors a vacuum; it is therefore filled from other sources. For example, events reported in the media; some of which are alarming, become the substantial basis of the public framing of these risks, or an interest group takes up the challenge and fills the vacuum with its own information and perspectives, or the intuitively-based fears and concerns of individuals simply grow and spread until they become a substantial consensus in the arena of public opinion, or the vacuum is filled by the soothing expressions beloved of politicians. Confused, complex messages about scientific risk, technical uncertainty, and prevailing climate of mistrust are just some of the factors that make effective risk communication difficult not impossible, but difficult. Covello et al (1988)-261 have summarized the seven cardinal rules of risk communication, as follows:

- **A**ccept and involve the public as a legitimate partner
- **P**lan carefully and evaluate performance
- **L**isten to your audience
- **B**e honest, frank and open
- **C**o-ordinate and collaborate with other credible sources
- **M**eet the needs of the media
- **S**peak clearly and with compassion

Scientists and journalists both use explanatory devices to convey the meaning of their work. Science is about models, explanation, and representation, while journalists often resort to metaphors. According to Layoff and Johnson (1980)-138, a metaphor is not just a rhetorical flourish, but also a basic property of language used to define experience and to evoke shared meanings-138. Nelkin (1987)-155 argues that the use of metaphors in science writing is particularly important in the explanation of technical detail, to define experience, to evoke shared meanings and to allow individuals to construct elaborate concepts about public issues and events.

Public communication about issues of technological risk often involves messages from diverse individuals or communities that are translated and synthesized by media outlets and other members of the public. At each step, message providers, journalists and audience members are framing a specific event using their own value systems, constraints and the filters of experience and expectation in a way that makes the most sense to a particular individual. Different people use different sources to collect information related to issues of scientific and technological risk. It is therefore incumbent on the provider of risk messages to determine how a specific target audience receives and perceives risk information.

Managing Agri - Food Related Risks:

There is a growing realization that there will be no quick fix to the inherent difficulties in communicating about food safety risks. Fischhoff and Downs, (1997) note that the food industry, like many others, has a risk communication problem, manifested in the public's desire to know the truth about outbreaks of food borne diseases; ongoing concern about the safety of foods, additives, and food-processing procedures; and continued apathy regarding aspects of routine food hygiene. Because citizens are ill equipped to discriminate among information sources, the food industry as a whole bears responsibility for the successes and failures of its individual members[74].

Powell and Leiss (1997) stress the need for a long-term institutional commitment to the gradual development and application of good risk communication practices, using the following guidelines[163].

Risk Communication Cost: Risk communication has typically been an area of vulnerability. Risk threats can be dramatic, with catastrophic implications, irritating, or disruptive. All these add to the cost for a timely management to avoid severe health implications.

In Canada, few observers complained that Canadian public health authorities have not communicated fairly the risks associated with infection from West Nile Virus. The resulting failures by citizens to understand the magnitude of the risk may contribute to excess cases of severe illness, death, and multidimensional increase in cost.

Similarly, the discovery in May 2003 that a northern Alberta cow had Mad Cow disease was bad for beef producers and consumers in North America. Canada faced a potential economic blow from its first case of mad cow disease in a decade. However, Canada is traditionally known for producing meat that is high quality and safe for human health, it is important that consumers remember mad cow disease, properly known as Bovine Spongiform Encephalopathy, or BSE, is not contagious. It is not spread animal to animal with contact between them. The one thing we know about BSE is that it's spread when animals eat contaminated feed. The human form of mad cow disease, known as variant Creutzfeldt-Jakob disease, is believed to be transmitted through eating infected meat. More than 100 people, mostly in Britain, have died from the human form of BSE, known as variant Creutzfeldt-Jakob disease, believed to be caused by eating infected meat. However, the United States, Japan, South Korea, Taiwan, and Mexico had all closed their borders to Canadian beef and cattle in the event of the BSE threat, forcing Alberta's C$4 billion (US$3 billion) industry to a halt. The only previous case of BSE in North America was in 1993, involving a bull imported from Britain.

The financial cost of the BSE crisis in the U.K. is currently pegged at more than $5 billion, a cost, which could have been substantially, reduced with more effective risk management and communication practices. However, It is estimated that BSE cost in the UK beef industry had a range of about US $6.4 billion between March 1996 and March 2001. Outbreaks of food borne illness routinely cost food industry millions of US dollars.

The on time risk communication to public and those concerned with food safety would save millions of dollars of tax payers' money in advance of a possible catastrophic damage. This will not only prevent the damage but it would develop awareness and confidence on public health authorities. Though critics point out timely awareness and attract the attention of Canadian public health authorities over risk communication, Canadian public health authorities have been pro-active in risk communication and have made Canada the safest place to consume food. Two essential components to risk communication are trust and perception Building trust is the pivotal focus of risk communication, which is problematic for government and government agencies as the public tends to see government as a less-than-trusted source of information. Canadian food supply chains are safest in the world. Thanks to a better risk communication system.

Food Regulators Responsibility: Risk communication has also been defined as an interactive process of an exchange of information, involving multiple messages about the nature of risk. Informing the public is a very important type of risk communication. Governments ministries, and in particular those agencies of governments which have regulatory authority over a broad range of health and environmental risks, who are capable of acquiring through enabling legislation the legal authority to manage risks are responsible. Evolution of risk communication from one-way to two-way communication is critical in cases where scientific uncertainty is a predominant characteristic. If public confidence is to be maintained, coherent communication from both risk assessors and regulators is of fundamental importance, particularly in an emergency.

In Canada, CFIA is the agency responsible for enforcing food safety regulations. The complexity of today's food chain means that responsibility for food safety must be shared, which the CFIA does through partners in provincial/territorial governments, other federal departments, food producers, industry, distributors, retailers, and ultimately every consumer of food in Canada.

Risk communication goals should reflect a two-way exchange of information leading to a common approach to discussion of issues and a common influence on risk decisions. If the public perceives it is being manipulated, loss of trust and even public outrage will be the outcome. In food safety issues, risk communication should be totally based on facts so the real perception remains trustworthy and practical. Successful risk communication is not about giving out information or about making stakeholders understand. Today, successful risk communication can result only when the quality of debate among government, the public, and all stakeholders is improved for a better understanding of the threat and preventative measures taken.

Risk communication, the science of understanding scientific and technological risk and how it is communicated within a socio-political structure, is a relatively new scientific endeavour. A successful model for risk communication must reconcile the views of scientists, the public, and politicians in order to achieve a common understanding of complex risks leading to credible management options and credible policy development around risk. The interface between science (or technology), politics and horizontal government priorities and the public, including socio-economic dimensions, is critical. As many as one person in three in industrialized countries may be affected by food borne illness each year and the situation in most other countries is probably even worse.

Food Safety Agency in United Kingdom does lots of work to help ensure the safety of the food consumers eat, from the drive to bring down food borne illness, to the regulation of pesticides and research into GM food. The agencies risk communication is a prime source of information to consumers.

In the United States, food safety regulations are not only confined to FSIS but at least a dozen federal agencies implementing more than 35 regulatory statutes make up the federal part of the food safety system. Three agencies play major roles in carrying out food safety regulatory activities: Food and Drug Administration (FDA) within the Department of Health and Human Services (HHS), the Food Safety Inspection Service (FSIS) within the U. S. Department of Agriculture (USDA) and the U. S. Environmental Protection Agency (EPA).

U.S. Environmental Protection Agency (EPA), and the Food and Drug Administration (FDA) together evaluate food supplies to determine if they are safe and free of toxins and allergens. Similarly, the primary mission of the U.S. Food and Drug Administration's Center for Food Safety and Applied Nutrition (FDA CFSAN) is to safeguard public health by ensuring the safety of food products in the United States. In the United States, communication is considered a key element to successfully conduct a risk assessment within a risk analysis framework. A body of knowledge has been created over the past decade, which can assist in the understanding of public perceptions of microbial food safety risk, how the media translates this information, and how government, industry and other organizations can better relate risk information over a wide range of disciplines. The need for exchange of information and opinions also extends beyond the risk assessment and risk management teams to stakeholders including consumers, industry, and other interested parties. The Food and Drug Administration (FDA)/Division of Human Resource Development (DHRD)/State Training Team (STT) has developed a satellite broadcast course on communication skills for regulators. The outbreak of Bovine Spongiform Encephalopathy (BSE, or mad cow disease) in the U.K. and the well-publicized 1993 outbreak of _E. coli_ O157:H7, known as the Jack-in-the-Box outbreak, have dramatically changed the public discussion of food safety and risk communication in North America.

States are also enthusiastically involved in activities designed to provide consumers with the appropriate information about identifying and managing risks in their purchasing, transporting, handling, preparing and serving food to their families and friends. State regulators are willing and able to assist with the content of consumer communications, but are looking to access the capacity and expertise of others in packaging and distributing behaviour-altering information to consumers.

In conclusion, the bottom line for states is summarized in the adage "think globally but act locally". State and local food safety agencies need to have the conceptual knowledge about risk assessment, management and communication for the primary purpose of converting that knowledge to concrete, risk-lowering food safety improvements in their states, cities, counties and towns.

In order to decrease the risk of future acute food safety problems, food control authorities should assign resources to the detection of emerging risks. The follow-up and reporting of food borne disease outbreaks should be improved and intensified in order to provide a better base for risk-based food control priorities and remedial measures. The results of food inspections and other food control activities should be made public. Improve contacts at the local, national, and international levels between those responsible for food safety and those responsible for environmental protection and pollution control.

Industries Responsibility: It is now generally accepted that industry must take primary risk communication responsibility for product-related risks and workplace hazards, as well as for community awareness in the vicinity of facilities where hazardous materials and processes are employed. Primary responsibility for food safety lies with those who produce process and trade in food - farmers, fishermen, slaughterhouse operators, food processors, wholesale and retail traders, caterers, etc. It is their duty to ensure that the food they produce and handle is safe and satisfies the relevant requirements of food law and they should verify that such requirements are met. However, with the rationalization of government services, industry is assuming more responsibility for the delivery of food inspection services (under government auditing) and therefore is assuming more of the risk communication responsibility.

The food industries in Canada are very ethical in communicating risk to its consumers through labelling, processing technology, packaging technology, trained staff, and a laid quality policy. In case of any quality failures, monitoring of food products immediately isolates the suspected product and banned for human consumption. At the same time, industry communicates immediately with CFIA to trace back all supplies to the market and risk communicated to the consumers through media for prevention and control. The basic aim is prevention and failure to communicate in time through proper channel may lead to health risk to public and subsequent punitive actions.

The main task of the supervisory authorities is to lay down food safety standards and to ensure that the internal control systems are well communicated and operated by food producers, processors and traders are appropriate and operated in such a way that these standards are met.

Consumers Responsibility: Public attitudes about risk are an important aspect of risk management-182 and communication. Timeliness is everything in effective risk communication: overcoming entrenched perceptions that are broadly dispersed in the social environment is a thankless task with almost no chance of succeeding. Further, doing good risk communication early is of little benefit if it not also done often, as often and as long as is needed to prevent a risk issue from being put into play by other interested parties. Consumers are responsible for food hygiene in the home and for ensuring that food storage and preparation recommendations are followed.

Public perceptions, values, and opinion all enter into characterizations of risk. The public tends to assess risk based on specific context, and where food is concerned, risk is not well tolerated because the public is more dependent on food than on any other commodity. In the absence of media coverage, for example, or public messages about food risk, the public tends to be lethargic about risk on a day-to-day basis.

The potential for stigmatization of food manufactured in factories or produced by genetically alteration are enormous. Well-publicized outbreaks of food borne pathogens and the furor over Agricultural biotechnology are but two current examples of the interactions between science, policy and public perception. One goal of risk communication on food safety issues is communication between risk assessors and risk managers and the average citizen. The public or segments actively concerned about food safety and seeking to influence the risk-management process, need to communicate their own scientific interpretations, as well as their criteria for decisions and their priorities, to decision makers. Protect them, they feel responsible for their own safety, and therefore are less likely to demand that government protect them. If indeed these risk perceptions explain the public's "concern" with assorted food safety problems, the public's priorities are actually rather sensible and less likely to misallocate resources than one may have perceived them to be.

The differing perceptions of risks on the part of experts and average consumers are just one reason why the two groups have often found it hard to communicate effectively about food-related risks. Risk communication is a matter of process for consumers but it depends on one's own urgency. They often feel no need to be "educated" on that score, but approach communication with the goal of ensuring that decision-makers pay adequate attention to their concerns about a risk—often such things as whether the benefits justify accepting the risks, or whether there is adequate information for consumers to make choices in the marketplace and to manage their own risks in the case in question. Consumer activists' goal in risk communication is typically to have these concerns taken seriously.

Consumers often have reasons to distrust the institutions that make food safety decisions. When the way the problem is defined and the ways in which agendas for debate are structured effectively exclude perspectives that are central concerns of consumers, members of the public understandably don't believe the institutions have their interests foremost in mind. Food safety decision-making processes that lack openness to public participation, and the lack of transparency about the basis for decisions, are additional reasons why consumers mistrust the food-safety risk-management process, and those who take part in it. In assembling scientific risk assessments, more explicit attention should be paid to identifying uncertainties, and their significance. So what are the consumer's responsibilities towards effective risk communication and food safety?

Consumers need to pay more attention to defining the value judgments that are enmeshed in their views on food safety questions; they are often at least as inarticulate in this respect as experts are. Consumers should give much thought to food safety and not to wait until a food-related illness prompts concern. The Food Safety Initiative by consumer is extremely important in reducing food-borne illness in the household as well as in a corporate status. Consumers must impart knowledge about the food they consume by reading the text on products, observing label, organoleptic perception, seminars, media coverage, audio-visual documentaries etc. For immediate consumption, a food sampling is the one way to make sure food is safe but there is no guarantee unless its back check of storage and processing are known. Consumer's knowledge about the nature of food, it's cooking, its storage requirements, knowledge about the impact of food-borne infections can be beneficial risk communication.

Consumers should take a view of their food and taking advantage of the healthful benefits of fruits and vegetables Studies by the U.S. Department of Health and Human Services, U.S. Department of Agriculture, and the National Academy of Sciences suggest that the nutritional goodness of fruits and vegetables, with a diet that is low in fat, saturated fat and cholesterol and that contains plenty of whole-grain breads and cereals, may decrease the risk of heart disease and cancer. Fruits' and vegetables' potential to help improve the health of Americans led National Cancer Institute (NCI) to begin a multi-year public education campaign in 1992. Its goal is to increase consumers' awareness of the importance of fruits and vegetables and to give consumers ideas on how they can increase their intake. This is the way of communication to consumers.

Science & Policy: Almost any type of risk issue can turn into a seemingly intractable risk controversy, and it is the nature of such controversies inevitably to give rise to demands on governments to "do something" about controlling or eliminating the risks in question. In other words, although the scientific description of the hazards and probabilistic risk assessments can be matters of widespread public interest, in the final analysis the competing choices among risk management options—banning or restricting a substance, say—make up the contents of letters and calls to politicians. This means that the contents of effective risk communication cannot be limited to the scientific description of hazards or the risk numbers. Rather, the science should be put into a policy (action) context, which in the early stages of an emerging risk controversy might take the form of forecasting a range of policy options—including the "do nothing" option—and of exploring their consequences in terms of implications for economic and social interests, international developments, and obligations for environmental protection (all in the context of the risk management cycle, mentioned earlier). Responsible agencies and industries ought to begin discussing the possible policy responses to emerging risk controversies as soon as they arise, and continue to do so throughout their life history.

Educating the Public:

Sanctimonious urgings for new programs designed to increase the public's awareness in the inner mysteries of scientific research are encountered. What appears to sustain this mission is the curious belief that the citizenry's ignorance of scientific method can best explain the observed differences between the expert assessment of risk and the public perception of the same. Technology promoters in discussions of technological risk for the past 200 years have advocated this rhetorical strategy. More recently, promoters of Agricultural chemicals in the 1960s and nuclear energy in the 1970s have embraced the public education model. Today, the notion of public education is the basis of dozens of communications strategies forwarded by government, industry, and scientific societies, in the absence of any data suggesting that such educational efforts are successful.

What is known is that levels of perceived trust in technology promoters and regulators are a better predictor of consumer support. Several surveys in North America and the U.K. have found that perceptions of trust in government regulation (and industry), regarding either pesticides (Dittus and Hillers, 1993) or the products of Agricultural biotechnology are the strongest predictor for consumer support. People either trust that pesticides and the products of Agricultural biotechnology are adequately regulated or they do not. Those with low trust have the highest concern about possible risks. Those with high trust perceive greater benefits from both products. Van Ravenswaay (1995) concluded that trust in government and industry may be a more important influence on risk perception than the inherent safety or the danger of a particular agrochemical. There is no reason to believe that the same would not hold true for microbial food safety risks.

If trust is a better predictor of consumer support, then what factors influence perceptions of trust? Lynn Frewer and colleagues at the U.K. Ministry of Agriculture, Fisheries, and Food's Institute of Food Research in Reading have conducted the most comprehensive work toward understanding food-related risk perception. Frewer et al. (1996) conducted two sets of in-depth interviews with about 45 people each, and then a larger quantitative survey to better understand the formation of trust. Overall, there were many findings of relevance to effectively communicating about food-related risks, including:

- The most important and frequently cited source of information about food-related information was the media, far ahead of any other source.

- While scientists and medical sources were rated as trusted but not distrusted (media were often trusted and distrusted), they were infrequently named as sources of food-related information.

- The single most important determinant of gain or loss of trust in a source is whether the information is subsequently proven right or wrong, and that the source is subsequently demonstrated to be unbiased.

- Information about natural toxins, genetic engineering, and pesticide residues was more distrusted than information about high fat diets, microwave ovens, etc.

- Medical sources are likely to be viewed as expert in medically related areas, but to have little knowledge in technological risk assessment and therefore poor sources of information about technological hazards.

- Trust is clearly multidimensional and cannot be predicted by single items or psychological constructs (i.e. surveys, which ask respondents to rank social actors -- doctors, farmers, environmentalists, government -- in terms of levels of trustworthiness, are somewhat meaningless in the absence of context).

- Trust appears linked with perceptions of accuracy, knowledge, and concern with public welfare.

- If government sources and risk regulators are seen to be proactive in their interactions with the media and other trusted sources -- including discussions of risks -- this may positively influence the way in which risk information is reported, as well as increasing trust in government regulation.

- **A**dmitting to uncertainty or facilitating public understanding of science as a "process" could increase communicator's trustworthiness.

- **P**eople seem to be adverse to ambiguous risks and trust is all the more likely to be important where there is a perception that accurate estimates of risk are not available, like genetically-engineered foods.

If trust is the key component in public perception of risk scenarios, what other guidance exists to build trust and credibility? Hance, et al. (1988)-112 offers the following:

- Be aware of the factors that inspire trust;
- Pay attention to process;
- Explain agency process;
- Be forthcoming with information and involve the public from the outset;
- Focus on building trust as well as generating good data;
- Follow up;
- Only make promises you can keep;
- Provide information that meets people's needs;
- Get the facts straight;
- Try to co-ordinate with other agencies
- Make sure to co-ordinate within your agency;
- Don't give mixed messages;
- Listen to what various groups are telling you;
- Enlist the help of organizations that have credibility with communities; and,
- Avoid secret meetings.

Eliminate "No risk" Slogans: Ironically, although citizens and environmentalists are often taken to task by government and industry officials for advocating "zero risk" scenarios, pronouncements of the "there is no risk" variety are a favourite of government ministers and sometimes of industry voices as well. In fact, at least some business sectors—the chemical industry in particular—do this less and less, which is a sea-change from what used to be their standard public relations practice.

W. Edwards Deming's best-known contribution was his 14 points for the transformation of western management. He advocated elimination of slogans, exhortations, and targets for the workforce. He also pointed out the importance of breaking down barriers between staff areas. These two points of the fourteen are keys to a proper communication in any given manufacturing situation.

Contest of Opinion: There is a curious reluctance, especially on the part of government risk managers, to avoid addressing directly the alternative representations of risk issues as they form and re-form in dialogue among interested parties in society. Quite simply, if government regulators and industry have the primary responsibility for effective risk communication, these officials cannot avoid confronting the issues as they are posed in the society. In every food safety question, there are experts with very different viewpoints about the actual risk to human health. Yet some food-related risks create greater public concern than others.

Critics of any subject are most likely energized by emotions rather than facts. The public food safety concern believes there is a serious risk; expect that initially the strength of their feelings will make them deaf to any discussion of figures from food business. Contest of opinion is best seen in the Internet. The Internet offers a very promising, though demographically still incomplete, new path for risk communication. There is often an attempt to recruit credentialed scientists at odds with the majority opinion in the relevant field of assessment science. This plays to the recommendation that "information must come from various, credible sources". The information coming from risk activists is consistent and repeated in many different media, which is an outlet to get information into the hands of those actively looking for it. Risk activists; have often used the Internet to amplify or to attenuate risks in public perceptions with an eye to generating public pressure on risk management policy makers. Food safety activists have been the most successful users of the Internet's advantages in the entire hazards community. It is wise for Government agencies to seek understanding of public perception then strive to be understood. A common understanding is the best way to minimise contest of opinion and it is best for the risk communication.

Every argument is a performance of communicative reasoning. Public is an audience that claps or boos the activities of the policy makers and then every two or four years decides whether they want to pay to see it again. Public is the subject and the subject acts by answering a survey or acts by voting, and that political science is about trying to predict their actions either in the future or predict it backwards by explaining why they gave the answer on the survey that they gave and why they gave the vote that they did. When public opinion really supports the policy then that policy is relatively cheap for the policy makers to pursue, but when the public opinion is strongly opposed to that policy then that policy's expensive. Public opinion then influences policy making by affecting the price or the cost that the policy maker receives for a course of action. Policy makers do anticipate "perceptions" of particular actions. Anticipating media reaction does have consequences for policy. Contest of opinion on food safety issues will continue to be debated and the issues like genetically modified food products, use of bovine growth hormones and unsystematic use of chemicals in Agriculture will draw more attention in future as importance of organic food is recognised and realised.

Good Risk Communication Benefits: Good risk communication practice should be regarded as of equal importance to the other key elements—risk assessment and the evaluation of risk control options—in the overall risk management process. In fact, good risk communication practice can be regarded as the causeway that links all the organizational elements in a well functioning risk management process, especially in the face of scientific uncertainty.

The current state of risk management and communication research suggests that those responsible with food safety risk management must be seen to be reducing, mitigating or minimizing a particular risk. Those responsible must be able to effectively communicate their efforts and they must be able to prove they are actually reducing levels of risk. As Slovic (1997) has noted, "We live in a world in which information, acting in concert with the vagaries of human perception and cognition, has reduced our vulnerability to pandemics of disease at the cost of increasing our vulnerability to social and economic catastrophes of unprecedented scale. The challenge before us is to learn how to manage stigma and reduce the vulnerability of important products, industries, and institutions to its effects, without suppressing the proper communication of risk information to the public."

Certainly the outbreak of bovine Spongiform Encephalopathy (BSE, or mad cow disease) could be characterized as stigmata using the evaluative criteria listed above. There have been dozens of other, well-publicized outbreaks since Jack-in-the-Box. For example, in the spring and summer of 1996, some 1,465 people across North America were stricken with *Cyclospora cayetanensis*, a parasite initially linked to the consumption of California strawberries. However, the common vehicle was later thought to be Guatemalan raspberries (Hoffmann, et al., 1996)-265. Most citizens did not hear the correction, and the California Strawberry Commission estimates it lost $20 to $40 million in sales. Yet despite increased surveillance and risk management of Guatemalan raspberries,

Cyclospora cayetanensis emerged again in 1997, associated not only with consumption of fresh fruits but with mesclun lettuce in Florida and fresh basil in Washington, D.C. Sales of fresh herbs immediately dropped (Masters, 1997)-[143].

In these cases and dozens of others, there is an enormous potential for economic damage, even damage to health as consumption of nutritious foods may decline. The potential for stigmatization of food is enormous.

The same criteria can be applied to other outbreaks. For example, in the Odwalla outbreak, the increased and more effective attention of the Seattle-King County Health Unit -- the same one involved in the Jack-in-the-Box outbreak -- toward _E. coli_ O157:H7 resulted in rapid identification of the Odwalla outbreak. The company exercised exemplary risk communication. Odwalla officials responded in a timely and compassionate fashion, co-operating with authorities after a link was first made on Oct. 30, 1996 between their juice and an illness, which was eventually linked, to 65 people in four U.S. states and B.C. Upon learning of the child's death, company chairman Greg Steltenpohl issued a statement which said, "On behalf of myself and the people at Odwalla, I want to say how deeply saddened and sorry we are to learn of the loss of this child. Our hearts go out to the family and our primary concern at this moment is to see that we are doing everything we can to help them" (Odwalla, 1996)-[26].

Yet despite the comforting words, the company failed to acknowledge the existence of risk, let alone efforts to reduce levels of risk. Steltenpohl told reporters at the time that the company did not routinely test for _E. coli_ because it was advised by industry experts that the acid level in the apple juice was sufficient to kill the bug. Because they are unpasteurized, Odwalla's drinks are shipped in cold storage and have only a two-week shelf life. Odwalla was founded 16 years ago on the premise that fresh, natural fruit juices nourish the spirit. In addition, the bank balances: in fiscal 1996, Odwalla sales jumped 65 per cent to $60 million (U.S.).

Odwalla insisted the experts in this case were the U.S. Food and Drug Administration. The FDA isn't sure who was warned and when. However, researchers from the U.S. Centers for Disease Control and Prevention wrote in the May 5, 1993 Journal of the American Medical Association that a 1991 outbreak of _E. coli_ O157:H7 which struck 23 people in Fall River, Mass. -- and was well-publicized at the time -- was caused by unpasteurized, unpreserved cider. The story received national media attention and noted that researchers had found that _E. coli_ could survive for 20 days in unpreserved, refrigerated cider. Further, the authors cited two previously reported outbreaks of illness associated with drinking apple cider.

In Dec. 1994, the Columbus Salami Co. of South San Francisco recalled 10,000 pounds of salami after health officials linked the product to at least 18 cases of *E. coli* O157:H7 in California and Washington. The bacterium was not supposed to survive the acidic environment of salami, and again the story received national coverage. In this case, the industry immediately pledged to test whether *E. coli* O157:H7 could survive the process used to make dry sausages like salami, which only involves meat curing, not cooking.

In addition, earlier in Oct. 1996, fresh (unpasteurized) apple cider produced at the Notch Store and Cider Mill in Cheshire, Connecticut was linked to an outbreak of *E. coli* O157:H7 in at least seven people. For Odwalla to say it had no knowledge that *E. coli* O157:H7 could survive in an acid environment is simply unacceptable in a global food manufacturing and distribution system, especially one becoming increasingly vulnerable to outbreaks of food borne illness.

Similar challenges face those promoting the adoption of Agricultural biotechnology. For example, genetically engineered Bt-containing corn has been widely adopted in Ontario and throughout North America. There is a potential risk that the use of Bt-corn will accelerate the development of resistance in the target pest, the European corn borer. Regulatory agencies in Canada and the U.S. have required companies seeking regulatory approval of Bt-corns to file and adhere to resistance management strategies designed to delay the onset of resistance in the corn borer, usually related to the use of refugia, whereby 20 to 30 per cent of a producer's corn crop would be planted in non-Bt corn to provide an area for the corn borer to intermingle. While many companies demand that farmers enter into contractual commitments to a minimum of 20 per cent refugia, there is a need to demonstrate, for public, regulatory and scientific reasons, that producers are indeed responsibly managing the introduction of the new, genetically engineered Bt-corn. To better understand the perceptions of Ontario producers regarding genetically engineered Bt corn, a survey was mailed to 2,400 Ontario corn producers selected at random in the spring of 1998.

Stigmatization is becoming the norm for food and water linked to human illness or even death. That is because stigma is a warning-system -- one that is often erroneous but in these cases extremely valuable -- that something is wrong. If trust is the most important component of consumers' confidence in the food supply then let us find how to establish trust? For a while, in the early 1990s, right after the Alar episode, many producers sought public salvation in the language of persuasion: that if we talk nice to people, we can establish trust; we can resolve conflict. Happy talk is important, but as Nancy Donley, president of Safe Tables Our Priority, and whose six-year-old son died from _E. coli_ O157:H7 in 1993 says, "We need sound science rather than soundbites." How then to reduce stigma? The components for managing the stigma associated with any food safety issue seem to involve all of the following factors:

- Effective and rapid surveillance systems
- Effective communication about the nature of risk
- A credible, open and responsive regulatory system
- Demonstrable efforts to reduce levels of uncertainty and risk
- Evidence that actions match words.

Producer-led risk management programs are an action, an appropriate risk management strategy, to demonstrate to consumers that producers are cognoscenti of their newfound concerns about food safety, and to demonstrate that producers and others in the farm-to-fork continuum are working to reduce levels of risk. When the next outbreak or crisis of confidence comes -- and Microrganisms can adapt and evolve to any food production and distribution system that is created -- producers need to demonstrate due diligence to minimize potential losses.

Risk communication has been described by Dr. Ortwin Renn, a leading researcher in the area of risk communication, as being characterized by three main elements: informing (changing knowledge), persuading (changing attitude and behaviour) and consulting. Risk communication is required to adequately address and respond to needs for criteria, hazards, risks, safety, and general concerns about food. People in Canada want to play an active role in the decisions that affect their lives. Citizens are no longer deferential to authority and unquestioning of information from government. Even scientific authorities come into question today.

There are certain very specific conditions and constraints applied to communications from government, which in turn determine the range and scope of activities that a regulatory agency of government can undertake in the area of risk communication. Now the relationship between governments and citizens has evolved and taken a better perspective. Citizen engagement is seen as a means to involve the public in government decision-making.

The complexity of today's food chain means that responsibility for food safety must be shared, which the CFIA does through partners in provincial/territorial governments, other federal departments, food producers, industry, distributors, retailers, and ultimately every consumer of food in Canada. The mandate of the Canadian Food Inspection Agency is to deliver all federally regulated food inspection and quarantine services as well as plant protection and animal health programs. The CFIA reports to Parliament through the Minister of Agriculture and Agri-Food.

Risk communication has evolved from the field of risk analysis and thus has a limited basis in the field of communications as such. Risk communication has been defined as an interactive process of an exchange of information, involving multiple messages about the nature of risk. Risk communication will not, even when effectively used, solve all problems or resolve all conflict on issues. On the other hand, poor or absent communication will almost certainly lead to a failure to manage risk effectively. Two essential components to risk communication are trust and perception. Building trust is the pivotal focus of risk communication, which is problematic for government and government agencies, as the public tends to see government as a less-than-trusted source of information. Perception, which emerges from a combination of complex factors, is an area under constant study.

Communicating about science poses a particular challenge for risk communicators. In a public risk management framework, input from both the scientific and the public contexts ensures a more complete range of information. The evolution of risk communication from one-way to two-way communication is critical in cases where scientific uncertainty is a predominant characteristic.

Theories on communication and risk communication are plentiful, but communication about food can have very specific characteristics. The public tends to assess risk based on specific context, and where food is concerned, risk is not well tolerated because the public is more dependent on food than on any other commodity. In the absence of media coverage, for example, or public messages about food risk, the public tends to be apathetic about risk on a day-to-day basis.

Dr. Ortwin Renn of Germany, a leading risk communication's theorist, has developed a model of policy-making that incorporates the concept of deliberation and the principles of deliberative processes. He identifies four key elements: markets, expertise, regulatory regimes, and, last, public discourse. The essential concept behind the model is that mutual understanding and consensus building are the best ways to address the elements of values and fairness in risk decision-making.

Theory dictates that a successful model for risk communication must reconcile the views of scientists, the public and politicians in order to achieve a common understanding of complex risks, leading to credible management options and credible policy development around risk.

The CFIA has adapted a model prepared by the Assistant Deputy Minister Working Group on Risk Management, highlighting communications as an integral aspect within each phase of decision-making. The communications challenges identified were:

- The importance of perception or assessments;
- The degree of public tolerance of risk;
- The role that pro-active risk communication can play in building public understanding of risk and management of risk; and
- The need to gain/maintain public trust, and its impact on the credibility of government messaging.

Developing a single model to embrace all aspects of the nature of decision (from single food recall situations to policy-making decisions to high visibility and controversial issues management) and all aspects of communication strategy is an impressive challenge.

The CFIA risk analysis model shows a natural flow of risk communication decisions. Having decided on the level of risk debate, the risk communicator must then turn to the mechanics of the risk communication process and focus on methodology, tools, and channels and communications products.

Much of the effectiveness of the CFIA's food risk communication is based on the alliances forged between the agency and its many partners, including stakeholders, governments at all levels and special interest groups.

Risk communication is a complex and emerging field. Practitioners are quick to point out that no one form of risk communication will satisfy everyone, but it is possible to align theory in a predictable way and thus, build an effective communication strategy.

As the authors explored theory and practice in risk communication, a single point appeared repeatedly—the issue of trust and credibility. Clearly, the relationship between the source of the communication and the recipient must be acknowledged as an important factor in effective risk communication, if not the most important factor.

Successful risk communication is not about giving out information or about making stakeholders understand. Today, successful risk communication can result only when the quality of debate among government, the public and all stakeholders is improved-18.

The HACCP system is a well-established and tested program that was pioneered over 43 years ago and has become a principal food safety program around the world, recognized by many governments and Codex Alimentarius. HACCP is best when applied to every step in the food chain from raw material production through processing to retail sale and consumption by the consumer. Benefits of HACCP revolve around it being a preventative system, fully compatible with Total Quality Management and ISO 9000, a systematic approach to increase assurance of safety in a cost effective fashion recommended by regulatory agencies, encouraged by food processors and suppliers.

Microbiological criteria when appropriately applied can be a useful means for ensuring safety and quality of foods, which in turn, elevates consumer confidence. It also can provide the food industry and regulatory agencies with guidelines for control of food processing systems. Internationally accepted criteria can advance free trade through standardization of food safety and quality requirements.

We as consumers make ourselves more and more vulnerable by making diversified food choices, through national import policies and local encouragement of diverse food processing, and we are often unaware of the consequences of our initiatives. A risk communication concerning different foods of different sources must be evolved for better safety. The area of risk communication research has its roots in the need of a better understanding of what kind of information consumers actually require and want in circumstances of risk, hazard, crisis, or catastrophe. Risk communication is linked to risk perception research in that it is necessary to know how, when and why people perceive risk in a certain way, and to the area of crisis communication, which deals with ongoing crises as well as follow-up evaluations. The dimension of risk communication on food safety issues includes both communication with the citizenry as a whole, through the mass media and other widely disseminated information, and communication with consumer organizations that participate in the risk analysis/risk management process.

Dietary habits have evolved along with the socio-cultural development of our countries. Food production is no longer purely about satisfying basic dietary needs, and processed food products account for a growing share of the market, thanks to the advances made by the agro-food industry. Eating a balanced diet should be considered as the main message to the consumer. Harmonisation of legislation on food safety for any new food category like GMF or OF would be legal, justified and easily understood, and presented in the context of an overall balanced diet and other healthy lifestyle factors. Consumer confidence could be enhanced if food products are communicated clearly, truthfully and in a way that is easily understood to the consumer, disclosing comprehensive information on product labels (quantities of functional ingredients, target population, length and quantity of optimum consumption, interaction with other components or drugs, side-effects, impact of cooking methods, etc.).

Food safety concerns are the scars of fear that should be eliminated through risk assessment, risk management, and risk communication. An approach to adequate nutrition and food supply as a human right for all citizens and an issue of governance since the foundation of a productive life is dependent on the quality of food we consume. Local governments and communities should be encouraged to develop partnership and solve nutrition and food safety problems towards the collective rallying the public and private sectors to support the quality of affordable staples and complementary foods to raise the prospects of making Canada a source of safest food supplying country.

A good communication example can be best served in the field of biotechnology. One of the first products of biotechnology to make a significant commercial impact in Canada has been insect-resistant corn, genetically engineered to contain the delta-Endotoxin produced by *Bacillus thuringiensis*, generally referred to as Bt-corn.

Bacillus thuringiensis (Bt) is a gram-positive soil bacterium that produces an insecticidal protein in the form of a crystal. The insecticidal proteins are commonly designated as *cry* proteins and the genes encoding the proteins are known as cry genes (Lambert and Peferoen, 1992). The Bt toxin is regarded as an environmentally friendly insecticide because of its target specificity and its decomposition to non-toxic compounds when exposed to environmental factors (Gould, 1995). *Bacillus thuringiensis* 'Berliner' is the most commonly used Biopesticide (Wearing and Hokkanen, 1995). Bt has been widely used in both conventional and organic farming operations as an insecticidal spray with some drawbacks. In order for the Bt Endotoxin to be effective, the insect must ingest it (Webber, 1995), before it is broken down by environmental factors such as ultraviolet light. One advantage of genetically engineered Bt-corn is that the insecticidal protein has been incorporated into the plant, limiting environmental exposure. Insecticidal properties of Bt can vary in activity against insects within a single insect Order. The toxins encoded by the *cry*I genes are toxic to Lepidopterans such as the European corn borer (ECB) [*Ostrinia nubilalis*].

Response	Percentage responses
• Yes	46.5 %
• No	52.5 %
• DK/NA	1.0 %

Figure 04(04): Ontario farmers growing Bt-corn varieties, 1999 (n = 874) -52

To preserve the functionality of genetically engineered Bt-containing field corn, scientists and regulators are recommending the planting of minimal refugia of 20 per cent non-Bt-corn per individual farm. Of the 400 Ontario corn producers who were growing Bt-corn this year and completed the survey, 53 or 13.5 per cent were planting in excess of 80 per cent of their acreage with genetically engineered Bt-corn. In 1998, approximately 15 percent of the Ontario crop was planted to Bt-corn varieties. One-third of the field corn in Ontario in 1999 was Bt-corn. As the percentage of the Ontario field corn crop devoted to Bt hybrids continues to increase, the importance of compliance with Bt-refugia guidelines also increases.

In 1998, approximately 15 percent of the Ontario crop was planted to Bt-corn varieties. One-third of the field corn in Ontario in 1999 was Bt-corn. As the percentage of the Ontario field corn crop devoted to Bt hybrids continues to increase, the importance of compliance with Bt-refugia guidelines also increases. The 400 Ontario corn producers who were growing Bt-corn in 1999 and surveyed here demonstrated a large level of compliance with Bt-refugia guidelines, particularly amongst those with more than 100 acres of field corn. Nevertheless, recommendations for Bt refugia need to be clarified and communications efforts expanded, especially for growers of less than 100 acres of field corn.

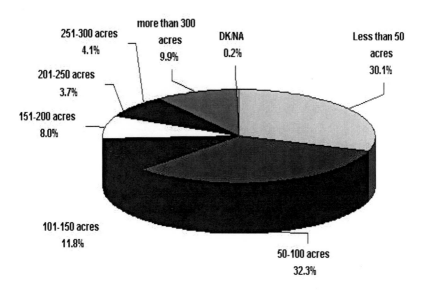

Figure 04(05): <u>Acres of corn planted in Ontario, 1999 (n = 943)</u> -52

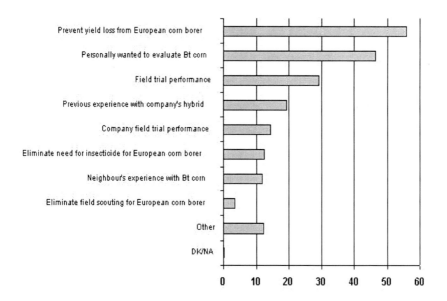

Figure 04(06): <u>Ontario farmers' reasons for planting Bt-corn hybrids, 1999 (n = 400)</u> -52

Chapter: 05
HACCP PRINCIPLES

Overview:

Safety of the food supply is a key to the consumer confidence. Sometimes the human common sense plays a vital role in solving scientific complexity. Food safety hazards are not different than any other hazard, which are faced by human. All hazards faced by humans can be prevented well in advance of its occurrence rather than reacting to it when it has already inflicted its blow to human health. Such a system known worldwide is Hazard Analysis Critical Control Point (HACCP). In the past, periodic plant inspections and sample testing have been used to ensure the quality and safety of food products. Inspection and testing provided information about the product that is relevant only for the specific time the product was inspected and tested. From a public health and safety point of view, these traditional methods offered little protection or assurance. New concepts have emerged which are far more promising for controlling food safety hazards from production to consumption. This system is designed to prevent risks from producing hazards by eliminating those risks to such an extent that does not cause harm to human health. HACCP functions effectively when all preventive measures, Good Manufacturing Practices (GMPs), Good Hygiene Practices (GHPs), Standard Operating Procedures (SOPs), Standard Laboratory Procedures (SLPs), Customer Specifications (CS), Regulatory Requirements (RR) and Qualified Manufacturing Personnel (QMP) are incorporated with in the seven principles of HACCP process. The system fits in well with modern quality and management techniques. It is especially compatible with the ISO 9000 quality assurance system and just in time delivery of ingredients.

The HACCP process requires its implementers to be trained and provided with adequate facilities with motivated support from the management of the food manufacturing organization. We should always remember that HACCP is a preventive process and must be continuously reinforced. HACCP was introduced as a system to control safety, as the product is manufactured, rather than trying to detect problems by testing the finished product. This new system is based on assessing the inherent hazards or risks in a particular product or process and designing a system to control them. Specific points where the hazards can be controlled in the process are identified. The allocation of resources and designing of the HACCP system must consider motivational commitment, removing the communication barriers, institute leadership, remove barriers that rob employees of workmanship pride and take actions to accomplish smooth transformation. The success of the system is also dependent on the processing, packaging, monitoring, analytical, detection and transportation equipments. The likelihood of the occurrence of a hazard in a finished product is definitely influenced by the facility, equipment design, and construction of production building, sanitary facilities and plant installation, which play a key role in any preventive strategy.

The contamination of food may be inherent from the raw materials, added during the initial recombination, processing or from the packaging materials during packing. No matter whether contaminants are inherent, occurred in the processing establishment, all lead to short illness, prolonged illness or death. HACCP contributes to the process of saving human lives by providing safe food.

Hazard Analysis and Critical Control Points (HACCP) is a process control system designed to identify and prevent microbial and other hazards in food production. There are hazards, which include contaminants of microbiological origin like bacterial, parasitic, viral, bacterial toxin, or cross-contamination. There are many potential physical contaminants, which may enter food chain from the farm to any stage of processing until packed and sealed in food packaging. Such contaminants are numerous and may include: stones, glass fragments, metal fragments, human hair, insects, and products charred particles from the packing machines, any foreign body or part of the packaging materials used. The same applies to Chemical contaminations which are more cause of concern when cross contamination of cleaning compounds occurs due to faulty pipe work in Cleaning In Place (CIP) systems or a spill over to final product reservoir. Sometimes the non-food grade lubricants fall during the packing of products. Insecticides and herbicides may contaminate the food products at raw stage in the farms. Sometimes antibiotics and hormones could reach human systems through meat and milk. The list is very long and screening and monitoring of levels are highly sensitive.

Leaving aside last two contaminants, microbial agents are the leading cause of laboratory-confirmed outbreaks and that the main reasons for the outbreaks and illnesses are improper holding temperatures, poor personal hygiene, improper cooking temperatures, lack of pasteurization, foods from unsafe sources, uncontrolled ingredients resourcing, contaminated equipment and very lately Bioterrorism. HACCP includes steps designed to prevent problems before they occur and to correct deviations as soon as

they are detected. Such preventive control syste
documentation and verification are widely recognized by
authorities and international organizations as the most
approach available for producing safe food. The HACCP sy
been successfully applied in the food industry.

It is the creation of a system, which is based on a perfect
objectivity to earn a safe, smooth running, profitable food
manufacturing or trading business. Managing for food safety must
be as fully integrated into the operations as those actions that one
might take to open in the morning, ensure a profit and manage
cash flow, oversee personnel, or any other aspect of the business.
Only by putting in place an active, ongoing system, made up of
actions intended to create the desired outcome, one could improve
food safety. Application of the HACCP principles provides one
system that can meet that criterion. The HACCP plan that one is
going to develop is to one's factory specific. One may seek
knowledge, help, consultancy from external sources such as quality
consultants, regulatory authorities but the design, implementation,
and success of the plan rests with the implementer of the food
safety system.

IDEA-CVD: HACCP systems must be based on the seven
principles. In the United States, the National Advisory Committee
on Microbiological Criteria for Foods (NACMCF) articulates it. In
Canada, Canadian Food Inspection Agency (CFIA) and Agri-Canada
recommend it. The seven principles are:

(1) **I**dentification of hazards (Conduct a hazard analysis)
(2) **D**etermination of critical control points (Determine CCPs)
(3) **E**stablishment of critical limits (Establish CCLs)
(4) **A**ppropriate monitoring of CCPs (Establish CCP procedures)
(5) **C**orrective procedures establishment (Establish corrective action)
(6) **V**erification procedures establishment (Establish verification procedures)
(7) **D**ocumentation of HACCP system (Establish effective record keeping Procedures)

1. Identification of Hazards:
Potential hazards associated with a food and measures to control
those hazards are identified in a food manufacturing set up. The
hazard could be Physical, Chemical, Microbiological, Environmental,
and Bioterrorism. Physical hazards are solid, foreign, visible, or
minute bodies, which are considered contaminant to the food
product. Examples may include human hair, machine parts falling
in product during production, even unwanted edible food

ngredients which are not desired in the under process items of food. Chemical Hazards could be detergents that may cross contaminate food during parallel CIP operations, seafood may be found contaminated with hazardous materials spilled in sea, unsuitable packaging materials may react with the product like unlacquered tin plate reacts with acidic juice concentrates etc. Microbiological hazards include Food pathogens, Food spoilage, and Toxin producing bacteria, Yeasts, Moulds, Protozoans and Viruses.

Environmental hazards could involve chemical or biological hazards where pollutants may enter food production chain. The number of possibilities as how the release of Genetically Engineered Organisms (GEO) into the environment may upset the ecology is very large. The possible complications are extremely difficult to identify and evaluate. Some of the substances get into our bodies after being emitted by industrial facilities as pollutants; others come from the foods we eat, from natural sources, from past pollution, or a combination of all three. Research suggests that over 40% of the global burden of disease due to environmental risk factors may fall on children under five, even though they constitute about 10% of the world's population.

Bioterrorism is an emerging source of critical point for human health and food safety. Bioterrorism can be described as the use, or threatened use, of biological agents to promote or spread fear or intimidation upon an individual, a specific group, or the population as a whole for religious, political, ideological, financial, or personal purposes. These biological agents, with the exception of smallpox virus, are typically found in nature in various parts of the world. They can be, however, weaponized to enhance their virulence in humans and make them resistant to vaccines and antibiotics.

How to Conduct a Hazard Analysis:

a) The hazard analysis and the development of the HACCP Plan is conducted by a HACCP team, including at least one member who has the knowledge of HACCP from either formal training or experience.

b) The hazard analysis is conducted at each process step for every product type. Process steps where a significant hazard may be introduced or where a hazard may increase to an unacceptable level must be identified.

c) The hazard analysis includes the identification of all potential hazards (biological, chemical, physical etc.), the determination of the significance of the hazard identified, i.e., consideration of its severity and the likelihood of occurrence and, if applicable, justification for a determination of non-significance of a hazard.

d) The processor demonstrates that they have considered all process steps in conducting their hazard analysis. A Hazard Analysis Worksheet, or equivalent, is used to organize and document the hazard analysis.

e) The processor shall consider all activities and materials in the establishment, including incoming fish, raw milk, food raw materials, food ingredients, packaging materials, establishment personnel, establishment itself, product descriptions, the process flow diagram, consumer complaint information, epidemiological and technical literature available when conducting the hazard analysis.

f) For some food establishments, it is possible that the hazard analysis will not identify any significant hazards to record. The HACCP component of the Plan would therefore only include the hazard analysis and other applicable documentation. The determination of CCPs and associated controls would not be applicable in such a case.

2. Determination of Critical Control Points:

These are points in a food's processing and production - from its raw state through ingredients receiving – to recombination - processing – packaging, storage and finally shipping to consumption by the consumer – during all these transitional stages, the potential hazards shall be controlled.

a) For each significant hazard identified in the first step, there is an appropriate preventive measure in place to prevent or eliminate the hazard or reduce it to an acceptable level as per the regulatory and scientific recommendations.

b) The method and results of the CCP determination are documented and CCPs are to be indicated on the process flow diagram. Which include?

1.   Resourcing of ingredients
        Receiving of ingredients as per specifications
        Inspection and evaluation for acceptance
        Proper recording and labelling
        Storage of ingredients at recommended temperatures
        Storage of ingredients in segregation and pest free store
        Storage of ingredients in dry store for ambient requirement
        Non-conforming items stored at isolated and labelled place
        Prompt communication of inferior product delivery
        Proper stock rotation
2.   Food manufacturing planning and execution
3.   Ingredients recombination system

4.   **P**otable water supply checks; parameters, continuity etc.
5.   **S**tandard functioning equipments with data recording
6.   **S**tandard heat process temperature time combination
7.   **S**tandard chilling temperatures after heat treatment
8.   **R**e-processing for corrective product quality
9.   **P**rotection from air borne contaminants
10.   **S**tandard packaging materials
11.   **F**inished food packing process
12.   **S**torage of finished products in time
13.   **S**torage at correct temperatures
14.   **C**onsistent use of properly calibrated thermometers
15.   **C**onsistent use of properly calibrated valves and graphs
16.   **S**toring food/ingredients beyond danger zone as per requirement
17.   **F**ood Personnel hygiene
18.   **D**isease monitoring
19.   **H**ygiene monitoring
20.   **A**ttitude monitoring; subversive activities etc.
21.   **S**afety issues monitoring; trained personnel for job task
22.   **S**tandard Cleaning and sanitizing system
23.   **G**arbage disposal system
24.   **G**eneral manufacturing place sanitation
25.   **P**est control system; insects, rodents etc.
26.   **C**ross Contamination Elimination
27.   **P**roduct monitoring in the market; shelf life, temperature etc.

3. <u>Establishing Critical Control Limits:</u>

Preventive measures and its establishment with critical limits for each control point is the third principle of HACCP. For a cooked food in catering, for example, this might include setting the minimum cooking temperature and time required to ensure the elimination of harmful pathogenic organisms.

The critical limit may be defined as "the maximum or minimum value to which a physical, biological, or chemical hazard must be controlled at a Critical Control Point (CCP) to prevent, eliminate, or reduce to a legally acceptable level the occurrence of an identified food safety hazard". A Critical Control Point (CCP) is a step or procedure at which control can be applied that is essential to prevent, eliminate or reduce a hazard to a limit. It may not be possible to prevent a hazard in some processes and with some degree of hazards minimisation could be the only reasonable goal of the HACCP plan. A critical limit is used to distinguish between safe and unsafe operating conditions at a CCP.

In UHT treatments, a time temperature combination may be fixed as 137 °C for 3 second etc. An upper limit of 140 °C and a lower limit of 135 °C are fixed to compensate variation in equipment operation and to safeguard the product from over or under heating during the process[01].

Milk that is processed in this way by using temperatures exceeding 135 °C permits a decrease in the necessary holding time from 5-2 seconds enabling a continuous flow operation. A control limit could be again fixed to compensate increase or decrease of time temperature combinations. Thermograph automatically records the processing temperature inputs. Establishment of Critical Control Limits (CCLs) in equipments is easily done by adjustments in control system. UHT processor's temperature, liquid flow and flow diversion CCPs are controlled by settings in computer.

The aseptic packaging system protects the product from atmospheric contamination and microorganisms in the product are not present in the form to develop or cause spoilage or diseases to human. Because of these guarantees product keeps with long shelf life without the need for refrigeration. Under normal storage condition, the shelf life of UHT Milk ranges from 6- 10 months (unopened) depending on existing regulations in different regions of the world. Complexity of equipment and plant is needed to maintain sterile atmosphere between processing and packaging; packaging materials, pipe work, tanks, pumps; higher skilled operators; sterility must be maintained through aseptic packaging. The most critical point in UHT process is the absence of viable bacteria and spores from the finished final product. The original quality of milk, processing equipments sterility, processing temperatures, packaging physical condition, packaging sterility, plant sterile system control and package integrity are the CCPs where control limits are required. When it comes to sterility, a zero tolerance is mandatory control limit.

Sealing of the long life milk packages under the sterile condition during the packing process is a critical control point. Although proper selection of packaging material, incoming component inspection, a validated sealing process and control of key sealing parameters may positively impact seal strengths, only a test or observation of sealed packages can effectively monitor integrity.

Manual addition of bacterial culture for the inoculation of yoghurt milk in small-scale production is an important CCP. Bacteriophages from surrounding environment, hygiene of outer surface of culture container, exposure of pasteurized milk for the addition of culture, manual technique of adding culture and the personnel hygiene of operator are the factors which impact this CCP. Tests results for

Bacteriophage in culture and microbial evaluation of environment would impact this CCP. A limit of phage contaminants in inoculated yoghurt milk is critically needed otherwise yoghurt milk may stand more than ten hours with out proper fermentation and subsequently culture bacteria eaten up by bacteriophages. A zero Bacteriophage tolerant limit is ideal.

In some cases, critical limits have already been established in regulatory requirements, scientific literature, or through expert consultation. One can establish critical limits, which are, different than regulatory requirements, however they must be based on sound scientific data and assure they result in a better production results than the minimum regulatory requirement for the product.

The control limits for microbial count is mandatory to safeguard food and human health. For example Canadian Milk Protein Concentrate (MPC) must be free from _Salmonella, Staphylococcus aureus, Escherichia coli_ and other Coliform. MPC-75 must not contain more than 10 000 Colony-Forming Units (CFU) per gram, in terms of Total Bacteria Count (TBC), and a maximum count of 50 CFU/g for yeast and mold. The number of microorganisms capable of developing spores under aerobic conditions must not exceed 500 CFU/g. Microorganisms capable of sporing under anaerobic conditions must not exceed 700 CFU/g-150.

a) Critical Control Limits (CCLs) are established for each CCP identified. A critical limit shall be fixed with the maximum or minimum value to which a hazard must be controlled at a Critical Control Point (CCP). For example, a temperature or time which must be achieved to ensure destruction of a pathogenic bacteria, a specific pH to prevent the growth of unwanted bacteria, a level of a preservative, a size of detectable shell pieces, or the presence of acceptable product analysis documentation from a supplier of raw materials would guide to fix CCL.

b) The Critical Control Limits (CCLs) are validated to demonstrate that they are effective and the validation is documented.

4. Appropriate Monitoring of CCPs:
Monitoring is a planned sequence of observations or measurements to assess whether a CCP is under control and to produce an accurate record for future use in verification. Monitoring will allow tracking trends, identifying deviations, and providing a record for verification. Continuous monitoring is ideal, but non-continuous monitoring frequency could be determined from historical knowledge of the product or process, which could be in acceptable intervals of 30 to 60 minutes. The frequency should not exceed an

acceptable risk level. If a deviation is found, corrective actions shall be taken appropriately.

The CCP of package sealing in liquid food products require that strength and integrity of packages be monitored so that failures can be detected quickly and early corrective actions taken. There is currently no standard test equipment to monitor the package integrity rapidly and reliably. Few manufacturers of packaging machines do provide a pressure grip at the outlet of machine to check and harmonize the paperboard brick packages, which is an important step towards package integrity. A similar monitoring for gable top packaging could also help reduce leakage. At Present, monitoring is by time consuming random dye testing on packs, which is an essential check.

Monitoring by line personnel and equipment operators can be advantageous because they can readily observe changes from the norm. However, the detection rate observed remained approximately 51% of seal defects[186].

Although it is appropriate to rely on monitoring devices to indicate operation within the validated seal parameters, and thus strength, it is difficult and unreliable to use the visual test for seal integrity. In a slow speed packing machine like 1200 cups an hour, individual aluminium heat sealed plastic cups could be checked with >80% success. A high-speed machine with >1800 cups per hour would require automatic device to monitor the integrity of packages.

Monitoring of time and temperature through thermographs in pasteurizing and sterilizing units is the best example of continuous monitoring. However, each thermograph chart must be used for a single day pasteurization operation, be dated, specify the operations to which it refers, be initiated by the operator and be eventually filed in chronological order.

Online foreign body detection in the finished and sealed product packages is another example of continuous monitoring. Foreign body detection by human eye is only possible during the filling and sealing of the pack. Later, opaque packs cannot be seen inside by the naked eye. However, multi detection points in the chain of food manufacturing and sales, a satisfactory result could be achieved. Sometimes a combination of metal detection device and visual monitoring during filling and sealing could provide safety from other foreign bodies too. However, a preventive metal contamination arrangement should be given more importance and should run parallel to metal detection devices.

Metal detection machines are very sensitive and detect different variables of metals. Conventional X-ray systems are limited in their detection of soft foreign body contaminants in food products. There is a growing pressure on the food industry to eliminate foreign bodies in food. Automation and consumer eating habits are leading to an increase in Critical Control Points (CCPs) in prepared foods so is the demand of a foreign body free product package. A zero limit of foreign bodies in most of the product is sought.

The human ability to detect light and synthesize an image is one of human's miraculous senses. Humans rely on sight to gather data that allows making decisions. Machine vision emulates this process in order to automate repetitive tasks or interpret complex information in an image. The heart of machine vision is the electronic camera, which employs a light sensitive detector known as a Charge Coupled Device (CCD). Colour cameras are specifically designed to limit sensitivity to the visible wavelengths (400-650 nm) in order to more closely mimic the human eye. However, the CCD sensor can detect light beyond the visible into the near infrared (650-1100 nm), allowing it to detect things the eye cannot. The colour of an object is determined by the wavelength of light reflected from it's surface. In biological materials, the light reflected varies widely as a function of wavelength, especially in the near infrared (NIR). These spectral variations provide a unique key to automated vision in food production-153.

Monitoring will go much more smoothly if the manufacturing management monitors Critical Limit Values (CLVs) for **W**hat, **H**ow, **F**requency, and **W**ho. When management identifies clearly the employee positions responsible for monitoring, trains employees monitoring the CCP in the testing procedures, establishes the critical limits, sets the methods of recording test results, sets the actions to be taken when critical limits are exceeded, ensures that the employees understand the purpose and the importance of monitoring; the purpose of monitoring will be well served. It is imperative to clearly identify the individual responsible for monitoring, train thoroughly on process requirements, and assure they understand the importance and purpose of monitoring. An appropriate monitoring of CCPs shall be followed with these sequences:

a) At each CCP, the processor shall establish monitoring procedures to determine that the system is operating within the critical limits identified. It is important to have monitoring procedures, which produce immediate measurable results to which action can be initiated since there may be potential food safety implications.

b) The monitoring procedures include what will be monitored, if applicable how the critical limits and preventive measures will be monitored, how frequently monitoring will be performed, and who will perform the monitoring.

c) For each monitoring activity, the processor shall establish that personnel performing the monitoring have the knowledge and ability to conduct the procedure. Where specialized skills are required in order to adequately monitor a process or perform an activity which is critical to ensure product safety, appropriate training requirements, experience, and/or skills are identified. For example, the following positions are recognised as requiring specialized skills: Pasteurizer operator, Tetra-Pak packaging machine operator, packaging dye testing operator, and container integrity inspector etc. Personnel in these positions require special knowledge and experience.

5. **Corrective Procedure**:

If a food item is not processed according to the standard procedures, failures occur in the final quality. In such a situation, reprocessing or disposing of food are the alternatives. We may define Corrective Action (CA) as "procedures to be followed when a deviation occurs." A deviation is a failure to meet a Critical Control Limit (CCL). Thus corrective action is a documented design, process, procedure or materials change implemented to correct the cause of failure or design deficiency. When limits are violated at a CCP, the predetermined, documented corrective actions should be instituted. Unfortunately, we do not operate in an ideal world so defined corrective actions are necessary. These include isolating and holding product for safety evaluation, reprocessing, or destruction. Corrective actions should determine and correct the cause of non-compliance, determine the disposition of non-compliant product, and record the corrective actions that have been taken.

An important purpose of corrective actions is to prevent foods, which may be hazardous from reaching consumers. HACCP is a preventive system to correct problems before they affect the safety of the food. The corrective actions are considered to ensure that the cause of the deviation is identified and eliminated. The CCP will be under control after the corrective action is taken. Measures to prevent recurrence are established.

The Corrective Actions may be included in forms that are created to address the cause of the deviation so that it can be identified and eliminated. Therefore, the CCP will be under control after the corrective action is taken. The establishment of appropriate measures takes place so that a recurrence is avoided. The affected food is not allowed to enter commerce that would be injurious to health or otherwise adulterated as a result of the deviation.

The HACCP Plan must identify what must be done, who is responsible, and what records must be completed in the event a deviation occurs. Some examples of corrective actions are to empower employees to stop the process, retain product that is not in compliance, adjust the process while holding the product, or implement an alternate process that can be substituted. If corrective actions become necessary frequently, the HACCP plan may need to be revised to be more effective thus preventing recurrence. In a typical food-processing establishment the corrective procedure shall pursue the following guidelines: -

a) Corrective action procedures are established to be initiated when monitoring indicates that the process is operating outside the defined critical limits. The corrective action procedures are established in advance so the personnel conducting the monitoring will have direction on the steps to take when a deviation is identified.

b) The corrective action procedures addresses: the correction of the deficiency that gave rise to the problem; the identification and segregation of all affected product; the culling, re-working, and/or disposition of affected product in an appropriate manner.

c) The corrective action procedures address the prevention or reduction in likelihood of reoccurrence of the problem by investigating how the problem developed? The review of Quality Assurance Plan (QAP), QMP, and HACCP is established to determine whether changes in procedures, control measures, standards, etc., are needed. The identification and implementation of necessary changes in the plan are recorded in procedures as well as in an amendment log.

d) The corrective action procedures include a record system to document at least the details of the problem, including the date the problem was identified, the corrective action taken, the person(s) responsible for the action, the date the action was taken and the changes needed to eliminate or prevent re-occurrence of the problem.

6. **Verification Procedure:**
Accomplishment of a task as well as its verification ensures confidence. "Verification is defined as confirmation by examination and provision of objective evidence that specific requirements have been fulfilled." The purpose of verification is to provide a level of confidence that the plan is based on solid scientific principles, that adequate hazard controls are available, that the process and the controls are being followed.

Package-sealing verification involves the maintenance of the equipment, trained personnel, recorded calibration and targeted sampling and testing of incoming materials and finished packages. This testing must be based on a sound statistical rationale and be conducted by employing validated test methods and by trained personnel-124.

Verification is concerned with those activities, other than monitoring, that determine the validity of the HACCP Plan and that the system is operating according to the plan. There are different types of verifications that must take place within this principle. First, there are verification activities for CCPs to determine the personnel responsible and frequency to verify the results of those performing monitoring activities. This would typically be completed by supervisory or quality control personnel several times per shift.

Second, there must be a verification that the entire HACCP Plan is performing as expected and written. This is critical to complete following the initial implementation of the plan and at least annually thereafter. An external auditor who is unbiased during the review often performs this task. Third, there must be a plan validation completed upon implementation and annually thereafter. The validation process is defined as the scientific and technical process for determining that the Critical Control Points (CCPs) and Critical Control Limits (CCLs) are adequate and sufficient to control likely hazards -186.

For example, testing time-and-temperature recording devices to verify that a heat-processing unit is working the way it is expected to work. HACCP team needs to verify that the HACCP system is working. By doing these verifications, the establishment will initially evaluate the operation of the HACCP system and then maintain an updated and effective HACCP system.

Verification process can be categorized down into three steps:

- ❏ **V**alidation
- ❏ **V**erification
- ❏ **R**eassessment

Validation — it tests that the process with the Critical Control Limits (CCLs) prevents, eliminates, or reduces the hazard to an acceptable level. If a hot deli-serving table is to maintain food above 140ºF (60ºC), then validate that it does.

Verification — it assures that all required information is written down and documented. If cleaning of equipment is stated in the Hazard Analysis, then check that cleaning is done. Do what you say and say what you do. Verify the written statements.

Reassessment — Do at least annually. Consider potential new hazards. Examine changes in the preparation, raw materials or raw ingredients, personnel, packaging of the finished product, or any other changes that could affect the hazard analysis.

Verification procedures may include evaluation of CCPs and CCLs to determine if they are still appropriate; confirmation that monitoring alerts staff about hazards; and visual inspections to ensure that corrective actions are always taken.

HACCP Verification ensures that HACCP plan is running smoothly day after day, week after week, month after month, and year after year. Verification has several steps. The scientific or technical validity of the hazard analysis and the adequacy of the CCP's should be documented. The unparalleled performance of HACCP offers one's valuable facility can be easily monitored with annual verification. The results are cutting-edge food safety. HACCP verification could be best done by an audit. The HACCP Verification Audit is a comprehensive review of how HACCP plans are being implemented in a food manufacturing facility. The HACCP coordinator receives a thorough verification to help determine if HACCP plans are working as written. The external HACCP auditor reviews current plans, past records and makes on-site observations. The system should be subject to periodic internal audits, periodic revalidation using independent audits, or other verification procedures.

HACCP offers continuous and systematic approaches to assure food safety. From a regulatory point of view, there is a renewed interest in HACCP due to vulnerability of people to food safety related incidents. Both Agri-Canada and USDA are continuously monitoring affectivity of regulations through HACCP plans for the food industry. In addition to CCP monitoring, verification is the assurance and shall be conducted with following guidelines: -

a) Verification activities are an additional level of control and monitoring to ensure the HACCP plan is operating as it was designed. The verification activities are conducted in addition to the CCP monitoring, but on a less frequent basis, in order to review the implementation of the plan through the records or through additional tests or analysis. For each monitoring activity, the processor must establish and document verification procedures to ensure that the CCP is working as designed.

b) The verification procedures include what will be verified, how it will be verified, how frequently verification will be performed, and who will perform the verification.

c) Verification activities are performed by qualified personnel and usually by personnel not associated with monitoring of the CCP.

7. Documentation of HACCP System:

This would include records of hazards and their control methods, the monitoring of safety requirements and action taken to correct potential problems. Each of these principles must be backed by sound scientific knowledge: for example, published microbiological studies on time and temperature factors for controlling food-borne pathogens. Maintaining proper HACCP records is an essential part of the HACCP system. Good HACCP records — meaning that the records are accurate and complete.

Records serve as written documentation of the establishment's compliance with its HACCP plan. Records allow the retail facility to trace the history of an ingredient, in-process operations, or a finished product should problems arise. Records help identify trends in a particular operation that could result in a deviation if not corrected. Records could help identify and narrow the scope of a recall in the event a product recall becomes necessary. Records that are well maintained are good evidence in potential legal actions against an establishment. There may be new HACCP team members and the rationale for certain decisions is forgotten.

Record keeping is absolutely critical to a good Hazard Analysis and Critical Control Point system. It is imperative that required records be available and is complete, accurate, and timely. The consequences of not maintaining good records in a HACCP environment demand that companies meet the challenge of establishing efficient record-keeping procedures.

There are several types of records that must be maintained. Six Types of Records are normally maintained to satisfy the HACCP system. First is the written Hazard Analysis along with supporting documentation. Second is Records of practices that keep hazards from likely occurring are Cleaning Procedures, Manufacturing procedures, Employee training and Medical Records. Third is, the written HACCP Plan, which includes the decision-making, documents regarding critical control points and critical limits. Fourth, the production records relating to the monitoring of the critical control points. These forms should also include columns for documenting verifications and corrective actions, unless one elects to record these on another form. Fifth is HACCP plan and reassessments include Validations and Verifications. Operating Records may include Operating records of Critical Limits, Records of preventive maintenance, Records of quality analysis, Calibrations record, Cold stores temperature records etc.

Sixth and last type of record involves the pre-shipment approval testimony. This record must include verification that the critical control points have been properly monitored and met to release the product for shipment. The timing of this document is extremely critical to assure completion before the shipment of product. Without this step, product may be considered adulterated and subject to recall. This step is not fully clarified from a procedural or interpretation standpoint at this time. More information will follow in later chapters regarding this subject.

Individuals with record-keeping responsibilities need to be well trained. Complete records must include specified information such as the date, time, product, lot, monitoring data, and signature. Information must be recorded in ink. Records cannot be recorded in pencil, nor should white out or complete erasure be evident. Erroneous information should be lined out with initials and the correct information recorded. Records must also be timely. Production records should be completed throughout the day at the time of processing. These cannot be completed at the end of the shift from memory.

The training for HACCP should include a section on the importance of complete, accurate, and timely records. Furthermore, individuals with CCP responsibilities should go through an additional training session detailing their exact requirements. Laminated SOP's should also be established at each workstation to document the responsibilities associated with the CCP.

One last note on record-keeping responsibilities involves the organization of the record-keeping system. Records need to be maintained in an organized fashion and be available for review on request. It is helpful to have a centralized location to maintain the records.

There is new technology available to ease the burden of record keeping. Many systems have remote units to input CCP monitoring information. This information resides in a central computer, which maintains the information and alerts the user in the event of a deviation. These systems are moderately priced and offer many benefits to organize your record keeping system. They also simplify the process of pre-shipment approvals.

Records have to be maintained for specific periods of time. Slaughtered and refrigerated product records have to be retained for a period of one year. Frozen product records have to be retained for a period of two years. Records may be stored off site after six months, however they must be available to CFIA/FSIS within 24 hours of request. Electronic records are permissible. Such records should be designed with adequate security measures and be routinely backed up.

The last aspect is the protection of your Quality Assurance HACCP records. It is advised that all of your HACCP Plan and related records be designated as "Trade Secrets". Monitoring records should be designated as "Confidential Commercial Data". These steps will limit access to the documents through the Freedom of Information Act. Accordingly, the company must treat the documents as such to afford this protection. Companies should not make the documents available for public review-124. The records of established process and HACCP implementation records shall be maintained as per the following guidelines: -

a) Processors keep two types of records associated with HACCP, "documentation", and "records". Documentation refers to those records, which are created as a result of the development of the HACCP Plan, and records, which are created as a result of the implementation of the HACCP Plan.

b) Documentation is maintained as a record of HACCP Plan development, recognising the support and input from many individuals and usually over a considerable period of time. During this phase there are numerous decisions taken and authorities referenced. This information is essential to justify, if necessary, to regulatory agencies or customers why certain actions or activities are taken and also to assist in future development and evolution of the plan. Documentation includes the QAP, QMP and HACCP Plans as well as component parts such as SOPs. It also includes the hazard analysis, product attribute data, CCP determination, CCL validation data, personnel training records, calibration records, manufacturer specifications for operation and maintenance of specialized equipments.

c) Records are generated by the procedures or activities performed and any corrective actions taken. The processor establishes a record-keeping system that ensures that CCP monitoring records, corrective action records and verification records are complete, accurate, legible, and available for review. These records include all information required in the QAP, QMP and HACCP and are initialled or signed and dated by the person responsible for monitoring and by the person responsible for reviewing to verify the monitoring or corrective actions where this review is identified in the Plan as a verification activity. A blank copy of each record is included in the HACCP Plan for reference.

The complete solution to Food Safety Management is available from innovative services all over North America. HACCP modules allow the coordinator to rapidly create complex HACCP plans that may include unlimited number of HACCP 'Projects, multiple process flow charts per project, flow chart/process step linking, multiple hazards per process with Hazard Risk Analysis (HRA), multiple preventive measures per hazard, with "remembered" decision tree for each multiple CCP types for integration with quality and safety systems, five or more Critical factors for each CCP, monitoring methods, records, corrective Actions and verification for each CCP.

Documentation interface allows associating text files, spreadsheets, or even databases with each preventive measure and CCP, full reporting capability, including automatic generation of SOPs for each CCP.

For the supplier's materials and products, these modules enable the coordinator to maintain details of approved suppliers and supplier reviews, maintain details of materials and commodities used (for normal production and for hazardous materials), maintain details of products manufactured, generate HACCP-based recipes, apply "Flow-through" recipe costing, with automatic price updating for all materials price changes, set margins and selling prices, scale recipes, and carry out basic Material Review Plan (MRP).

The module could also maintain a "Batch Register" of products manufactured, including details of each supplier batch number used. One can quickly locate isolate all production containing a faulty supplier batch in the event of a recall.

Checklists function helps quickly set up key checks needed for prerequisite programs like pest control, cleaning and sanitation, internal audit, etc. Checklists may be generated for any subject, checklists can be printed for offline processing where needed check results may be recorded and retained in the database

The Document Control can be maintained which keeps HACCP description and revision details of all system documentation, including policies and procedures, work instructions and control forms. Each document record can be linked to the actual text or spreadsheet file created by the user, making HACCP module your central documentation source. If distributed, records of document holders will be maintained, and both filing details and document archives can be recorded if desired.

Calibration record can be maintained in the module. The module helps track calibration for all measuring and testing instruments: Individual record maintained for each item of equipment, users set calibration frequency, checkpoints and tolerances, program automatically extends next calibration date, schedules may be generated at any time, calibration data may be entered for all equipment, history is maintained, HACCP modules automatically reminds when calibration is overdue.

Problem Management can be recorded to trace back incidence in manufacturing plant. The Incidents module could have a profound effect on the success of food safety system. It is intended to be used to record every food safety or quality related problem, including supplier performance, raw material defects, processing deficiencies, customer complaints, operational problems, quality defects, audit deficiencies requiring corrective action. Information may be entered for each incident, including remedial and long-term corrective action.

Users can nominate a person responsible for rectifying each incident, and the expected completion date. HACCP module automatically tracks each problem through to closeout, and reminds when unresolved by the nominated date. Detailed analysis and reporting should be available.

Personnel and training is an integral part of HACCP. The HACCP coordinator shall be aware that part of the responsibility is to demonstrate that food-manufacturing employees have received adequate training. These modules should be able to track competency or outcomes-based training provided to entire workforce. Specify competency requirements for each employee, maintain details of all training programs and course modules, with outcomes per module, maintain records of attendance at all internal and external training, including costs, record skill assessment tests and schedule certification renewals and track current and past employee training.

Internal audits are the corrective factor of the Food Safety Operation (FSO). Module recommended should be able to schedule and record all internal audits needed to verify that the system has been implemented and that is effective. Set up an audit schedule for all user-defined elements of the food safety system. HACCP modules available in the market are designed to automatically track audits due and remind you when not completed by the scheduled date, enter results each time an audit is conducted, generate and print audit findings and generate Corrective Actions for audit deficiencies.

Qamrul A. Khanson

Chapter: 06
HACCP: THE ULTIMATE SOLUTION

Overview:

The Space-age technology designed to keep food safe in outer space became standard for the food manufacturing industry in North America and all over the world. The countries in oil rich Gulf countries have simultaneously introduced and adopted HACCP principles in their food production. Canada, United States, and EU have been in the forefront of HACCP revolution.

USDA, FSIS and US-FDA, in the United States, Health-Canada, Agri-Canada and CFIA in Canada have already adopted a food safety program developed nearly 43 years ago for astronauts and is being applied to dairy food, meat products, seafood, bakery, beverages and juice. These agencies have developed pilot programs with the cooperation of food industry and intend to eventually use it for much of the food supply in North America. The program for the astronauts focused on preventing hazards that could cause food-borne illnesses by applying science-based controls, from raw material to finished products. Those involved with food production and safety will follow the suit by eliminating pathogens and food spoilage microorganisms from ready to eat food.

Traditionally, industry and regulators have depended on spot-checks of manufacturing conditions and random sampling of final products to ensure safe food. This approach, however, tends to be reactive, rather than preventive, and can be less efficient than the new system. The preventive system is Hazard Analysis and Critical Control Point (HACCP). Many of its principles already are in place in the government-regulated food industry. US-FDA established HACCP for the seafood industry in a final rule December 18, 1995 and for the juice industry in a final rule released January 19, 2001. The final rule for the juice industry has taken effect on January 22 2002 for large and medium businesses, on January 21, 2003 for small businesses, and the final rule for very small businesses took place on January 20, 2004.

In 1998, the U.S. Department of Agriculture has established HACCP for meat and poultry processing plants, as well. Most of these establishments were required to start using HACCP by January 1999. Very small plants had until Jan. 25, 2000. USDA regulates meat and poultry and FDA all other foods. FDA now is considering developing regulations that would establish HACCP as the food safety standard throughout other areas of the food industry, including both domestic and imported food products.

To help determine the degree to which such regulations would be feasible, the agency is conducting pilot HACCP programs with volunteer food companies. The programs have involved cheese, frozen dough, breakfast cereals, salad dressing, bread, flour, and other products. The National Academy of Sciences-USA, the Codex Alimentarius Commission an international food standard-setting organization, and the National Advisory Committee on Microbiological Criteria have endorsed HACCP for Foods. A number of U.S. food companies already use the system in their manufacturing processes, and it is in use in other countries, including Canada-[87].

Necessity of HACCP:

Microbiological hazards took a lead in risk factors and challenged the food manufacturers and regulators. There are many challenges to the food industry in present times. North American cultural diversity adds value to food system. New challenges to the food supplies have prompted US-FDA to consider adopting a HACCP-based food safety system on a wider basis. The most challenging task for food regulators is to control microbial contaminants, which cause panic and hazards to general public health. In eighties, bacteria not previously recognized as important cause of food-borne illnesses--such as _Escherichia coli_ O157:H7 and _Salmonella enteritidis_, became more prevalent.

Chemical contaminants are second in line to challenge the natural food resources and its usage as ingredient in factory manufactured food. There is also increasing public health concern about chemical contamination of food: for example, the effects of lead in food on the nervous system. Exposure to a chemical in food approach or exceed the acceptable level of intake, maximum levels for chemicals in food may be set by Codex often based on at the lowest level achievable as shown by data submitted by countries. Chemical contamination of food may lead to toxic or allergenic reactions in humans and animals.

Diversity in food manufacturing and consumption is posing challenges of its own importance. This important factor is that the size of the food industry and the diversity of products and processes have grown tremendously in the amount of domestic food manufactured and the number and kinds of foods imported. The three key issues– "Diversity, Quality, Safety" – must be central to our whole approach towards Agriculture and food production. We must fundamentally review the Community role in relation to food safety. In Canada, diversity in food and Agricultural systems needs to be protected and promoted. Local systems of production and traditional products are fundamental to this diversity. We must, collectively, seize this opportunity in the interests of our citizens and our responsibility to maintain a diverse, high quality and safe system of food production. Today, HACCP is more needed to protect and expand the diversified Canadian food system.

International trade is creating necessity to unify and evolve a common food safety system for better international food safety. The need for HACCP in Canada and the United States, particularly in the seafood, dairy and juice industries, is fuelled by the growing trend in international trade for worldwide equivalence of food products and the Codex Alimentarius Commission's adoption of HACCP as the international standard for food safety. The future trend in HACCP can be moulded today and we must understand few facts about the HACCP concept.

HACCP does not stand alone in the food safety system. It is interlinked and it embeds, GMP's, SOPs, Plant design, Recalls, Preventive maintenance, QC Programs, Training and Prerequisite programs that are the building blocks to HACCP.

HACCP is a hazard preventive and food safety system for the food manufacturing industry. The system is based on seven declared principles under which the system works.

HACCP is Plant and product specific, a systematic approach to food safety, hazard preventive, adaptive, dynamic, flexible, only as good as those found and identified hazards and a predictor of what can go wrong.

HACCP is not a total quality control system, a tool to manage the entire facility, an absolute guarantee of food safety, and a static system. However, it is amalgamable with ISO-9000 systems to provide a total quality system.

HACCP is needed because of Technological advances in food processing and packaging, Diversified food pattern, Diversified cultural requirements in North America, Emerging food borne pathogens, Diminishing inspectional resources, New food distribution and consumption patterns, Increasing public health safety concerns and promotion of Global food trade.

HACCP is recognised internationally. The system is designed to remove food trade barriers among nations and it is designed to promote diversified food with human health safety objectives. All food safety conscious food-manufacturing units voluntarily adopt HACCP and simultaneously the system is being enforced by regulatory agencies in Canada and the United States of America.

HACCP is economically viable system, concept, and a process that can be applied to a product when it is innocuous, nutritive, appetizing, and if it satisfies the expectations of the consumer in national and international markets alike.

HACCP Advantages:

Knowledge is an important tool to succeed. The past-current system of food safety offered some protection but guarantees were more verbal than comprehension. A passion for safe food is a necessity but its achievement requires scientific approach to latest production technology, hygiene, and quality monitoring. Thus a system, which has number of advantages over the past-current system, requires implementation with conviction. The International Dairy Foods Association (**IDFA**) launched a comprehensive Hazard Analysis and Critical Control Point (HACCP) certification and training program that will train food technologists with operation to fully meet the requirements for U.S. dairy and juice plants. With the advent of a HACCP pilot program from NCIMS and the US Food and Drug Administration's (US-FDA) mandatory program for juice plants, HACCP is, more than ever, the best food safety choice for food manufacturers. Such initiatives create better understanding; advancement of knowledge and food manufacturing becomes a specialized field. How HACCP impacts our food safety drive and how it is comparatively advantageous, must be learnt.

The HACCP concept calls for identifying those points in an operation, which are important in the prevention of significant food borne hazards, and identifying the hazards associated with each such point. Controls are then established at these critical points and systematically monitored to prevention of a hazard.

HACCP focuses on identifying and preventing hazards from contaminating food. It is based on scientific reasoning and it permits more efficient and effective government oversight. It is primarily because the record keeping allows auditors to see how well a firm is complying with food safety laws over a period rather than how well it is doing on any given day. This system places responsibility for ensuring food safety appropriately on the food manufacturer and all those who are involved in its distribution and handling.

Implementing a single, more-focused method for product safety, efficiency and cost savings would create confidence among factory workers, quality assurance, vendors, and profitability in the business. HACCP endorses all matters, which are related to food safety in a factory.

By implementing HACCP in ones food plant, one would improve relationship with state and federal officials and will be commended for better quality standards nationally and internationally depending on the size of business.

HACCP implemented food plants are better prepared for inspections by potential clients, regulatory agencies, and government officials.

HACCP criteria can be measured through reductions in *Salmonella* prevalence and Food borne Illness. This is judged by improvements in food safety as measured by prevalence data on *Salmonella* and reductions in food borne illness. The data demonstrate that all sized plants show improvement in all categories of product over baseline studies conducted prior to HACCP implementation. For example, 50 percent reductions have been achieved in broilers and ground beef. Overall reductions in *Salmonella* prevalence demonstrate the success of the performance standards in conjunction with HACCP in improving the safety of meat, poultry, fisheries, dairy, and bakery products.

Regulatory reforms in the Canadian and U.S. food industry were possible because of food safety concerns. HACCP brought success in this direction by updating sanitation requirements, performance standards, encouraged innovations, legalizing certain preservatives to improve food safety and finally eliminating non-result oriented regulations.

Farm-to-Table Strategy worked in United States by implementing HACCP. Food safety strategy addresses every step in the process of producing animals on the farm, converting them into food products, distributing the products to consumers, and preparing these products for consumption. Safety of foods during distribution is governed by government standards regulated by FSIS and FDA.

HACCP introduced efficient system for ensuring safety of seafood than had previously existed. The Seafood HACCP regulation does not replace the need for seafood manufacturers to comply with GMP Regulations. It is an additional measure. HACCP differs from GMP for foods in that it requires a proactive approach to food safety. While the food GMP maintains that food must be manufactured, processed, held, and packaged in sanitary conditions, it does not require any record keeping.

Regional foods and its trade are now impacted by HACCP. In every region of the world, people are addicted to their own delicacies. There are traditional processors who can provide a better taste food but safety remains an issue. By respecting the food diversity, modern techniques could bring safety and expand these regional and traditional foods in the world market. The commercialization of food trade has necessitated the adoption of HACCP not only in North America but Europe and rest of the world. HACCP helps food manufacturing companies to compete more effectively in the world market because it help advance the safe food trading by reducing barriers to international trade.

Voluntary recalling of suspected food products from the market has become the standard with food manufacturers in North America, Europe, and GCC. First of all, these recalls are instituted because of HACCP system, which systemises the recalls in case of suspected contaminants in marketed food. To help prevent future outbreaks, stricter HACCP regulations and HACCP corrective actions are implemented to eliminate recurrence.

Refrigerated transportation is a key to expanded food trade. HACCP studies indicate that human error accounts for up to 80 percent of cargo losses during transportation. Luckily, major contamination outbreaks have not yet been the result of ineffective transport temperature control. Most often, as is the case in many outbreak incidents, the contamination source is the result of manufacturing and/or processing errors. Thus a cleanest possible environment for the transportation of perishable foodstuffs is part of HACCP system. In addition, uniform temperatures throughout the load ensure product integrity. The worst problem is to deliver perishable cargo of inconsistent quality." An inclusion of HACCP system in refrigeration of food products in factory stores and in refrigerated truck transports enhances food safety and confidence.

HACCP software tools, which are available in the market, can assist users in creating a systematic food safety environment by managing the many details of a HACCP system. Such tools could ease the work for food processors, food service institutions, food sellers, educational institutions, consultants, and food handlers to ease HACCP education, plan creation implementation, and plan maintenance. Assist in the development of a complete HACCP system based on emerging world HACCP standards and the NACMCF92 standards (National Advisory Committee for Microbiological Criteria in Foods, 1992). Such software enables the formation of a HACCP system around any food production or distribution system by providing an easy to use "drag & drop" method of building the flow of materials-[87].

Enhanced public health has been very well impacted by the application of HACCP system. In past many years, public concern regarding food safety had build-up as a consequence of the outbreak of bovine Spongiform Encephalopathy (BSE) in cattle, the prevalence of *Salmonella* serotype *enteritidis* illnesses (from poultry, meat, eggs), and the more localized outbreaks of illnesses associated with _Listeria monocytogenes_ (from dairy products, pâté, salads) and _Escherichia coli_ O157:H7 (from ground or minced beef, unpasteurized apple juice, vegetables). Emerging pathogens and the appearance of problems such as BSE have resulted in enactment of specific controls in many countries, while the general heightening of interest internationally has prompted health professionals and the food industry in many countries to scrutinize the control of emerging infectious agents by following HACCP principles.

Adherence to good manufacturing practices and good hygienic practices and application of the HACCP system can result in food safety and ensure food quality. Food safety is the shared responsibility of governments, academia, the food industry, and the consumers.

Control over the occurrence of potential hazards in the food supply is the nucleus of Food safety. HACCP is a prevention-focused food safety tool that requires identification, monitoring, and control of specific food borne hazards that are biological, chemical, or physical in nature. HACCP allows the user to focus hazard control efforts on specific critical points in a process. The processor gains efficiency and a greater assurance of food safety. When combined with a good hazard analysis technique, it allows safety and quality to be built into each step in the process from product formulation specifications to product distribution.

Increased consumer confidence in the safety of the food supply has been noticed after the HACCP introduction in the food industry. Trends in consumer perceptions of risk in foods and of individual responsibility in preventing food borne illness provide one indication of consumers' receptivity to food safety knowledge. The percent of consumer's complete confidence or mostly confident in the safety of the food supply increased from a low of 72 percent in 1992-93 to a high of 83 percent in 1996. The percent of consumers who consider bacteria in food a "serious health risk" increased during 1995-97. Consumers' sense of their own responsibility for ensuring food safety may increase their motivation to follow food safety recommendations-[36].

Better oversight and use of resources by governing parties in different countries have been noticed. In 1995 U.S. Department of Agriculture proposed to require new food safety procedures in meat and poultry plants are the first step in a long-term strategy that will fundamentally transform the Food Safety and Inspection Service and its food safety program. Michael R. Taylor, USDA acting under secretary for food safety mentions "To achieve our food safety goal, we must also reinvent the existing FSIS regulations to make them compatible with an entirely new approach to regulation. And we must reinvent FSIS itself--how it defines its regulatory roles, allocates its resources and organizes itself to do its food safety job, Our food safety strategy for the future goes beyond our rule making to implement the HACCP".

Beyond the obvious benefits, HACCP provides to minimizing food borne illness, there are significant economic benefits. The USDA Economic Research Service estimates - in a period of 25 - years an average of 4.6 to 22.19 billion dollars will be saved with the implementation of HACCP. Social Account Matrices (SAM) were developed to incorporate the cost of implementing HACCP and the benefits of reducing food borne illnesses.

Every dollar of income saved by the prevention of premature death caused from food borne illness results in an economic gain of $1.92.
 The Net impact of costs and benefits of HACCP is increased in production output of $7 billion. There is an increased factor portion of $5.6 billion. There is an increased household income of $9.33 billion. If the benefits of reduced work were to be included, net benefits would be greater.

Canadian Food Inspection Agency's Food Safety Enhancement Program (FSEP) developed to guide Canadian food manufacturers has many advantages and benefits, which are either, equal to or additional to generic benefits of HACCP.

Benefits Internationally and Nationally

a) International Acceptance: Internationally, FSEP principles are consistent with the principles and application of the Hazard Analysis Critical Control Points (HACCP) system, developed by the Working Group of Codex Alimentarius. International markets will be maintained or expanded as HACCP based programs are accepted worldwide.

b) National Acceptance: The introduction of FSEP meets national expectations to include HACCP principles in food inspection. Nationally, FSEP principles are consistent with Good Manufacturing Practices (GMP) regulations proposed by Health and Welfare Canada, Fisheries and Oceans Canada's Quality Management Program (QMP) and with HACCP initiatives in the provinces. FSEP will provide the means to apply HACCP principles uniformly across all commodities.

To start with FSEP, back in 1994, many Canadian companies started inputting HACCP-based food safety program following the guidelines of the FSEP Manuals, Volumes 1 and 2 plus the appropriate models. The following two years a number of revisions were made to the existing volumes, Volumes 3 and 4 were written, other models for a variety of products were developed, and the hazard database started. It is interesting to note that this activity was taking place before the Jack-in-the-Box incident in January 1993 and the panic situation facing the U.S. over the lack of development of food safety programs. Many companies at that time were reviewing finished product and trends on with Agriculture and Agri-Food Canada (**AAFC**) and other regulatory jurisdictions at a yearly review meeting. Such a practice is a part of Total Quality Management (TQM) and led to the industry government cooperation towards food safety.

c) Responsibilities Defined: FSEP enhances the principles of shared responsibility for food inspection in Canada. By clarifying the respective roles and responsibilities of both government and industry regarding inspection activities, this sharing of responsibility can occur without loss of assurance of food safety. The policy and regulatory environment within which the services are delivered and implemented continue to be progressive at the same time subject to punitive actions if the compliance leads to or probability of leading to food poisoning.

d) Improved Marketability: The use of special logos or symbols, which are recognized nationally and internationally, may have a significant impact on the marketability of product produced under FSEP. To maintain and/or expand our international markets it will be essential to have inspection processes in place acceptable to those countries to which we export. The Canadian Food Inspection Agency, in cooperation with industry, wishes to be proactive with regard to this reality and will maintain effective contact with these countries to ensure their acceptance of FSEP.

As domestic markets are maintained or expanded, Agri-food products will have to meet the expectations of the Canadian consumer who demands a safe and high quality food product. Producers and processors from federally registered establishments will have to demonstrate that their products meet this demand. Knowing this, the consumer can be assured of safe and wholesome food products. FSEP is constantly looking to expand its activities to all food sectors by developing links and partnerships with individuals and companies, particularly in the area of food safety assistance and implementation.

e) Standardization of Food safety: HACCP regulators also benefit from the standardization HACCP brings. Benefits for the industry in terms of harmonization within the North American and EU regulatory bodies have been recognised as well as the improvement of practices and controls for the food industry.

Benefits to Industry and Government:

a) Positive Communication: Closer communication will result between inspection and industry staff. This communication will permit informal, as well as formal, exchange of information related to safe handling of food products.

The CFIA, working in collaboration with other levels of government, producers, processors, and distributors has developed a food inspection system that Canadians have confidence in, and is respected worldwide. During the past year, CFIA inspectors, veterinarians, and scientists regulated the food system to enforce provisions of the federal food safety and quality statutes.

The CFIA shares responsibility for food safety with producers, processors, distributors, retail outlets, and consumers, as well as with other government organizations and jurisdictions. As an agency responsible for enforcement of federal legislation, the CFIA uses data on compliance rates and other quantitative and qualitative information to measure its success in achieving the objectives of the Government of Canada.

b) Resource Impact: Government will have the ability to direct its resources towards those plants not currently able to produce product under HACCP. This will permit government to direct its resources in a sequential fashion, from high risk to low risk, depending on product type, establishment compliance, or plant complexity.

Focusing on food processing establishments or production lines considered to be higher risk areas will permit a more efficient use of inspection resources for both the industry and government allowing both to achieve maximum effect at minimal cost.

Four key management commitments form the basis for vision of how the Government will deliver their services and benefits to Canadians in the new millennium. In this vision, departments and agencies recognise that they exist to serve Canadians and that a "citizen focus" shapes all activities, programs and services. This vision commits the government of Canada to manage its business by the highest public service values. Responsible spending means spending wisely on the things that matter to Canadians. Finally, this vision sets a clear focus on results - the impact and effects of programs.

Over the coming years, the Agency will continue to assess its priorities and examine resource options in order to meet program standards prescribed by legislation and increases in demand for CFIA services due to growing market conditions. Agency has a positive impact on Canada's food industry, which contributes approximately $45 billion annually to the Canadian economy. By bringing about industry compliance with federal regulations, the CFIA helps the Canadian food industry maintain and strengthen its excellent national and international reputation for safe, quality products. As a result, the industry continues to support the social and economic well being of Canadians.

c) Strategic Partnerships: The CFIA's success in protecting the food safety system, the health of animals and plants depends upon the expertise and support of other federal departments, provincial/territorial/municipal governments, producers, industry, distributors, retailers and consumers.

The production of meat provides a good example of collaboration and working together as partners. Provincial governments regulate how an animal is raised and the CFIA provides inspection services at slaughter and processing plants that move product interprovincially or internationally. The provinces provide inspection services at smaller plants that sell within their jurisdiction, and municipal authorities enforce public health standards at restaurants that serve the final product.

Although the three levels of government are working together to maintain a safe food supply, food safety is everybody's business. In the final analysis, successful collaboration among all the players is vital in protecting food safety system and the health of Canada's animals and plants. Ongoing efforts by the Government of Canada and the provincial and territorial governments to improve effectiveness and efficiency are contributing to a more integrated and harmonized food inspection system for Canada.

d) Reduced Recalls/Product Destruction: Increased plant employee awareness and responsibility will result in rapid and efficient response to deviations at critical control points in the process. Not only will minor problems be corrected in an efficient manner, but the enhanced on-line monitoring of product will result in reduced recalls and/or product destruction due to compliance deviations with respect to safety concerns.

This will have a direct impact on the processor while having an indirect impact on the processors' clients. Sometimes products listed in the food recall archive have been subject to removal from the marketplace for appropriate corrective action. Food recalls or allergy alerts are not an indication of the food safety status of products produced at a later date.

The mandate of the food Safety Program is also to regulate and monitor compliance of the advertisement, sale and importation of hazardous products that are not covered by other legislation and to provide clients with safety information.

Benefits to Government:

a) Relationship with Other Programs: Implementation of FSEP by an establishment may permit a streamlining of other programs currently requiring inspection services, e.g. export certification. Special agreements may be possible with specific trade partners, which will reduce the need for direct inspection control over certain products. In such an endeavour, Guelph Food Technology Centre (GFTC) completed part of its ongoing training programs in Good Manufacturing Practices (GMPs) and Hazard Analysis Critical Control Points (HACCP) implementation with Japanese companies. The program is run for Keiran-Niku Joho Center. This ongoing relationship underscores Canada's international reputation as a leader in HACCP implementation, and GFTC's position as Canada's largest HACCP trainer."

Similarly the government of Alberta emphasized Canada's high safety standards and HACCP compliance while making a pitch for Alberta canola oil and Alberta beef in Japan through HACCP related business seminar in Japan's southern island of Kyushu. Such cooperation's and relationships with other internal and external food safety programs strengthen Canada's resolve in this sector.

The Canadian government and the fish processing industry developed and implemented a close relationship with HACCP and fish specific safety plan the Quality Management Program (QMP). Its introduction represented the first time that five of the seven principles of the Hazard Analysis Critical Control Point (HACCP) inspection system were incorporated in a mandatory food inspection system. This was a critical step for the industry to remain competitive in a global market. Indeed, this program has served the industry well and has kept Canada in a leadership role. Later Canada had to develop up-to-date training, which would address all seven HACCP principles and stand compatible with U.S. and the European Union inspections' new protocols. New partnerships were created to develop standards and curriculum and the program's modified new name became a Quality Management Program Revised (QMPR). The new partnerships involved educational institutions, the federal government, regulatory agencies, and the Sector Council, which includes representatives and experts from within the industry.

The collaborative work of various stakeholders during the developmental and implementation phases of QMPR, HACCP, and other courses, and with the Youth and Science Technology Internship Program, has resulted in concrete and successful outcomes. These initiatives were innovative, timely, and specific to industry's requirements.

Many on-farm food safety programs in Canada are aligned with the CFIA's Hazard Analysis Critical Control Point (HACCP) system. HACCP and HACCP-based systems are meant to complement and build on traditional methods of food safety assurances such as good production practices and inspection programs.

b) Response to the Increases in Inspection Demands: The implementation of FSEP by industry compliments the increased inspection resource demands within the food inspection system, e.g. imports. The Canadian Food Inspection Agency will be in a better position to respond to new priorities and the increased requirements within its existing resource base.

Canadian citizens expect their federal and provincial governments to formulate and implement regulations and to ensure compliance with regulations in the public interest. There is a need to general monitoring against set standards conducted on a multi-year planned basis.

The Canadian Food Inspection Agency is mandated to enhance the efficiency and effectiveness of federal inspection and related services for food, animal, and plant health. Health Canada's Food Safety Assessment Program (**FSAP**) assesses the effectiveness of the CFIA's activities related to food safety. This includes reviewing the design and operational delivery of CFIA's programs related to food safety, assessing compliance with health and safety standards and evaluating the results achieved.

The Therapeutic Products Program (**TPP**) is a regulatory authority that manages the benefits and risks of products intended for therapeutic use in Canada, with the goal of ensuring that the public has access to safe, effective, and high quality products that adhere to quality and safety standards.

The Product Safety Program (**PSP**) administers the Hazardous Products Act (**HPA**), which provides the authority to control, restrict, or prohibit certain materials, as well as the sale, importation and advertisement of other dangerous or potentially dangerous consumer and industrial products. On behalf of the employer in the Public Service, Health Canada takes the responsibility for co-ordinating health and safety programming across departments.

Benefits of these programs, agencies, and departments go beyond their target jobs. The targets of regulatory and inspection activity vary. The work of CFIA is largely one of regulating an on-going activity in the market place. Health Canada does post-market surveillance (i.e., monitoring the manufacturing, distribution and use of the product in the market place for any indications of adverse effects that could necessitate changes in the product or the marketing regime). The two areas offer some potential for improvement between CFIA and Health Canada with respect to food safety, and between HRDC and Health Canada with respect to occupational health and safety.

c) FSEP and the Market place: To maintain and/or expand our international markets it will be essential to have inspection processes in place acceptable to those countries to which we export. The Canadian Food Inspection Agency, in cooperation with industry, wishes to be proactive with regard to this reality and will maintain effective contact with these countries to ensure their acceptance of FSEP.

As domestic markets are maintained or expanded, Agri-food products will have to meet the expectations of the Canadian consumer who demands a safe and high quality food product. Producers and processors from federally registered establishments will have to demonstrate that their products meet this demand. Knowing this, the consumer can be assured of safe and wholesome food products.

Current State of HACCP

Hazard Analysis and Critical Control Point (HACCP) began as an assurance of safety for the food, it has strong academic roots, and many books and courses exist for scientific HACCP. As originally developed, HACCP was strictly a food-safety program, and quality was not a part of the program.

The early food laws put a great emphasis on chemical adulteration; filth; insects, rodents, the use of rotten or decomposed raw materials; product composition and economic violations, short fills, drained weights etc. To help combat such problems, the FDA has had a program of surprise inspections of food establishments and random sampling of products from the trade since its inception. Anyone familiar with sampling plans recognizes that random sampling of a very small portion of a company's production only uncovers problems that are very common to that company. Continuing economic violations and mislabelling would be easy to discover due to the ongoing nature of such problems, but random bacterial contamination and inadvertent adulteration with allergens would be difficult to discover.

Infrequent inspections of a plant only affect the most blatant operators. For an effective inspection, the inspector needs to know the plant. Even if an inspector visits a plant on a frequent basis, there's opportunity to try and slip something by him or her. In addition, with closed records, how can an inspector know if there are problems with process controls and infrequent environmental contamination?

HACCP puts the burden of control where it belongs - on the people making the food. However, proper use and storage of food by consumers is also a problem. No one can protect consumers from themselves, so there's a need for consumer education on the proper storage and preparation of food, even beyond label statements.

Implementation issues:

The Hazard Analysis and Critical Control Point (HACCP) system has now become generally accepted as the key safety management system for the food industry worldwide. HACCP programs are based upon the Current Good Manufacturing Practice (cGMP) for the Manufacturing, Packing, or Holding of Human Food. The GMPs are changed as the state of the industry and knowledge changes, and the proposed changes are published in the Federal Register for comment prior to being changed. Under the GMPs are the "defect action levels" for naturally occurring defects that do not exempt a company from operating a sanitary facility.

In some cases, the US-FDA has promulgated current GMPs for specific industries. For example: quality control procedures assuring the nutrient content of infant formulas (21 CFR 106); current GMP regulations for thermally processed low-acid foods in hermetically sealed containers and for acidified foods and current GMP regulations for bottled water.

In other cases, industry associations have used a combination of industry and academic experts to develop industry-specific current GMPs. A recent example of this is the *Guidelines for Developing Good Manufacturing Practices and Standard Operating Procedures for Raw Ground Products*. These guidelines were coordinated for the National Meat Association by the Institute of Food Science and Engineering at Texas A&M University, College Station.

The lack of reference, however, by the USDA/FSIS (Food Safety Inspection Service) to the current GMPs has been cited as a problem with that agency's program. It should be noted that all USDA-inspected meat and poultry plants are required to have a "Standard Sanitation Operating Procedure" in place for all lines prior to implementing HACCP.

Prerequisite programs are essential. It is impossible to implement a HACCP program without the prerequisite programs in place, but it is possible to write a HACCP program without them. Lack of prerequisite programs and lack of company understanding of the HACCP principles have proven to be a problem. Another problem, according to Jeffery Brown, consumer safety officer with the FDA, is wrong and false information being dispensed by consultants and other 'experts.'

Verifying the control points of a HACCP plan - and validating that the plan actually controls the critical control points - is of paramount importance. Bill Smith, assistant deputy administrator, USDA/FSIS, states that there has to be a scientific reason for the control point, and that the control limits must be deliverable every day, and for each step, for the system in question. Consider, for example, that a company writes a cook time of 160°F (71.20 C) for 30 seconds as the critical limit for their process. Once in operation, however, the heat distribution and loading of the equipment make it impossible to maintain 160°F (71.20 C) in all parts of the product, and worse, the company finds a pathogen in the product after processing. Variation in the system prevents the maintenance of the critical temperature. Thus an upper and a lower limit shall be in place to control such variations.

Ken Gall, seafood specialist with the New York Sea Grant Extension Program, says that the major problems encountered by industry are: sanitation programs that are in place, but not being monitored and verified that HACCP plans are being implemented correctly according to the knowledge of the HACCP principles. He also observes that, overall, training has eased implementation and that compliance by the industry is good.

HACCP implementation process should use relevant scenario exercises. It allows industry to do what is best with minimal regulatory interference. Environmental medicine and infectious disease practitioners are also finding benefits from the HACCP pathogen management system. The environmental health, holistic and preventive medicine clinicians, and Agriculture veterinarians have been using parts of HACCP principles for years. Law in many industries for food safety purposes requires HACCP. HACCP concepts have been used for a number of years to prevent drug residues in food products. Many Agriculture commodities have seen their competitor lose markets because of residues. All the industries, which provide appetite for human alimentary canal, are striving for far-reaching HACCP benefits with out reservation. The implementation issues are not impediments to its application.

Prerequisites to HACCP:

The National Advisory Committee in the United States has recommended that HACCP be based upon a solid foundation of prerequisite programs. These programs include:

- ❑ **F**acilities design and maintenance
- ❑ **L**abel control
- ❑ **F**ormula control
- ❑ **P**est control
- ❑ **T**raceability and recall
- ❑ **Q**uality-control procedures
- ❑ **S**upplier control
- ❑ **P**rocess procedures
- ❑ **S**pecifications
- ❑ **C**alibration of instruments
- ❑ **P**roduction equipment
- ❑ **C**leaning and sanitation
- ❑ **P**ersonal hygiene
- ❑ **C**hemical control
- ❑ **T**raining
- ❑ **R**eceiving, storage and shipping

HACCP for Bakery: Organoleptic quality is the secret ingredient in every bakery product and the safety of bakery product is the life of the consumer attracted by that secret ingredient. The HACCP approach in bakery takes isolated quality control procedures at various points in the process and puts them together as a system thus enhancing shelf life, organoleptic quality, and safety on the shelf. HACCP points interrelate in such a manner as to prevent situations that are outside standards and specifications, therefore could cause a major hazard without the information being picked up through the monitoring system. Thus, preventive techniques in bakery are not unique but specific to individual segments of the bakery, which require same treatments as other ingredients like meat and milk when used with the final bakery products.

Ingredients play a decisive role in post-baked bakery products. The full potential of HACCP in the bakery industry could only be realised when Meat, Poultry, Fish and Fruit industry are fully mandated with HACCP program because these segments interlink the applied bakery products like pastries, stuffed baked patties, and bread with mince and cake with cream, fruits and nuts. The ordinary loaf, Greek bread, and French bread are well taken care due to their non-involvement with post baking stage. Thus the fate of the HACCP system with bakery is directly linked and adoption of the system would require more and clear emphasis on the supplies of ingredients for post baking additions, seasoning and patting.

CFIA monitors the bakery products, its ingredients list, and its recall whenever need is materialised. Consumer's sensitivity to ingredients and its non-declaration is closely watched by the agency. The operators of the industry are warned to notify immediately if and when an allergen is added to the product incidentally, intentionally but not declared or unintentionally and not investigated in time. The Canadian Food Inspection Agency (CFIA) administers the federal labelling requirements for pre-packaged foods. The CFIA is monitoring the effectiveness of the recall whenever the calls are initiated with perfect reason. Such an example could be traced to a recall in Januray-2003 when Canadian Food Inspection Agency (CFIA) and Grain fields Bakery warned consumers with sensitivities to sulphites not to consume Grain fields Bakery Granola Deluxe. This product was expected to contain sulphites, which were not declared on the label. This alert was initiated due to concern of those individuals who had sensitivities to sulphites.

Rheology could also become a safety issue in bakery and confectionary products. The monitoring of products where rheology plays a decisive role in causing illness to consumer has been traced and recalled by CFIA. According to information obtained by the CFIA (2001), mini-cup jelly products are traditionally manufactured in South-east Asia and sold under various brand names. Individual jellies are about the size of coffee creamer (16 - 17 g), with rounded edges. These products usually contain a flavoured centre enclosed in a shell of konjac jelly. These mini-cup jelly products may become lodged in the throat and may be difficult to remove due to their consistency. There have been fatalities reportedly linked to these products, including several recent deaths in the United States. One fatality in Canada was reported in the year 2000. It is important for consumers to heed the warning on the outside package stating that children and seniors should not consume these products without supervision-113.

Antibiotics in bakery ingredients are to be watched by CFIA. As a part of CFIA's testing program, the test provides consumers with an assurance that Canadian honey is free of harmful residues. The HACCP drive by CFIA also checks antibiotics in imported honey, which is also used as an ingredient in bakery products. A recent case was caught when chloramphenicol residues were found in imported honey. This antibiotic also called "Chloromycetin" was discontinued for general use in North America many years ago because of the health risk.

Ingredient suppliers in Canada are not behind the race when it comes to HACCP. The bakery ingredient suppliers are also encouraged to get HACCP certification by CFIA so that their market image improves and that image turns to increased profits. Well known ingredients producers and suppliers in Canada are switching to HACCP system, which follows strict regulatory guidelines to prevent potential errors, which may impact on food safety.

HACCP for Beverages: Juice industry took a beating from the safety issue when unpasteurized juices were found to contain microorganism-causing illness to the weaker immune people and children. It is a case of science that bacteria belonging to Enterobacteriaceae dwindle their multiplication under lower pH values if stored for a particular period and storage temperature. That will all depend on their numbers per ml of juice. If the count is < 10 per ml then it is expected that it will take at least ten days to reduce that number to <01 per ml. The pattern of counting the benefit of that science missed the other variables and stuck to the theory, which failed the test causing illness to many.

Acidity in juice is nourishing but may play a bactericidal role under certain circumstances. HACCP implementation does not allow that chance to be taken at the cost of some ones life. When it is proved that _E. coli_ survives lower pH and do not die when the juice is in the market then something should be done to make the juice free from such contaminants. If the standards are kept at absent in 100 ml juice then achieving even <0 per ml of juice is absolutely accepted. Let us always plan a standard better than regulatory requirements so that any odd sample will also be within the regulatory limits.

Principles of HACCP and their application in juice industry mean a critical approach to safety. The critical control points and fixation of critical control limits with juice products should be seen with proper processing technology and proper packaging. Unpasteurized juices would require much more stringent measures to achieve an Enterobacteriaceae free beverage. The problem is the consumption of these unpasteurized juices will take place well ahead of any analytical results leaving complete and religious preventive techniques in the form of HACCP.

Water for commercial bottling plant would require much better standards to prevent any form of impurities in bottled water. At stake are the microbiological quality, mineral content, and the pH of the bottled water. The purest water with zero TDS could have a pH of 7 ± 0.1. Many health conscious people are switching to extremes and use distilled water for the purpose of drinking, though medical advice is necessary for such a decision.

HACCP in Dairy: Analysis of dairy products in Canada for conformity is strictly followed by CFIA. As of year 2000, the Canadian Food Inspection Agency (CFIA) dairy inspection program's objective is to help ensure that dairy products leaving CFIA-inspected establishments, or being imported to Canada, are safe, meet standards and are appropriately labelled to avoid fraud under the *Canada Agricultural Products Act*. Most program activities are delivered at federally registered establishments, with some laboratories being accredited to perform analyses of dairy products.

CFIA's dairy inspection program applies to any establishment engaged in the interprovincial or international trade or movement of all dairy products. The major activities undertaken by CFIA staff under this program include: Evaluating the overall manufacturing practices of processing establishments to ensure that dairy products are manufactured under sanitary conditions, Inspecting Pasteurizers and thermal processing equipment, Verifying product formulation; Verifying labels to assess compliance of ingredient and net quantity declaration for accuracy; and, Issuing export certificates for dairy products on request. CFIA staff activities also include inspecting Canadian Dairy Commission warehouses for sanitation and health and safety conditions-46.

Microbial contamination risks in dairy processing companies have seen the devastation that consumers concerns can have negative impact on their products and the dairy industry. The *Staphylococcus sp.*, contamination in Japan led to more than 10,000 people becoming ill and closure of many milk-processing plants due to milk safety issues. The company at the centre of the problem sought $280 million to cope with the devastating effect of the safety scare. In the United States, Good Agricultural Practices Program (GAPP) has prompted to seek third party assessments to verify its application.

Quality Assurance Program embedding HACCP is of paramount importance to Canadian Dairy Industry. The Canadian dairy Industry realises that without a QA program, preventive measures in the dairy industry cannot be verified. One of the encouraging factors in HACCP based QA programs is the consumer's attention towards dairy food safety in Canada. Consumer's awareness and expectations of safety have increased along with the ability to investigate and link food safety issues to a specific point of trouble. That specific point of trouble to food poisoning or contamination leads to bad publicity for the manufacturer and financial devastation. The launch of Canadian Dairy Farm Milk & Meat Quality assurance program in 2001 is the well-accentuated direction for the industry. This will meet the demand of consumer, processor, and retailer. To date more than 70 dairy processing plants have certified HACCP programs that indicate how well consumers impact the safety related issues in the dairy industry.

HACCP for Meat and Poultry: Meat industry is highly sensitive but highly important food sector in Canada and United States. The USDA chose to implement HACCP in the meat and poultry industry over a period of three years. During the first year, 1998, the largest meat and poultry plants came under the program.

In January of 1999 the next tier of plants, numbering about 2,300, came into the program. These were the medium-sized plants, with between 11 and 499 employees. In January of 2000, the remaining small processors came under the program, with 3,000 federal-inspected and 3,000 state-inspected facilities. According to Keri Harris, International HACCP Alliance, "the meat and poultry industries continue to use HACCP as one tool to improve food safety and maintain process control. The remainder of the industry, the smaller processors, are moving forward with final preparations toward implementation. Snags in applying HACCP are not new. There have been snags along the way to implementation in the meat and poultry industry, which is not surprising, given the size of the industry. One of the problems is the nature of the Federal Meat Inspection Act. There are two types of infractions - adulteration and misbranding. Yet, subsection m (8), under adulteration, would appear to belong to misbranding. In addition, the USDA has used a command-and-control regulatory approach for a long time, and on-site inspectors are an industry norm. However, the USDA chose not to include current GMPs as part of the regulation, and with initial implementation came notice from the USDA that there were regulatory issues that had to be addressed in the HACCP plans. However, while the industry was trained in HACCP plan development, the inspectors were trained in HACCP plan enforcement, and had little training in plan development.

Technical service centre of the USDA has been established in Omaha. If an inspector has a question, he or she can call the centre for a decision on whether the plan in question is compliant. An expert technical team is available to handle the really difficult questions. There's an appeals process in place as well, which is monitored to make sure that appeals do not take too long.

Table: 06(1) - The Bacterial Spoilage & Pathogenic Risks from Meat

No	Meat	End Result	Spoilage Organisms	Pathogenic Organisms
1.	Beef, Mutton	Gas and acids	Saccharolytic Organisms, Proteolytic Organism,	*Clostridium thermosaccarolyticum* *Clostridium botulinum*
2.	Beef Liver	Turbidity and gas	Thermophillic anaerobes	*Clostridium thermosaccarolyticum*
3.	Liver, raw meat	Colour change of lever and spoilage, Some bacteria may reduce additive nitrate,	Saccharolytic Organisms, Proteolytic Organism,	*Clostridium perfringens* *Streptococcus faecalis,* *Proteus vulgaris,* *Proteus mirabilis,* *Proteus morganii,*
4.	Poultry	Meat colour defects, Bone darkening Discolouration, putrid smell and obnoxious odour	*Bacillus sp.* *Pseudomonas mallei,* *Spirillum lunatum*	*Salmonella sp.* Faecal streptococci *Shigella* sp., *Yersinia* sp., *Staphylococcus aureus, Listeria monocytogenes, Clostridium perfringens, Bacillus cereus*
5.	Sea foods, Fish etc	Discolouration, slime production. Lesion swelling, Pathogens may cause cellulitis, muscle necrosis or septicaemia, ulcers, abdominal pain; diarrhoea; nausea; vomiting	Proteolytic Organism *Piscirickettsia salmonis* *Renibacterium salmoninarum,* *Flavobacterium psychrophilum,*	*Clostridium Botulinum,* *Aeromonas hydrophila,* *Edwardsiella tarda,* *Erysipelothrix rhusiopathiae,* *Mycobacterium marinum,*
6.	Rabbit meat,	Spoilage results in discolouration, putrid smell and obnoxious odour	Proteolytic Organism,	*Vibrio haemolyticus,* *Vibrio cholerae,* *Aeromonas punctata* *A. hydrophila*
7.	Oysters, Meat, Mussels	Spoilage may result in discolouration, slime production.	Proteolytic Organisms, Saccharolytic Organisms,	*Yersinia enterocolitica*
8.	Frog	Slime production, unhealthy smell or none	Proteolytic Organisms, Saccharolytic Organisms,	*Aeromonas hydrophila*
9.	Meat Products	Spoilage results in discolouration, putrid smell and sour odour	Proteolytic Organisms, Saccharolytic Organisms,	*Proteus vulgaris,* *Clostridium sp.*

All finalized appeals are published in quarterly reports and are available from the USDA and on its website. The findings are recorded in a database, which is reviewed regularly, and all USDA personnel have access to technical support 24 hours a day, 7 days a week.

Modification of food safety programs according to the new knowledge and research is the norm in USA. To the credit of the USDA, it has chosen to modify its program to address new hazards as they have become known or have become widespread. This has just occurred, in fact, in response to the _Listeria monocytogenes_ problem in packaged RTE meat products. On May 25, 1999, the USDA posted regulations for the control of _L. monocytogenes_ in these types of products in the Federal Register. As new hazards become known, notices will come out to re-access existing HACCP plans with the new hazards in mind.

Training in HACCP is like equipping self with tools to win the battle against risk factors. Within the meat and poultry industries, training has taken a different track from that of the fisheries. The poultry industry uses a uniform HACCP training plan that is administered by the U.S. Poultry and Egg Association, according to Steve Knight, director of training for the organization. This includes the basic principles of HACCP and plan development, as well as compliance issues. The people currently going through training are from plants that already have HACCP plans in place, which is helpful, because it gives them a little exposure before they arrive. Inconsistencies in training should be removed. The lack of a single course guide and list of generally recognized hazards accepted by the industry and regulators has led some to believe that there is inconsistency in training and understanding of HACCP. The sheer quantity of people to be trained is a problem, and the last-minute inclusion of regulatory compliance into the HACCP scheme did not help matters.

An article in the July 5, 1997 Food Chemical News entitled "Congress Seeks Explanation for FSIS regulatory reform delays, _Listeria_ requirements" illustrates the tight scrutiny from Congress under which the USDA operates. There is criticism of USDA sending the _Listeria_ notice to the trade, while the FDA includes a list of hazards in its Fish and Fisheries program and updates this list on a regular basis. Of more concern to the House Agriculture Committee was "the length of time it is taking USDA Food Safety and Inspection Service to review its regulations and remove those that are not HACCP-compatible. While the agency originally promised to remove unnecessary, outdated command-and-control regulations before HACCP was ever implemented, very little progress toward that goal has been made".

The good news is that according to the USDA, the portion of the meat and poultry industry covered by the program is 90% compliant with the program. The problem is the lack of understanding of the seven HACCP principles, especially validation of the program. Table: 06(1) describes the Bacterial Spoilage & Pathogenic Risks from Meat. A study on available microorganism with reference to their incubation temperatures, their susceptibility to processing temperatures and permitted preservatives, required water activity in meat products, drying of meat, fixation of storage temperature and prescribed shelf life would help prevent bacterial hazards in processed meat more scientifically and confidently.

In Canada, under the guidance of CFIA two poultry processing plants in Quebec and Ontario volunteered to pilot the Modernized Poultry Inspection Project (MPIP) with all HACCP process controls in place. MPIP was designed and introduced to modernize the Canadian poultry inspection system by further introducing Hazard Analysis Critical Control Point (HACCP) principles into the existing inspection program. The pilots were run for six weeks. The purpose of the pilots was to test the modernized inspection system to determine if it meets or exceeds strict federal food safety standards. At the time, the implementation of MPIP set the stage for further integrating HACCP into poultry production, which ultimately enhanced the safety of poultry products-[151].

The Meat Hygiene Program (MHP) introduced later to ensure that meat and poultry products leaving federally inspected establishments for interprovincial and export trade or being imported into Canada is safe and wholesome. It also monitors registered and non-registered establishments for labelling to avoid fraud and audits the delivery of a grading program based on objective standards of meat quality and retail yield to facilitate the marketing of meats from producer to consumer. MHP includes Poultry Slaughter Inspection; Meat Processing Inspection; Red Meat Slaughter Inspection, Meat Imports and Exports; and, Surveillance of Canadian Poultry Grading.

In the year 2001, Canadians produced beef, pork, poultry, and other meats valued at an estimated $14 billion. On average, Canadians consume 23 kg of beef, 33 kg of poultry, and 22 kg of pork per capita, per year. In total, 2.4 million tonnes of meat were consumed domestically and 1.6 million tonnes were exported to 116 different countries. The CFIA enforces the *Meat Inspection Act* so that meat products leaving federally inspected establishments for domestic and export trade or being imported into Canada is safe and wholesome-06.

HACCP for Seafood: The Fish and Fisheries HACCP program went into effect for the entire industry on December 18, 1997. The Seafood HACCP Alliance for Training and Education developed a standard training manual - *HACCP: Hazard Analysis Critical Control Point Curriculum* - the primary manual used for training. *Fish and Fishery Products, Hazards and Control Guide*, published by the FDA, accompanies the former, and the two publications are used together. These publications have solved the problem of confusing information by presenting a unified program that all operators and inspectors are required to take. The training is a standardized three-day course, and all trainers have been briefed on how to teach the course outline.

All participants go through the general training, including FDA inspectors. The FDA inspectors then go through a supplementary training at the agency. This is similar to the Better Process Control schools, which have been in use by the FDA since the 1970s. Everyone covers the same material - from operator to inspector - and the general hazards are pointed out to each person during the course. It should be noted that the FDA inspectors carry badges, and are law-enforcement officers, while USDA inspectors cannot make arrests.

In a follow-up study entitled "Seafood HACCP Implementation Survey Evaluation Report," Gall solicited input on all phases of the implementation process, and reports that "the most frequent changes in equipment to meet HACCP requirements of the FDA regulation were to thermometers, delivery trucks, truck refrigeration units, coolers, other monitoring devices and shipping containers".

Another striking finding was that "smaller firms invested as much money as medium-sized firms, and the investment made by the largest firms was significantly higher." Ninety percent of the respondents felt that the HACCP training had benefited the industry, but only 47% thought that the benefits of implementing HACCP would outweigh the cost to the company. Only 58% of respondents thought that the program would benefit consumers, and a striking 79% felt that consumers were not aware of the program. Only 70% of respondents reported having had an FDA or state HACCP inspection since the start date of the program.

Historic HACCP:

So how did the current programs of food inspection begin, and why do so many people think they are less than ideal? (After all, wouldn't it be better if industry and government worked together to produce a wholesome, affordable food supply?) Just as Rachel Carson's *Silent Spring* eventually galvanized the birth of the Environmental Protection Agency and the Endangered Species Act, Upton Sinclair's *The Jungle* was the straw that broke the proverbial camels back in the case of food laws. In this situation, the "camel" was a Congress resistant to passing a national food law, but in 1906, the Food and Drugs Act and the Meat Inspection Act were finally passed.

Initially, the FDA was part of the U.S. Department of Agriculture (USDA). In 1940 it was moved to the Federal Security Agency, the predecessor to the Department of Health, Education and Welfare. (So at one time, one part of the Federal Government was responsible for food inspection.)

The USDA has done a very good job over the years of improving crops and Agricultural methodology and helping the American farmer feed the world. Research programs and state/federal extension programs have helped make the U.S. population the best and most cheaply fed in the world. However, many ask: Is the USDA still the best agency for meat and poultry inspection?

The original HACCP system was developed at Pillsbury in the 1960's. HACCP was first conceived when Pillsbury was asked to design and manufacture the first space foods for Mercury flights. As they moved onto Gemini with its more complex foods and longer flights, the problems were magnified. By the time the Apollo program landed on the moon, HACCP was developed. Within two years of that first moon landing HACCP was in commercial use in the manufacture of consumer foods at Pillsbury.

Pillsbury concluded, after extensive evaluation, that the only way they could succeed in having safe food would be to have control over the raw materials, the process, the environment and people, beginning as early in the system as possible. In using this approach they developed the Hazard Analysis Critical Control Points concept for food safety.

In 1973-74, the first preventive program within the FDA - Low-Acid Food Processing Regulations - was adopted. This program is very similar to a HACCP plan.

In 1985, a Subcommittee of the Food Protection Committee of the National Academy of Science (NAS) recommended that HACCP be used as the most effective means of controlling the safety of our food supply. This report was issued after a study to establish the microbial criteria for foods.

In late 1994, the FDA announced a HACCP pilot program. This study was aimed at eventually expanding HACCP to the entire food industry regulated by the FDA. Since then, both the FDA and USDA have enacted a number of HACCP programs, such as that for Fish and Fisheries, and several more are in progress.

Canada, the European Economic Community (EEC), the United States, and other countries are being guided with regard to the HACCP approach by the deliberations taking place at the Food and Agriculture Organization (FAO) and the World Health Organization (WHO) of the United Nations and the pertinent Codex Alimentarius Committees.

Codex has initiated a working group to formalize a worldwide approach and application of HACCP principles. The concepts incorporated in the Canadian model, FSEP, are consistent with the Codex approach towards HACCP.

Chapter: 07
FUTURE OF HACCP SYSTEM

Overview:

The Hazard Analysis and Critical Control Point (HACCP) system has now become generally accepted as the key safety management system for the food industry worldwide. Whilst there are numerous publications on its principles and methods of implementation, there is relatively little on the future course of action on implemented HACCP systems and what can be learnt and done more from that point.

Food safety requires full time attention by all. It's a pleasure to discuss food safety, HACCP, and future directions for food safety regulations. This is a perfect time to be addressing these issues because North Americans reached a milestone in the strategy for change, and it is appropriate to reflect on future directions. The future of HACCP is expanding beyond the seafood, poultry, and beef industries into a wide range of facilities for quality and food safety.

Expanding HACCP to the entire food industry would be good for all concerned. In the United States, the implementation of the Pathogen Reduction and HACCP rule are milestones. As of January 25, 2000, all meat and poultry plants--large, small, and very small--must operate under all of the requirements of the rule. Just as a quick review, the rule requires plants to implement HACCP, sets standards for _Salmonella sp.,_ that plants must meet, requires plants to test for generic _E. coli_ as a measure of process control, and requires plants to follow Standard Operating Procedures for sanitation. Implementation of the Sanitation SOP's began in 1997, while the rest of the requirements were phased in over 3 years, with large plants having to meet the requirements first. Let's briefly review how we reached to this point, so we can turn to directions for the future. As evidenced by the meat, poultry and seafood industries, the safety of the food being shipped has improved. The number of reported cases of food borne illnesses has declined.

Pilot programs sponsored by FDA have played a vital role in HACCP diversity to different food segments. The companies in the FDA pilot program went so far as to state that their product quality improved, as did their production process efficiency. HACCP may also eliminate the marginal operators who have consistently cut corners and who have driven those of us who want to make quality products-passionate.

Dairy industry is a highly vulnerable industry and food safety concerns are not less than meat or poultry. At this time, the National Conference of Interstate Milk Shippers (**NCIMS**) has a committee looking at HACCP as an alternative system for rating and auditing plants operating under the Pasteurized Milk Ordinance (PMO). They may have an easier time using HACCP, since all requirements under the PMO are based upon identified public health concerns. The committee has sent out applications to various states looking for participants in the pilot program. According to Claudia Cole, committee chairperson with the Washington State Department of Agriculture, they want plants from all regions of the country to participate in the pilot program. Once the plants are selected, personnel from the plants and the state agencies involved will train together. The plants will then have to develop HACCP plans and the states will have to create a monitoring scheme to determine how well HACCP is working. The pilot program has started in January 2000, so that it will have been in place for a year before final assessment of the pilot program.

Low acid foods are comparatively more safety risks prone than acidic foods. Like the PMO for the grade-A milk industry, other industry segments have regulations very similar to HACCP - thermally processed low-acid foods in hermetically sealed containers and acidified foods, for example. It would be difficult to see how a change in these programs would benefit public safety.

Restaurants and the catering agencies must come to the HACCP fold. The US-FDA is working in conjunction with the NRA (National Restaurant Association) to test HACCP use in restaurants as well as In-flight Food Service for use of the HACCP approach to the preparation and handling of foods used in air travel. Although HACCP is not mandatory for institutions and restaurants, organizations such as Joint Commission on Accreditation of Healthcare Organizations (JCAHO) is strongly encouraging HACCP implementation by offering strategies on how adopting HACCP guidelines can help increase JCAHO compliance.

Food equipments suppliers should design their processing and packaging systems according to the requirements of quality assurance and specifically HACCP. In fact, HACCP has impacted the future of foodservice, processing and packaging equipments. Equipment manufacturers are competing to ensure their product aids in HACCP compliance.

Juice industry is almost like dairy industry and sometimes dairies do manufacture juice products. Therefore, Juice and beverage industries will implement HACCP very soon. On April 24, 1998 the US-FDA published in the Federal Register (21 CFR part 120) proposed HACCP Procedures for the Safe and Sanitary Processing and Importing of Juice. It was originally set to go into effect for large processors in two years from date of publication, and to go into effect for all parties within four years.

Learning process is never ending. We can learn much from those who already have HACCP programs administered by the various governmental agencies. The basic problems that the industry faces are the lack of the prerequisite programs and monitoring systems. Many companies cannot verify at present that their sanitation plans are being followed or that other basic quality-control programs are being followed. In addition, not just small companies - recently a large, well-known company admitted to a lapse in basic quality-control procedures. Again, the key issues are verifying the critical control procedures and validating the processes that control them. Making sure these missions are effectively fulfilled will make HACCP implementation easier for everyone, and will ensure that HACCP works as it is intended - to make the food supply even safer.

US President's Council on Food Safety:

On January 25, 1997, the US President announced his food safety initiative by directing the Secretaries of Agriculture and Health and Human Services and the Administrator of the Environmental Protection Agency to identify ways to further improve the safety of the food supply. Those agencies held public meetings with consumers, producers, industry, states, universities, and the public, and reported back to the President. The Report, issued in May 1997, was entitled *Food Safety from Farm to Table: A National Food-Safety Initiative*.

The President's Council on Food Safety was established in August 1998 under E.O. 13100 to strengthen and focus on efforts to coordinate food safety policy and resources. The Council was directed to:

1) Develop a comprehensive strategic Federal food safety plan.

2) Advise agencies of priority areas for investment in food safety and ensure that Federal agencies annually develop coordinated food safety budgets for submission to the Office of Management and Budget (OMB).

3) Ensure that the Joint Institute for Food Safety Research (JIFSR) establishes mechanisms to guide Federal research efforts toward the highest priority food safety needs-165.

Impetus for Change: The 1990's were associated with significant food safety challenges as well as significant progress in our ability to meet those challenges. The outbreak of _E. coli_ O157:H7 in late 1992 and early 1993 attributed to undercooked ground beef patties was a turning point because it provided an impetus for real change to improve food safety. In fact, it changed the Nation's mindset about food borne pathogens. Less than a decade ago, the pervasive attitude among industry--and even among some regulators--was that pathogens are a natural part of the environment and can't be controlled. The idea that government would begin setting standards for pathogen reduction, and testing raw products--not just ready-to-eat products--for bacteria, was beyond belief.

In addition, the idea that industry would begin to embrace HACCP as good business was a reality only among the most progressive industry leaders. Although NASA and a large food processing company invented HACCP, it had not been widely embraced by the meat and poultry industry. However, that's exactly what happened. It didn't happen overnight. It was an awakening that began with emerging scientific data about pathogens and a growing realization that the meat and poultry industries had to change. Many factors have forced us to place more emphasis on food borne pathogens as a health risk.

First, of course, is the growing knowledge about pathogens, how they are transmitted in the food chain, and their role in causing disease. Now, there are more opportunities for larger outbreaks when contamination occurs, with a trend toward more concentration in the industry and greater reliance on convenience foods, as members of this association are well aware. We also have a population that is not as savvy as our grandparents when it comes to food preparation. In addition, there are more immune-compromised and elderly individuals in the population who are more susceptible to food borne illness.

The numbers speak for themselves. The cost of medical treatment and productivity losses associated with only four food borne pathogens is estimated at $9.2 billion to 11.2 billion annually in the United States of America. The latest estimates on the incidence of food borne disease in the United States from the Centers for Disease Control and Prevention are that 76 million people get sick, 325,000 are hospitalized, and 5,000 die each year. These statistics indicate that food borne disease is still a very serious problem and a threat to the public health. In addition, all of us are paying for the costs of treating these illnesses through our insurance bills and taxes that support Medicare and Medicaid.

Food Safety Accomplishments: Since the 1992-93 _E. coli_ O157:H7 outbreak, we have made great progress, with improvements in a number of key areas. Mandatory safe handling labels were first on the list and rightly implemented in 1994. The Pathogen Reduction and HACCP rule went in place in 1996, and it was implemented in phases beginning in 1997. In addition, in 1997, the President's Food Safety Initiative set in motion a number of activities that have contributed greatly to reducing food borne illness. Federal agencies have joined together with public and private organizations to fill gaps in the food safety system. Improved surveillance and outbreak response, the trend towards HACCP for many foods, new food safety research, and developments in the science of risk assessment are among these improvements.

In Canada, Canadian Food Inspection Agency has long excelled in implementing food safety standards in poultry. In January of 1996, the members of the Canadian Turkey marketing Agency established the Canadian Turkey Marketing Agency-Hazard Analysis Critical Control Point (CTMA-HACCP) Design team, with the mandate to develop a comprehensive bio-security and quality assurance program based on HACCP principles. In November 1996, the members adopted a manual, "Raising Turkeys . . . Producing Food", for implementation on Canadian Turkey Farms. A best example of cooperation and coordination is demonstrated in the recommendations outlined in the Code, which have been developed by producers, processors, government and mainstream humane societies to ensure that turkeys are raised and marketed humanely and responsibly. All aspects of turkey handling and care are outlined in the Poultry Code of Practice.

In Canada, during 1998-1999, the main objective for the Year was to launch a national food safety awareness campaign for consumers. After performing significant research, including a national safe food handling study done by the CFIA, the Partnership adopted the United States Partnership for Food Safety Education Campaign _Fight_BAC! ™, the key messages of which are: Clean, Separate, Cook and Chill. The _Fight_BAC! ™ Campaign was launched in five Canadian cities in November 1998. The events consisted of a press conference followed by kitchen food safety demonstrations. Speakers at the events included representatives of consumer, industry, health, environmental, and government organizations. A media analysis conducted in a two-month period following the launch proved the campaign's initial success with the press media. Over 10.9 million Canadians were exposed to the campaign and its messages. The media content was accurate, consistent, and positive.

The messages were also communicated by other means such as a Website, Supermarket/ Retail, and Community Action Kits, a portable exhibit, *Fight*BAC! ™ Bookmarks and the BAC! ™ Mascot.

During 1999-2000, the objectives of the Partnership for Year 2 were to communicate the messages of the *Fight*BAC! ™ Campaign to Canadian consumers and to develop food safety materials for children.

In Year 2, the Partnership developed communication tools and investigated the feasibility of adapting the United States Partnership for Food Safety Education Kindergarten to Grade 3 Education Program for use in Canada.

The Partnership felt that it required further effort to accomplish its goals. As a result, a number of Standing Committees were created and formalized; Education Committee, Consumer Tools Committee, Website Committee (www.canfightbac.org), Media Relations/Advertising Committee, Scientific Committee, Strategic Planning Committee, Sponsorship Committee, Nomination Committee, Communications Committee, Communications Committee, and 1-800 National Food Safety Information Line Committee. These committees pursued a number of activities throughout the year and proposals were developed for short and long-term funding requirements[176].

Ronald L. Doering, President; Canadian Food Inspection Agency's (CFIA) referring to activities for the period April 1, 1999 to March 31, 2000, described the Agency's accomplishments along three principal business lines – food safety, animal health, and plant protection. He emphasised about HACCP achievements, "our current direction is showing positive results. Canadians continue to benefit from one of the best food inspection and quarantine systems in the world".

The strength of the industry and its organization through the Canadian Meat Council, working together with its partners in CCA, CPC, CBEF, CPI, CSF, CFIA, AAFC, HC and DFAIT, facilitated an impressive list of Accomplishments during 2001: The most important aspect was Upgrade of Food Safety and Spread of HACCP in industry sector and support for on-farm HACCP and start in transportation and retail.

The Future Directions:

Canada already has a well-earned reputation for producing safe, high-quality food. Leaving aside over-cautious issue of BSE, which lacks substance, consumers will choose Canada because it sets the standard for food safety, for environmental responsibility and for innovation; and because a Canadian product is one you can trust and believe in.

When Mr. Ron Doering, President of the Canadian Food Inspection Agency (CFIA), stated in December 1999, the CFIA's intention to move towards the implementation of mandatory Hazard Analysis Critical Control Point (HACCP) in all federally registered meat and poultry processing establishments registered under the Meat Inspection Act. The future direction of HACCP in Canada was evident. It was not surprising to see HACCP being implemented in dairy, beverage and even in all catering institutions in very near future. Many dairy and juice-manufacturing units are voluntarily adopting HACCP because it saves them from the embarrassment of food safety failures.

Spurred by the success of HACCP efforts a new food safety program someday might be coming to us as an improvement. For the future, it is believed that science is the key to continual progress. It is important that regulators design policies and focus resources based on the most significant public health risks. Good Manufacturing Practices (GMPs) are the foundation on which a strong HACCP system rests. As we have learnt earlier, HACCP deals with five kinds of major hazards: physical, microbiological, chemical, environmental and Bioterrorism. However, even a good sanitation program with GMPs can't deal with problems such as sulphites on shrimp or naturally occurring histamines, to which some people are allergic. HACCP procedures include checks for such problems." Educating North American food processors about the resulting new food safety regulations and principles is the building foundation for future food safety drive. Would we head towards a quality and safety revolution? Well the evolution had begun back in sixties; a revolution in food safety is mandated by the consumer's consciousness towards healthy living.

It is calculated that five major directions for the future may take shape: Fine-tuning HACCP, New Performance Standards, Reliance on Risk Assessment, Better Risk Management, Continued Investment in Research, and Strategic Planning. However, HACCP is limited to manufacturing and service industries, a future role of HACCP in domestic manufacturing cannot be ruled out.

1. Cost of Safety System: The cost of improving food safety and quality at various levels of health risk reduction achieved by using different processes within different regulatory rapprochement regimes ranging from harmonization to coordination needs to be determined and compared over the next decade. This will allow governments to modify programmes toward the most effective approach. The most cost-effective techniques to satisfy consumers must be determined in order for government and industry to agree on the appropriate mix of regulatory and voluntary methods to use in decreasing the risk of contracting seafood-borne disease or illness. For further study please refer Economics of HACCP Application, Chapter: 03.

2. Benefits Determination and Publicity: In the International arena, the benefits to society of reducing risk levels associated with seafood-borne disease or illness in major seafood consumption areas; Japan, European Union, United States and Canada, need dedication, determination and devotion for greater benefits. Only then can governments effectively evaluate the net economic benefits of seafood safety and quality programmes to further expand seafood trade between these nations. Other nations like Bangladesh, Gulf countries and South American countries who heavily depend on fisheries products can take advantage and be part of safe fisheries trade.

3. Effectiveness through Training: One vision on food safety involves the concept that people in North America should not fear of their eating habits and places when all registered eating places, food manufacturers and food services would provide guaranteed safe food. That is possible when the food you eat is risk free and encompasses the farm to table concept with new controls put in place each step of the way to final edible food products. This will require a very diverse, educated workforce that will come from our existing employees and through attrition with new hires. HACCP is now implemented in approximately more than 6000 plants in the United States but we do not yet have a sense of the quality or effectiveness of the HACCP plans at these plants. An in-depth review process must be developed and trained employees with scientific and technical skills must be utilized to perform these reviews.

The right balance and mix of people shall be utilized in performing the review function and where it is determined that HACCP plans are ineffective, the appropriate enforcement actions should be taken. As in the December 1999, Mr. Billy of FSIS reiterated that they had only half of the compliance officers they needed in FSIS.

It is strongly recommended by CFIA in Canada that any provider that is considering the development of a HACCP / FSEP course should acquire the CFIA Food Safety Enhancement Program Implementation Manuals Volumes I, II, III and IV as well as the Reference Database for Hazard Identification and the appropriate generic models. The implementation manuals provide detailed descriptions of the Food Safety Enhancement Program (FSEP) as well as recommendations concerning the process and format for HACCP system development, and the use and application of generic HACCP models. Many types of courses may be offered according to the targeted population. The main courses are: [58].

❑ **H**ACCP/FSEP Orientation for Executive Managers -- Duration: 2 to 4 hours

❑ **C**ourses for HACCP Coordinators -- Duration: 2 or + days according to needs

❑ **C**ourses for Production Staff working at CCPs -- Duration: 1 or + days according to needs

In Canada almost all provincial and territorial governments have adopted training programs in food safety. One of the responsibilities of governments is to ensure that farmers, processors, distributors, and retailers provide citizens with safe and wholesome food products. One such example could be given of joint efforts by CFIA, Manitoba Agriculture and Food, Manitoba Health, City of Winnipeg Environmental Health Services, Health Canada and Canadian Grain Commissionaire jointly working and providing skills and services to Manitobans ensuring a Safe Food Supply for Manitobans[20].

Majority of rejections worldwide are for non-safety reasons and training could help reduce that level. Similarly "education increases the ability of the consumer to recognize safe food, and may influence him to bear part of the cost". The original quality, the storage conditions, and transitional strains are the three main factors influencing the food product rejections all over the world. In Canada, the Guelph Food Technology Centre Guelph-Ontario is Canada's only independent technology centre specializing in food technology and Canada's largest HACCP Trainer. Training-Based Implementation of Food Safety and Food Quality Systems work much effectively than implementation to fancy the name or please the regulatory authorities of regulatory implementations. Regulatory implementation requires effective steps with concrete results in the elimination of risks from the cultivation /breeding /procurement to blending and to processing till is packed and distributed for the final consumption.

4. Improved Communication: Lack of Communication paves the way for ignorance and wrong manufacturing practices. US-FSIS discussed the need for improved communication with Association of Technical and Supervisory Professionals (ATSP) and sought help to work in this endeavour. Extensive use of web site and Newsletter will enhance communication of food safety related literature and issues. Establishment of chat rooms for food technologists, microbiologists, food specialists and regulators will pave the way for more comprehensive expansion of HACCP and food safety.

The fear among employees from the management actions should not exist, as it will deprive them of their excellence and workmanship. Breaking down the roadblocks and barriers in communication will enhance clear understanding of the purpose for improvement of product and service. Food manufacturing organizations of multiple people working towards a common purpose cannot function without communication that may involve verbal message, data transmission, imparting information and training. It should be understood that communication is a transmitting and a receiving process that, for effectiveness, depends upon the receiver's perceptions.

An effective communication system in a food manufacturing organization will let employees understand organizational strategies, goals, and objectives, and their role in meeting them. That results in cost reduction as safety tasks are managed effectively, eliminating the wastages, time delays and preventive lapses associated with miscommunication. Thus communication in most understood languages of the manufacturing personnel or hiring the personnel who know the official languages of Canada fluently should be the important step in the risk based food manufacturing industry.

5. Common Legislative Base: Food legislation, regulation, and inspection are areas of shared jurisdiction. In Canada, A federal-provincial initiative is being undertaken by the Canadian Food Inspection System Implementation Group (CFISIG) to develop a Common Legislative Base for food law in Canada. The Common Legislative Base initiative is aimed at encouraging all jurisdictions to develop a similar legislative base for food safety and quality, thereby facilitating the adoption of harmonized regulations and standards.

At the international level, laws respecting the safety and inspection of food are evolving in response to a changing environment. The increasing influence of international standards setting organizations as a result of trade agreements like the World Trade Organization

(WTO) is having a significant effect on the domestic food law policies of all major food producing nations. In an increasingly globalized economy these international developments are an important consideration in any domestic review of policy or legislation. That will narrow the gaps in international food safety.

6. HACCP Model for All: New challenges arising from the growing size of the food industry and the diversity of products and processes have prompted US-FDA to consider requiring HACCP regulations as a standard throughout much of the remaining U.S. food supply. When adopted, the regulations would cover both domestic and imported foods. Any process that helps eliminate contamination in US food and beverages is a positive sign to expand and cover all other foods with HACCP principles-[40].

7. Fine-tune HACCP: Now that HACCP is already in place for all plants producing meat and poultry products, it is now time to fine-tune the HACCP system. For example, we need to reinforce the culture change that is so important to a successful HACCP-based inspection system. HACCP required major changes in the way that USDA inspectors perform their jobs, and periodic retraining and correlation sessions are built into our budget.

In addition, we are now in the process of developing an in-depth verification protocol that would be used to evaluate plant HACCP compliance. This would not be an everyday compliance tool, but a more intensive method that would be used by a multidisciplinary team or an individual inspector with extensive HACCP expertise.

FSIS emphasises the importance of reassessment. It conduct surveys of plants that produce ready-to-eat products covered by the Federal Register notice issued in May 1999 regarding the reassessment of HACCP plans for _Listeria_. The survey is designed to determine what actions plants have taken, and are now carrying out, in response to the Federal Register notice. FSIS also has extended HACCP concept to the slaughter line with its HACCP-based inspection models project. This project represents the next evolutionary step for HACCP. Volunteer plants are extending their HACCP and other process control systems to cover certain activities carried out before and after slaughter that are not currently covered under HACCP.

Plants are responsible for preventing meat and poultry that are unsafe or unwholesome from entering the food supply. They will carry out these activities under FSIS oversight inspection and verification. Inspection will be required to meet FSIS performance standards.

8. Additional Performance Standards: Revising and setting additional performance standards are another important part of strategy for the future. HACCP by itself is only a tool—it must be combined with performance standards in order to achieve results. Experience so far with HACCP shows that this combination of HACCP and performance standards works extremely well. With available two years of data on _Salmonella sp._, testing from the HACCP rule, and the data show significant reductions in the prevalence of _Salmonella sp_.

Work has been underway to collect baseline data on _Campylobacter_ in order to explore setting performance standards for that pathogen. There is also a need to develop performance standards for ready-to-eat products that will be designed to control pathogens, including _Listeria sp_. With the performance standards for _Salmonella sp._, plants will determine how best to meet the standards, using plant-specific processing procedures.

9. Risk assessment: The beauty of HACCP is that it is a flexible system that can be adapted as new risks are identified. That is where risk assessment comes in. Industry and government need to ensure that HACCP systems are addressing the most critical hazards associated with dairy, meat, poultry and fisheries products, and risk assessments provide us with this information.

Risk assessments have already completed for _Salmonella enteritidis_ in eggs and egg products and are using this information to develop and implement a food safety strategy for those products.

10. Research Work in Future: Food safety research also is extremely important to future progress. One of the limitations of risk assessments is that they are only as good as the data available. There is still much we do not know about the hazards in foods and how to reduce them. We need basic as well as applied research. The US President's Food Safety Initiative has very substantially increased funding for both pre-harvest and post-harvest food safety research.

USDA Agricultural Research Service conducts a shelf-life study on the pathogen _Listeria_. In fact, volunteers were invited to participate in the study. The goal of the study was to obtain a snapshot of _Listeria_ prevalence in ready-to-eat products specifically, frankfurters-over a 3-month storage period.

In Canada, The University of Guelph, along with the Canada Foundation for Innovation (**CFI**), Ontario Innovation Trust (**OIT**), and Brenda Chamberlain, MP for Guelph-Wellington, unveiled the results of a more than $8-million investment in the future of food safety by officially opening the Canada Research Institute for Food Safety (**CRIFS**). CRIFS allows scientists to perform multidisciplinary research to help improve the safety of the Canadian food supply at all points from farm to fork.

The Canadian Agri-food sector has always been a good provider but why settles for good, or even better, when best is a reachable goal? Food safety and quality, environment, by engaging in constant renewal, acquiring new skills, adopting new technology, making informed business choices, science and innovation, effective business risk management, should help protect food and its producers in coming years. Served with generous portions of these strategic priorities, Canada can become the world leader in food safety and quality, innovation, and environmentally responsible production to meet the needs of consumers at home and abroad.

US President's Food Safety Council: As these activities are carried out within USDA, the Federal food safety agencies are working together through the President's Food Safety Council to coordinate activities government-wide.

The Council is now involved with two major activities. First, it is developing a comprehensive strategic plan for Federal food safety activities that will help Federal agencies to address the most important food safety challenges. It is much broader than the Food Safety Initiative, which focuses on the risks posed by microbial pathogens only.

The strategic plan is closely tied to another important activity— developing a coordinated food safety budget. So while you may hear less about the Food Safety Initiative in the future, its activities in the United States will be reflected through the President's Food Safety Council.

Recall Policy: The recall is the last but decisive attempt to pre-empt any risk to consumers. None of the food manufacturers want to reach the stage of recall thus denting their image of a safe food manufacturer. At the same time, recall process shows the timely sincerity of food manufacturers in realising the risk in their manufactured food. That is the least and last attempt to eliminate the risk posed by their manufactured food. That should not be sufficient. The very needful stage of recall should be pre-empted by fine tuning HACCP process in the manufacturing set up.

Considering that recall stage cannot be eliminated as human errors and weaknesses in "determination" to apply food safety elements may result in risk transmission to the market, the recall policy is to be perfect to ensure minimum risk of consuming the recalled product. The change in the press release policy was the last in a series of changes undertaken after a two-year review of FSIS' recall policies. That review had produced a policy manual for the Agency, and it had resulted in improvements in the communication of results from the laboratories to the recall committee so that their deliberations can be speedier. The change in policy related to press releases was just one decision out of a series of decisions made related to recalls.

People have raised concerns that this change in policy regarding press releases is wearing out the public's interest and attention to recall notifications. Over the last several years, FSIS has conducted approximately 50 to 60 recalls, and press releases were issued in about 40 of them.

In addition, there have been some instances in the past, under the old policy, where press releases were not issued, these cases to be troublesome. A good example is the finding of *Listeria monocytogenes* in meals served on an airline. The product was recalled, but a press release was not issued because the meals were in HRI (hotel-restaurant-institutions) channels, and thus, the meals would not have been identifiable to consumers. This is troubling because *Listeria monocytogenes* has a long incubation period, so "at-risk" individuals could have been exposed to the organism in the meals while flying and not developed symptoms until a couple of weeks afterwards. These people should have been informed because if they had developed flu-like symptoms and had flown on the airline, they would have known to seek medical care.

In Canada, The Office of Food Safety and Recall (**OFSR**) is a part of the Canadian Food Inspection Agency and was created to coordinate food emergency response with CFIA staff across Canada and external partners. Once a company realized that they have a product that may pose a serious risk to consumer they must contact the Office of Food Safety and Recalls. A recall occurs when food that may cause serious harm if consumed is sold, distributed, or imported. When a recall occurs all of the food products that may cause harm are removed from store shelves immediately and disposed. Press releases are issued immediately to inform consumers of the unsafe products.

There is a legitimate need of guidance to consumers to refrain purchasing the suspected food, and instructions to producers and manufacturers of food to hold product in their stores until found free of contaminants and safe for human consumption.

11. Juice HACCP Regulation: In the year of 1998 in the United States of America, it was mentioned that once the HACCP regulation is finalized, implementation would allow a year for large manufacturers, two years for small businesses, and three years for very small businesses-38.

The CFIA already had the Processed Products Regulations (Canada Agricultural Products Act; **CAPA**) respecting the grading, packing and marking of processed fruit and vegetable products. To protect consumers from pathogens in juices, the US-FDA announced a rule on January 18, 2001, requiring juice processors to use Hazard Analysis and Critical Control Point (HACCP) programs for juice processing. This rule went into effect on January 2002 for large companies. Small companies had until January 21, 2003, to comply and very small companies must implement HACCP programs by January 20, 2004. Producers in Canada voluntarily followed the suit to make their products eligible for US market.

On October 30-2002, US Food and Drug Administration (US-FDA) officials and state field staff completed their training on how to conduct juice HACCP inspections; these staffs are now starting to inspect dairy plants that produce 100% juice beverages. While FDA has stated that a plant's first inspection is intended to be educational, it is possible that serious violations of the juice HACCP regulation could result in disciplinary action by FDA. As reported earlier in News Update, FDA's juice HACCP regulation became mandatory in January 2002 for most dairy plant producing juice. However, FDA delayed on-site enforcement while drafting additional guidance documents. The HACCP regulation would apply to juice manufacturers that sell products in the United States-39. Juice HACCP Hazards and Controls Guidance are in preliminary phase and finalization of juice HACCP regulation may take some time. However, urgency to finalize the regulation remains a priority.

12. Continuation of Dairy HACCP Pilots: The pilot program is intended to provide information that food science professionals can use in determining whether HACCP should be expanded beyond to dairy foods as a food safety regulatory program. The information is being gathered from firms that produce several different types of food products and from firms, which control a variety of potential food hazards. The pilot program is also intended to provide FDA with additional experience in working with the audit type inspection necessary for verifying a HACCP program. The pilot program is continuing at several additional firms, which are not covered.

13. <u>Continuation of HACCP Pilots</u>: US-FDA's role in the HACCP Pilot Program is to verify that the firm's HACCP program is effective and is being followed. Verification involves on-site evaluations of the firm's HACCP system as documented by the firm's HACCP records. The focus of the evaluations is to determine whether food hazards that are reasonably likely to occur are being properly controlled at critical control points (CCPs). Such programs are necessary and should be continued.

Two poultry processing plants in Quebec and Ontario volunteered to pilot the new Modernized Poultry Inspection Project (**MPIP**). MPIP has been designed to modernize the Canadian poultry inspection system by further introducing Hazard Analysis Critical Control Point (HACCP) principles into the existing inspection program-75. Such manufacturing HACCP pilots should form the basis of improvements for dairy, catering, and other food industries.

In preparation for the pilots, most poultry processing facilities across the country were reviewed to establish a base-line performance level for the current poultry inspection system. This level will be used to compare future microbiological and defect detection performances against the current ones.

14. <u>Initiate Retail HACCP Pilots</u>: Expanding on the Clinton Administration's initiatives to ensure the safety of America's food supply, the US Food and Drug Administration has asked for volunteers from the retail sector of the food industry to participate in a pilot program designed to reduce the risk of food borne illness. The retail sector includes restaurants, grocery stores, institutional food service, and vending operations. The retail food industry has expressed a willingness to work jointly with US-FDA on this pilot which will look at each food establishment's role in continuous problem solving and prevention, rather than relying on periodic facility inspections by regulatory agencies. The pilot will test the implementation of Hazard Analysis Critical Control Point (HACCP), a food safety system, in retail settings-97.

15. <u>HACCP for Supermarkets</u>: Supermarkets have a complex system of storage, distribution and selling of their goods. Many hazards which may be present are identical with those in food industry. The structure of a supermarket includes the head of the organization with the main delivery of food, their storage and the distribution to the branch stores. Supermarkets deal with stabilized food like tin cans and dried foods as well as frozen foods and perishable food like salads, dairy products; cheese, yoghurt, butter, meat and meat products as well as fish and derivates.

This means all efforts concerning distribution, storage, handling and processing have to be made related to cooling and freezing, in relation to cleaning of the machines and utensils, disinfection and hygiene of the personnel, Pest control, good condition of the building, hand washing facilities, toilets with no direct access to the area where food is stored, handled or sold. A timetable to establish HACCP in Canadian supermarkets need to be regulated.

16. HACCP for Domestic Production: The HACCP regulators have not yet given a thought that quite a substantial degree the domestic food production which is kept for next day consumption causes home borne illness. The food poisoning at domestic sector could result from over thawed meat, poorly refrigerated rice products; fungus infested bread and spoilt curry unnoticeable by sensory organs of the human nature. It is doubtful that government agencies will regulate home made food but certain thoughts and its implication on health department, human health, human resources and feasting guests at home should be considered. At least an educational drive to impart knowledge to home cooks, housewives, family members who cook and consume food mostly at home should be considered for the general interest of the public. The best start should be from primary schools.

The second concern is towards flourishing home made food business which is often catered to social events like marriages, cultural activities and religious gatherings. People love to eat such foods and keep in their bags to carry it to parks and picnics where the food is kept unrefrigerated for a long period of time under the sunlight and elevated temperatures. People do fall sick from such foods and get through with in a day or two. The attention is not being given to such a food poisoning because it is from home made food, it remains a home matter and no one wants to indulge in someone's problem unless it is brought to the notice of the government agencies. Hospitals would have more knowledge about such illnesses but they are limited to prescriptions, treatments and guidelines. The domestic food preparation needs food hazards preventive system so that common illness arising from home food source could be minimised and finally eliminated.

The home cooks do understand that eating fresh cooked warm food is healthy. The secret of eating fresh cooked hot food is scientifically not known to more than 90% of the people. If they know the flat scientific reasons, the number of people going to hospitals will be dramatically reduced. People know that refrigeration preserves food but they do not know why lower temperatures <4 °C preserves food. The "DANGER ZONE" is a range of temperature where all pathogenic disease causing bacteria and majority of spoilage bacteria multiply to increase their numbers and produce toxins. That temperature range is between 40° and 140°F (5-60°C). It means food items with higher water activity (not dry) should be kept either below 5°C or above 60 °C to preserve the food for a considerable number of hours or period. Even dry foods should not be kept at higher humidity to maintain almost nil water activity. Foods that could give you food poisoning should be kept below 5 degrees Celsius or, for hot food, above 60 degrees Celsius to prevent food poisoning bacteria, which may be present in the food, from multiplying to dangerous levels. If this knowledge is imparted to all domestic cooks, federal budget will have surplus due to reduced home food borne illnesses.

17. Pre-Shipment Review Requirements: FSIS has clarified "*shipping*" to mean that the pre-shipment review must be carried out while the producing establishment still has control of the product. The final rule requires record review prior to shipping. Failure to perform a records review could lead to product being designated adulterated. The purpose of this requirement is to provide the establishment a final check to be certain that no products are released without meeting the critical limits of the HACCP plan under which they were produced.

In order to prevent the introduction of quarantine pests, several directives are issued from time to time regarding the import of food products. Other Canadian Import Requirements include chemical residue standards as established under the Food and Drug Regulations, licensing and inspection requirements as established under the Licensing and Arbitration Regulations under the Canada Agricultural Products Act, regulatory inspection as established under the Fresh Fruit and Vegetable Regulations under the Canada Agricultural Products Act, and packaging and labelling requirements as established under the Consumer Packaging and Labelling Act and Regulations. It is the importer's responsibility to know and satisfy these requirements. Pre-sampling of products, manufacturers HACCP system audit should form the basis of future food products imports in Canada.

While performing the HACCP procedure, the requirement for the establishment is to complete the pre-shipment review before releasing the product for shipment. A records review component of the procedure could be used to verify the points like the documentation that reflects all critical limits were met at all CCP's, the documentation that shows all corrective actions taken were appropriate, all parts of corrective action were addressed, all process-monitoring records are complete and it is to verify that pre-shipment review is signed and dated.

18. <u>Scientific Data to Identify Potential Hazard</u>: Scientific data to support whether or not a potential hazard is a significant hazard is a crucial element of HACCP system. Uncontrolled application of Agricultural chemicals, environmental contamination, use of unauthorized additives, microbiological hazards and other abuses of food along the food chain can all contribute to the potential of introducing or failing to reduce hazards related to food. Scientific data would help realize in identifying a hidden potential hazards in food production and ingredients procurements from overseas.

19. <u>Scientific Data for Appropriate CCLs</u>: Scientific data to determine appropriate critical limits for critical control points is another crucial element in HACCP implementation and its success. Limit for critical control point is a criterion, which separates acceptability from unacceptability. It is the maximum or minimum value to which a physical, biological, or chemical hazard must be controlled at a critical control point to prevent, eliminate, or reduce to an acceptable level the occurrence of the identified food safety hazard. The level of particular hazards causing illness and toxicosis shall be studied and limits appropriately established through the use of historical and viable data collected.

20. <u>CCLs for Non-Thermal Processes</u>: Critical limits for non-thermal inactivation process how much reduction is enough though possibilities of reactivation or growth need thorough studies and research. The use of ultraviolet irradiation, sulphur dioxide and dimethyl bicarbonate as potential no thermal processes that will achieve a 5-log reduction of *E. coli* O157:H7 in fruit juices specially apple and related products. Similarly to eliminate the pathogens *E. coli* O157:H7, *Salmonella sp.,* and *Cryptosporidium parvum* in apple cider and orange, grape and cranberry juices, by treatments involving UV light and ozone, alone or in combination should be thoroughly studied, upper and lower limits identified for the safe application.

Scientific data to support whether or not a potential hazard is a significant hazard, scientific data to determine appropriate critical limits for critical control points, critical limits for non-thermal inactivation processes and investigative as how much reduction is enough should be studied for future course of safety actions.

Research should be conducted to support the development of new methods and improvement of existing methods to reduce biological and chemical contaminants in food systems. One of the methods is non-thermal preventative measures such as organic acids, irradiation, high pressure, UV light, ozone, etc. Research priority should be given to those projects that use methods to reduce contaminants that pose a severe threat to human health and for procedures that can be directly applied to food systems. Assuring that foods are produced and delivered safely and of high quality relies on development and implementation of effective food processes. Monitoring important parameters that affect food safety and quality is important during any food process. However, developing the most effective process and being able to adjust to processing deviations is critical. The focus should go to the research, which will be to optimize the non-thermal processing conditions, set critical limits for safety and quality, and adjust the process based on changes in ingredients or processing conditions.

Acidified sodium chlorite is being used at 26 chicken-processing plants, as a pathogen control strategy to treat 4.8 billion pounds of poultry, and Emmpak Foods will become the first beef processor to commercially apply the food-safety technology. Emmpak is installing a spraying system from Alcide Corp., Redmond, Wash., to treat beef trim with an acidic solution (pH 2.5 to 2.9) of sodium chlorite -- essentially salt and lemon juice -- in concentrations of 500 to 1,200 ppm. FDA cleared sodium chlorite for use with red meat in 1999, and in February USDA accepted the results of water solution uptake tests that determined no cellular changes result from treatment, thereby allowing processors to use the antimicrobial without a label declaration. The process results in a 2-log pathogen reduction, supplements existing food-safety systems and operates at modest cost: only 2 to 3 ounces of solution per pound of trim is needed. It is applied in 10 to 15 seconds as product passes through an auger with a spray manifold[132]. A CCL is needed to guide such non-thermal processing in the food industry.

21. Predictive Mathematical Modeling: Predictive microbiology should be considered in a food safety research area that focuses on estimating the growth or inactivation kinetics of microorganisms in food systems. It will involve the pooling of intelligence inputs from food scientists, microbiologists, processing specialists, engineers, and statisticians. The focus of this study should be based in the test of environmental or processing conditions that affect microbial growth or death. Kinetic models of microorganisms are then developed and used to estimate risk. These models are important to develop and use during product formulation development, when determining food processes and packaging, and during storage of foods.

22. Possible Future Codex Regulations: It is possible that the sale of dietary supplements in the United States could be additionally governed by international regulations. The GATT Treaty ratified by the U.S. specifies Codex regulations as a guideline for the U.S. dietary supplement regulation.

Codex Alimentarius formed in 1961 as an outgrowth of the World Health Organization and the United Nations. Its stated purpose is to improve world health by establishing guidelines for food safety for two purposes:

- ❏ **T**o provide safety standards for less developed countries that don't have any, and

- ❏ **T**o ensure artificial trade barriers are not set up ("harmonization").

All guidelines are to be based on valid science using principles of risk analysis. Codex policy is that consumer opinions and health should be overriding concerns. Some consumer groups believe, however, that pharmaceutical interests represented at Codex could encourage over-regulation that would run counter to consumer interests. Codex guidelines take many years to formulate and thus have been slow to have any impact in the United States. Furthermore, the FDA Modernization Act passed in 1997 forbids U.S. adoption of any Codex regulations that undo the freedoms established by the 1994 Dietary Supplements Health Education Act (**DSHEA**). Nonetheless, it is important to watch Codex regulations since there are various ways in which they could get adopted into US law.

Though on the surface HACCP may seem like a good idea, requiring HACCP for dietary supplements runs the risk of imposing costly procedures on the manufacturing process that are not necessary and not even helpful. The only serious outbreak of contamination ever found in a dietary supplement - tryptophan in 1989 -- would not have been caught by HACCP. The outstanding safety record of dietary supplements and the lack of benefit that HACCP would provide strongly suggest that such regulations are not needed[162].

23. <u>Future Trends in Quality Auditing</u>: In the past few years, discussion regarding the future importance of on-farm, Hazard Analysis Critical Control Point (HACCP)-based quality assurance (QA) programs in livestock and poultry production has been common. In a 1995 USDA report, QA was identified as a highly valuable service the Animal and Plant Health Inspection Service (**APHIS**) could provide production of Agriculture over the next decade. In the report, producer and practitioner leaders indicated that on-farm quality assurance (QA) and certification of quality parameters would become increasingly important. Furthermore, APHIS was recognized as an "on-farm" Federal agency with a field force of sufficient size and geographic location to provide QA services. APHIS leadership concurrently affirmed its unique position as a federal agency to provide QA services, and indicated a willingness to assist industry in this regard.

Though the future importance of on-farm QA is clear to industry and government, how to proceed in initiating and administering such activities at the farm level is somewhat unclear. Discussions on the topic are populated more by questions than answers. How will on-farm QA programs work? Will it be industry or government that owns and manages these programs? Why have uniform national QA programs when export requirements vary so dramatically? For what issues do we need to develop certification versus auditing programs? How pressing are the present quality assurance needs of producers? How many producers are likely to seek QA assistance for a given issue? Will each QA program require a new set of standards or will they share attributes? Will producers make more money if they receive certification? The list goes on. For QA efforts to move forward nationally, this ambiguity must be removed.

24. Quality Assurance Services: Discussion regarding the future importance of on-farm, Hazard Analysis Critical Control Point (HACCP)-based quality assurance (QA) programs in livestock and poultry production has been a common feature to discuss. QA has been identified as a highly valuable service the Animal and Plant Health Inspection Service (APHIS) could provide to Agriculture production over the next decade. The area of quality assurance and accreditation in the food business has been identified as a vital and integral component to an ideal food safety and quality system. Concrete recommendations for future can be put forward and implemented after convergence around the high level issues of quality assurance and accreditation agreement on their importance. Additional study, planning, and discussion may be required to satisfy the industry, regulatory agencies, and the customers. The future course of QA would define criteria of certification, auditing, service components, status, and further opportunities for quality and safety assurance for the integrated food manufacturing system.

Certification Defined: Regarding APHIS services to producers, on-farm QA is comprised of two activities... certification and auditing. When using the term "certification", we are referring to a process whereby a herd is conferred a status based upon the implementation of a series of Good Production Practices or other standards. Good Production Practices are the cooperatively developed uniform standards that, if applied, produce a product of known quality. Herds obtaining certification will have used the same set of standards for implementing good production practices and be uniformly evaluated... no matter where in the nation (or state, if a state program) they are located. More specifically, certification will refer to the process of verifying that a series of science-based production standards, known to result in a specific outcome, have been implemented at the farm level.

Certification standards may rely on scientifically supported criteria for status determination including analytic tests, production process controls, and other quality measurement tools. Certification activities may be undertaken as part of a state, national or marketing group activity. To initiate a certification program, the sponsoring group must provide the certifying body with a program description, standards, and verifiable procedures by which participants can be judged for compliance. Producer participation may be voluntary or required, depending on the certification objective. In some cases, certification may involve a company or producer group wishing to exploit a specific market niche. When voluntary niche programs evolve to become a national production norm, they may be rolled over into an on-going national program.

Auditing Defined: The term "auditing" refers to a process that transmits information within a buyer-supplier relationship. The buyer defines production specification for its suppliers, the supplier declares to have met those specifications in their production system, and a third party audits the suppliers to ensure that specifications have been met. Auditing standards are set through a process of buyer and supplier negotiations and must have characteristics that can be independently verified. No uniform national standards need be established. The audit simply determines that what the buyer expected, and the supplier provided, is one in the same, and provides a mechanism for transmission of this information within the commercial marketplace. Here, the validity of the audit only has meaning within the context of the buyer-supplier relationship. Bear in mind that the buyer may be a packer, state, supermarket chain, country, etc., and individual producers, cooperatives, networks, companies, and the U.S. meat industry the suppliers. Just as the size, scope, and distribution of buyers can be broad and variable, so can the specifications for the audits. Furthermore, the tools used to standardize the process and audit systems form the foundation for constructing the certification programs documented earlier in the HACCP manual.

Service Components: Auditing and certification are simply tools then for establishing and verifying processes at the production unit level that build quality into animal-derived food products. In addition, both require the application of techniques that are grounded in HACCP and ISO-9000 methodologies. It is in providing auditing and certification functions that APHIS is able to assist industry in achieving QA objectives. By providing auditing and certification functions, one is providing a QA service.

Status: There has been considerable discussion regarding the future importance of on-farm, HACCP-based quality assurance programs to national food safety efforts. Although expectations and rhetoric have been high, the appearance of, and market demand for, such programs have been small. With exception of a few poultry egg quality assurance initiatives and the national trichinae herd certification pilot efforts, APHIS Area Office reports of active involvement with multiple commodity groups in developing on-farm, quality assurance initiatives are relatively few.

The implementation of the Pathogen Reduction Act of 1996 by USDA Food Safety and Inspection Service (FSIS) has substantially changed the relationships between government and the packing industry and between the packers and their suppliers. Packers will increasingly look to producer-suppliers, and the QA programs they have implemented, as a means of strengthening the overall plant HACCP plan for reducing physical hazards, chemical residues, parasitic and microbial contamination. Additionally, market competition with other protein sources will require a mechanism for demonstrating continuous product improvement in quality and safety attributes to both domestic and international consumers. Having a successful plant HACCP program will ultimately require that the quality of process inputs be known and verified, both within and external to the processing plant. Specific quality attributes cannot be assumed, but must be described and documented. The impact of this dramatic program change is slowly working its way from the packers to producer-suppliers. It is inevitable, that packers will increasingly look to producer-suppliers, and the QA programs they have implemented, as a means of strengthening the overall plant HACCP plan.

A final QA driver is that Europeans have devoted considerable energy to developing quality systems that have raised the "quality bar" for the collective international community. Although the U.S. need not imitate these systems directly, integration of such key features as market responsiveness, strong process control, and production audits into a credible quality reporting system will be key to U.S. producer competitiveness.

Opportunities: The need for, and expectation that, QA programs be developed is not likely to diminish. Whether industry owned and operated, or industry designed and government administered, QA initiatives will require an ongoing, systematic investment of time, energy, and resources by all parties if successful programs are to be realized. Unlike regulatory programs that are traditionally hatched by State and Federal authorities with industry support, QA initiatives will be market and/or service driven and grown over time. National QA initiatives may not be conceived or implemented spontaneously, but will require the convergence of many technical, market, and partnering events over an extended time to be successful. The previous requirements by several packers that all pork producers be Pork Quality Assurance SM Level III by January 1999, illustrates how an accepted voluntary program, has become a means for ensuring supplier quality. The increased emphasis plant HACCP is engendering on process controls will accelerate the adoption of similar methodologies in all segments of the food chain.

As for APHIS, the ability to assist production Agriculture with QA will be evolutionary in nature, dependent upon several converging events. By developing national certification programs and providing audit services for buyer-suppliers, while concurrently developing a culture that includes HACCP and ISO as a skill set among its employees, the Agency will be able to deliver industry a QA service. Whether originating at the local, state or national level, experience tells us there are two constants to all successful QA initiatives. One is that they are industry driven, and two is that they are based on trust, partnership, and cooperation between a broad base of groups and organizations. Without doubt, if these criteria are satisfied, chances are maximized for successful QA efforts-211.

25. <u>Other Product Regulations</u>: Game farming and Specialized Livestock production is regulated in Canada, e.g., Animal Products Act of Saskatchewan. The Act provides the force for regulations that govern the licensing of domestic game farm operators, the species that are farmed, and the products that are produced from these animals, as well as the organizations that represent the interests of game farm operators and producers.

The existing regulatory structure does not serve specialized livestock product development, so regulations, standards or some type of branding of regional products will emerge in order to serve consumer needs for consistency, quality, or other particular product attributes. Across the United States, small meat processing facilities depend heavily on game processing season. In some states, more than half the plants depend on hunting business to get them through. In other states, nearly 80% of the plants need that season to survive. The spectre of hunting ranched and wild deer and elk herd populations, and the tandem of public fear and scientific inconclusiveness with reference to food safety is casting a pall on the hunting game.

At the heart of the problem is a highly contagious nervous system disease that afflicts elk, mule deer, and whitetail deer. Known as Chronic Wasting Disease (**CWD**), it is fatal to the animals but has not been known to be contracted by humans. Compounding the fear is the fact that it deteriorates the cervid brain in a manner similar to BSE, or the "mad cow" disease. USDA should take regulatory steps to harmonize game animals so that its hunting and meat consumption is regularised and human health secured scientifically. The problem is not new as for about two decades, it had been found in isolated areas of Colorado and Wyoming, and the treatment was to quarantine those areas and eliminate the indigenous herds. Farm raised deer and elk operations normally depopulate the entire herd when one animal is detected with CWD. The problem is that should CWD continue its spread, there is virtually no compensation or emergency funding for plants that would be affected.

There have been reports of the West Nile Virus in bird blood and in bird feces, but we have seen no reports of the virus appearing in deer. From a health standpoint, the normal precautions of gloves in field dressing and processing deer should take care of that concern. Questions have arisen regarding any effect Chronic Wasting Disease (CWD) may have on deer meat and its hide. It is understood that there should be no problem with deer meat and hides since they do not seem to be associated with the prion that carries CWD. However, HACCP guidance to hunted deer meat may be necessary and required in future as a lot of such meat could be donated to charity institutions for human consumption.

26. Nutrition labelling: The food products containing large amount of saturated fatty acids, heavy lactose, cholesterol and other constituents which may cause illness or aggravate health problems to immune deficient, diseased or weak humans. Health conscious consumers are well aware of the nutrient values in the food they eat and your products should carry a nutrition label to remain competitive in today's marketplace and to allow consumers to make choice on their health requirements. If you produce over 100,000 pounds of any one product in a year's time, (sausage, bologna, jerky, etc.) you are required by law to display a nutrition facts panel.

In the United States, Congress is now considering legislation that would require nutrition labels on all raw meat and poultry products. USDA's Food Safety & Inspection Service is also planning rule making on the same requirements. The labelling requirements containing sensitive constituents pertaining to different portions of meat should be properly labelled at least with a given range in content. Selection can include any raw beef; poultry, veal, pork, or lamb item listed, with all the variations based on bone-in or boneless, product, grade, or trim. The producers could give choice to consumers so that they can also choose from any exotic raw product item from species that are now being considered for inspection, such as farm-raised venison, bison, ostrich, and emus.

27. Emergency Future Operations: There are questions raised about the situations in the United States and Canada whether USDA and CFIA respectively grant emergency powers to meat and poultry plants to open and do business, if for some reason inspectors can't or won't come to plants to carry out their inspection duties, due to a domestic emergency due to terrorism or some other kind of major disaster. The concerns are genuine and a solution is to be found. FSIS has published in the form of a directive to both meat inspectors and meat processors to increase security of food producing plants due to the increased threat of terrorist attacks in the United States, because of the war in Iraq and ongoing war against terrorism all over the world.

However, at the same time, the business interests of the inspected meat and poultry plants must be protected. If something like that were to happen, it might be possible that FSIS employees might not be able to get to their assigned plant to carry out their inspection duties. If that were to take place, there is no reason that meat and poultry plants should not be able to operate as usual, and produce their products. For that reason, USDA needs to grant authority for plants to open on an emergency basis, to operate and produce their products as they usually do.

28. Comparable Data Analysis: Over the next decade, comparable data on the number of outbreaks and cases of seafood-borne disease or illness for Japan, the European Union, the United States and Canada must be collected and analyzed. Only then can the economic value and effectiveness of HACCP designed to reduce the risk of contracting food-borne disease or illness be properly evaluated worldwide.

With the influx of immigrants from Chinese, Indian, Pakistani and Middle Eastern origins, the comparable data on the number of all food related outbreaks must be initiated and collected for analysis for future safety measures. The comparative data will provide trends in resistance, control, and guidelines to import legislation for the food products imported from these regions.

29. <u>Future HACCP Knowledge Sharing</u>: The researcher in food industry, government funded institutions; educational institutions are busy in the development of technology for important food safety issues. The sharing of the researched knowledge, technology, its transfer to the needy, regulatory agencies, and transfer programs should include development of workshops and conferences or the development of computer-accessible information. Prioritising the sequence of projects that develops technology transfer programs support the research-focussed categories.

The fact cannot be ignored that HACCP knowledge sharing mostly comes from the Internet. The published research papers, reviews, and ongoing work are scripted in food safety journals and press releases. The most part, educational institutions have been instrumental in producing more knowledge based literature and industrial researchers have been contributing to the advancement of technology in practical field. Future knowledge sharing should be made easier; one cannot deny the fact that knowledge is generated after investment cost. The sharing of knowledge from each other would require funding and the role of media; industry, government, and the educators will be appreciated by the general public consciousness.

Chapter: 08
A Blueprint for the Future

Overview:

In the United States, during the era of President Clinton, U.S. administration had taken a number of important steps to improve food safety in the United States, such as mandating preventative controls for seafood, meat and poultry; the Food Quality Protection Act; and the President's Food Safety Initiative. While these improvements were important for the North American consumers, there is still a long journey ahead to improve the safety of food for the North American and other markets, which depend on US and Canadian food imports-22.

New hazards in food products are showing up without reprieve: parasites and viruses on imported berries; hazardous strains of *E. coli* on lettuce, on sprouts, and in unpasteurized apple juice; *Salmonella Sp.*, in breakfast cereal, in orange juice, and on alfalfa sprout etc., -157. Old hazards remain unaddressed: *Salmonella Sp.*, in eggs and poultry; harmful bacteria and viruses in shellfish remain a concern-80. Public health officials estimate that up to 33 million illnesses and 9,000 deaths occur each year from the contaminated foods in the United States of America-43.

Today, the federal government deploys an army of meat and poultry inspectors and a small squad of food inspectors for all other foods-43. It is using laws that were enacted up to 90 years ago, which are not proving adequate to address emerging hazards of the modern times or to encourage new technologies in near future. Food safety regulations need fundamental streamlining, and while this process has begun, it is nowhere near finished.

In the meat, poultry, and seafood industries, reliance on government inspectors to ensure safety is slowly giving way to a scientific system of preventative controls, known as Hazard Analysis and Critical Control Point (HACCP) system, which is implemented and monitored by the food industry-168. HACCP is a highly touted system developed by the food industry that has been adapted to regulatory programs. While the system may encourage greater responsibility for food safety in the food industry, there are no real models detailing how the government can best ensure that such systems reach their potential for maximizing food safety, such as what is the best use of government inspectors. The change in the government's oversight role over food plants that utilize HACCP systems is just beginning. With new food borne hazards, new process control systems, and new roles for government all on the horizon, US federal oversight structure is in dire need of streamlining. Responsibility for food safety is spread among a number of federal agencies, with the U.S. Department of Agriculture (USDA) and the Food and Drug Administration (FDA) playing the leading roles, with assistance from the Environmental Protection Agency (EPA), the National Oceanic and Atmospheric Administration (NOAA), and thousands of state and local agencies. Meat, poultry, and some egg products, which are regulated, by USDA, Food Safety and Inspection Service (FSIS) are subject to continuous oversight by government inspectors. All other foods are regulated by FDA, which has an average inspection frequency of once every ten years for food processors. FDA has jurisdiction over many high-risk foods, such as seafood and shell eggs, and foods that are becoming riskier, like fruits and vegetables.

The Acts that establish the food safety programs at USDA and FDA set up two entirely different regulatory schemes. The statutes governing the safety of meat and poultry products focus on preventing contaminated food from reaching the market, while the Food and Drug Act places the emphasis on removing contaminated products from the market. FDA and USDA also utilize entirely different inspection approaches; with USDA inspecting plants on an ongoing basis while FDA rarely even visits food plants unless there is an illness outbreak associated with a particular food product-[21]. Such discrepancies between the two agencies are already assuring inconsistencies in HACCP implementation and enforcement, which raises questions regarding the federal government's ability to address food safety problems proactively-[164].

This fragmented structure has given rise to a number of peculiar situations. While under such situations the process of inspection and preventive efforts still continue to comb the industry to minimize the possible hazards in locally manufactured and imported foods but the much greater task lie ahead to guarantee food safety in American and Canadian markets. Let us pinpoint here, few of the important examples, which need attention and corrections.

Jurisdiction Controversy: Under the current structure, food safety problems fall through the cracks of different agencies jurisdiction. Lettuce and other fresh vegetables and fruits are essentially unregulated for food safety to human consumption. The use of animal manure on food crops is also not controlled. These are problems that quite literally fall through the cracks of the current jurisdictional systems in the US.

Health Failure Problems: Under the current structure, multiple agencies fail to address glaring public health problems. Eggs are regulated both by FDA and USDA, but neither agency has developed an effective containment strategy to prevent the spread of *Salmonella enteritidis* (SE) in shell eggs. Instead, the agencies have acted like keystone cops, tripping over each other and bungling each attempt to control SE in eggs-50. In May 1989, six nursing home patients in Pennsylvania died from *Salmonella enteritidis* poisoning after eating stuffing that contained undercooked eggs. Today, over thirteen years since SE inside eggs was first identified as a public health concern by the Centers for Disease Control and Prevention, consumers still await an effective strategy to eradicate SE in shell eggs. *Salmonella enteritidis* (SE) remains an important cause of outbreaks and sporadic cases of gastroenteritis in the United States. When eggs are implicated; investigation of outbreaks, notification to state Agriculture departments and the U.S. Department of Agriculture are crucial in efforts to identify sources of contaminated eggs to develop and implement control measures.

Repeated Inspections: Under the current structure, the same food processing plant may get two entirely different food safety inspections. The classic example is a processing plant that produces both pepperoni and cheese frozen pizzas. The pepperoni line will get daily visits from a USDA inspector to check on conditions in the plant as workers slice the pepperoni and apply it to the pizza-171. The cheese line will be subject to FDA inspection on average once every 10 years. The minimal difference in hazard between the processing of cheese and pepperoni pizzas is not enough to justify the vast disparity in government inspection. Several situations warrant court action. The most serious is when an imminent potential health hazard is found to exist in a food establishment and the proprietor refuses to voluntarily close the operation until the potential hazard is abated. The Sanitary Inspector must convince the judge that the potential hazard is imminent and that a court order should be issued to close the establishment.

Lack of Federal Inspections: Under the current structure, some food processing plants may get no federal food safety inspections. Due to resource constraints, FDA has turned some portions of its regulatory responsibility over to the states. The best example of this is in the area of shellfish production, where FDA relies totally on state inspectors. In other instances, FDA is simply unaware of plants that it is supposed to regulate. A 1991 Inspector General investigation documented that FDA identifies food firms "by reviewing newspapers, magazines, phone books, industry publications, trade periodicals, surveillance reports and consumer complaints. Inspectors may also walk through stores looking for new products"-56. The Inspector General reported that, under this system, some food plants escape detection for long periods of time.

Frequency of Safety Inspection: Under the current structure, quality inspections occur more frequently than safety inspections. There are many shell eggplants that receive regular inspections from U.S. government inspectors, but the inspections are for quality, not for safety. All plants shipping eggs between states are visited by the Agricultural Marketing Service (AMS) each quarter and many plants also participate in a voluntary grading program where they receive continuous inspection by AMS. Under the voluntary AMS program, US government ensures that each has a yolk of the proper diameter, but nothing in the program checks for the presence of SE-56. FDA, the agency charged with food-safety oversight of shell eggs, also does not check for SE during its once-a-decade inspections-213.

The structure of FSIS needed to be reorganized to be more efficient and effective, to carry out our critical functions such as preventive inspections, and to serve as the management system of food safety issues for protecting the public health. This reorganization should increase accountability for all FSIS employees and refocus the duties of many employees with in the agency for improved results.

HACCP Difference: Under the current structure, HACCP is a different system at FDA and at USDA. The new HACCP systems for seafood, meat, and poultry share almost as many differences as similarities. For example, both frequent inspection and laboratory verification of product samples are essential to give the government appropriate oversight over plants utilizing HACCP. Otherwise, the HACCP program becomes little more than an industry honour system. While USDA requires both on-site inspection by government inspectors and two levels of laboratory verification of meat and poultry products, FDA requires neither for seafood products. FDA inspects seafood plants once every one to five years and made laboratory testing for HACCP verification optional for seafood processors. One should not see food safety problems as related to their personal food handling practices.

The National Advisory Committee on Microbiological Criteria for Foods (NACMCF) guidelines are consistent with and rely on more than 33 years of experience with HACCP that began with Dr.

Bauman's original introduction of the systems' principles in the 1960's. The NACMCF was established to provide scientific advice and recommendations on the development of microbiological criteria for foods for those topics requested by the sponsoring agencies. The Secretary of Agriculture appoints NACMCF members based on their scientific qualifications. To ignore the latest NACMCF guidelines would be to ignore the most current scientific advice on the true science-based application of HACCP from a committee co-sponsored by the agency. FSIS rule deviates from established HACCP principles and is based on the agency's perception of HACCP rather than established practices effectively used by industry. It is incumbent on FSIS to embrace concepts accepted by scientists, risk assessors, industry, and governments worldwide in order to maintain the integrity of the HACCP system. HACCP has been the most successful system when it is presented and implemented in the form envisioned by its founder; that is, one, which focuses on, the critical steps needed to protect public health during the manufacturing process.

The hazard analysis approach used by FDA currently differs from that used by USDA. This leads to considerable confusion and difficulty in achieving effective HACCP implementation in facilities that produce products subject to regulation by both agencies. Although product standards and program monitoring may vary between FSIS and FDA's regulation of food products, the underlying concept of HACCP, a preventive system of hazard control, should remain the same in both agencies. For example, in one processing facility, FDA expects a record of all hazards considered while developing the hazard analysis documentation. All potential hazards are listed and a rationale is required as to whether to control the potential hazard via a CCP. This approach assures that all potential hazards are properly considered, thus preventing the possibility of overlooking a potential hazard, and clearly documents how effective control is achieved. It is very useful for communicating the thought process used in determining CCPs.

In the same facility; the current USDA implementation approach severely limits this useful documentation because listing of any "hazard" in the hazard analysis requires control by a CCP in a HACCP plan. As a result, only those items requiring control via a CCP are listed in the hazard analysis for USDA products. Other potential hazards that were considered in the process are not listed, and the useful historical record of why they were not considered to require control via a CCP is lost. The FDA approach is much more powerful in promoting food safety. It reduces second-guessing and repetitive work, and is more aligned with internationally recognized HACCP principles. In addition, the existence of two different approaches to HACCP presents training and implementation difficulties. A harmonized approach is needed for a clear and consistent food safety message.

Single Food Agency: it makes sense to incorporate entire food inspection system under one agency's umbrella. Currently, there are two big players, USDA and FDA. There are, however, several other agencies with significant responsibilities: National Marine Fisheries Service, Department of Defence, Environmental Protection Agency, and Customs. While there are any numbers of Memorandums of Agreement between these agencies, in which they pledge mutual support and cooperation, communication and coordination do not always exist. Additionally, there traditionally has been a difference in regulatory philosophy between agencies, particularly USDA and FDA.

Communication with Customer: There is need to do a better job in communicating with consumers. Parallel to talking about zero risk, associated with food safety concerns, we need to be communicating the concept of risk minimization as well. As a veterinarian, one is cautious in making absolute guarantees and may have a high degree of confidence in such treatments. The same applies in the area of food safety. We all recognize that certain risk factors are small, even very small, but it is unwise and unethical to lead consumers to believe that all foods are free of food safety risks.

Benefits of New Technologies: Multiple agencies may prolong the time it takes to bring the benefits of new technologies to the consumer. Under the existing system there are at least 20 government agencies involved in food safety research-59. The industry recently netted the benefit from one of their projects when Agriculture Secretary Dan Glickman announced the commercial availability of a biological inoculation for young chicks against _Salmonella_-120. This product was developed by the USDA Agricultural Research Service and then spent years being considered for approval at the Food and Drug Administration. For several other heralded technologies, like trisodium phosphate (TSP) for poultry, irradiation for poultry and red meat, FDA approval is just the first step in implementation; there is often a public rulemaking process at USDA before products can be used in meat and poultry plants. This bifurcated process can take years to get through.

Trisodium phosphate (TSP) is fairly new to the market and is becoming more widely accepted and used, because the USDA is encouraging its use within the industry. There are negative aspects to using TSP in poultry processing plants that should be considered. Residual TSP on carcasses causes the chiller water pH to increase dramatically. In plants where TSP is used, the chiller water will generally be in the pH range of 9.7 to 10.5. This is extremely high and completely eliminates the ability of chlorine to become in its effective form, hypochlorous acid. Hypochlorous acid forms most effectively when water is in the pH range of 6.5 to 8.0. Thus, plants using TSP may as well be dumping their bleach down the drain. This is not a desired situation because chlorine is very effective against *Salmonella sp*.

Imports Not Regularised: Under the current structure, imported products are treated differently at FDA and USDA. Imported meat and poultry products are subject to a two-stage approval process by USDA. First, USDA must approve the exporting country's meat or poultry inspection safety system; then, USDA must inspect the individual plant before it can ship meat to the U.S. Even then, it is subject to random verification checks at the border. FDA meanwhile only has the authority to inspect food at the border but has the staff to check less than two percent of import shipments[63]. FDA can't send inspectors to foreign countries except by invitation, even when they are checking the source of food involved in an outbreak in the U.S.

Harmonization Required: Under the current structure, we risk exporting our irrational food safety system though it assures much of the safety we are concerned about. There is increasing international pressure to "harmonize" our food safety systems with the systems used in foreign countries. "Harmonization" is the process of assuring that the systems used in the United States and foreign countries provide an equally safe food product[64]. With international trade in food products expanding rapidly, tremendous energy are being devoted to identifying and eliminating unnecessary barriers to trade and simplifying standard setting internationally, using organizations like Codex and the World Trade Organization[140]. We shouldn't harmonize internationally before we have harmonized our systems domestically, and this alone should provide some urgency to developing a more rational basis for our food safety system today.

These problems are just some of the disparities that exist because of the fractured structure of food safety regulation, and they are the reasons behind why professionals called upon the President Clinton during his tenure to consider combining food safety oversight functions into a single independent food safety agency. Washington insiders doubted the idea of creating an independent food safety administration, which can't be done in near future. Apparently, combining the current hodge-podge of federal agencies in order to make food protections more effective would offend too many high-ranking government officials and Congressional committees. However, year-by-year, outbreak-by-outbreak, it is becoming clear that food safety issues can no longer afford to have government programs that protect Washington bureaucrats and special interests better than they protect consumers. The structure of federal food safety programs today is an obstacle to a safer food supply.

A combination of events has coalesced and convinces us that the time to combine food safety functions is especially good right now. First, HACCP systems are being implemented at both the FDA and the USDA for seafood, meat, and poultry. These systems are also being considered for juice, eggs, and egg products. However, FDA's weak regulatory program may be responsible for jeopardizing the credibility of HACCP with the American public. Seafood plants that have been inspected to date show that the compliance with HACCP implementation is distressingly low. Approximately 70% of seafood plants inspected by FDA so far this year were not fully in compliance with FDA's seafood HACCP rule. FDA has indicated in public meetings that their goal is to get compliance up to 50% next year-71.

Secondly, imports have increased dramatically in the last few years due to several trade agreements, which have expanded food trade with US closest neighbours. This is creating a tremendous problem especially for the Food and Drug Administration because of the acute lack of resources directed to food safety at that agency. For example, FDA has less than 200 inspectors devoted to food safety inspections of imports. Several major outbreaks in the last few years have demonstrated the weaknesses in FDA's system of inspecting imports.

Finally, there are many discussions in Washington about how to better utilize our existing inspection force. Technological innovation may make our current system of inspecting meat and poultry obsolete within the next few years. Those inspectors are urgently needed to provide inspections at the tens of thousands of food plants under FDA's jurisdiction. However, in Washington, you cannot simply transfer resources across agencies. Appropriate, efficient, and flexible utilization of the inspection resources in the twenty first century requires the reorganization of the government structure.

Congress has been debating with these questions. Both the House and the Senate have legislation pending calling on the President to develop a plan to consolidate the food safety functions into a single federal food safety agency. They have also appropriated money for the National Academy of Sciences to discuss several key questions. Legislation was introduced that is beginning to examine the ways that the current statutes could be modernized. For example, a bill filed in April 1998 by Representative Frank Pallone (D-NJ), with 25 cosponsors, set out a division of labour for food safety between industry and government. The food industry, for example, would have been responsible for implementing HACCP and other process control systems; for utilizing available technology to improve food safety; and for registering with the government. The government would have been responsible for doing appropriate inspection and enforcement activities; approving new technologies; inspecting imports; and monitoring the safety of the food supply. While these are not radical proposals, the bill had put the burden for food safety squarely on the shoulders of food producers and it mandated and encouraged the use of HACCP systems and new technologies. Compared to the 1906 law that provides the current underpinning for most of our food safety laws, perhaps that is essential.

Bioterrorism Threats: It is vitally important that US federal agencies take, and continue to play, a leadership role in the prevention of an attack on the food supply. The international implications of Bioterrorism dictate that, to maintain uniformity in a regulatory system such as we have in the U.S., the States and local food safety programs must be able to depend upon federal counterparts for advice, direction, and support. Since more than 40 percent of the foods we consume in this country today are imported, federal agencies such as the FDA must have in place a system to ensure that foods entering the U.S. from foreign sources are just as safe as foods grown or produced here. Our federal agencies must also have a good system in place for real time communications, both among themselves as well as with their State counterparts. This is one of the key elements of an adequate system to both prepare for, and react to, a Bioterrorism threat or event.

Congress, federal food inspection agencies and security agencies must help build up the infrastructure for Epidemiology, laboratory support, and surveillance within the States, in order to adequately prepare for, prevent, and respond to Bioterrorism threat or event - especially when any associated with food. The United States and Canada are vulnerable to Agricultural Bioterrorism and need a joint and comprehensive plan to defend against it. Biological agents that could be used to harm crops or livestock are widely available and pose a major threat to North American food and Agriculture. Sept.

11 terrorist attacks in 2001 give us a lesson to defend against Agricultural Bioterrorism; it should be to enhance our basic understanding of the biology of pests and pathogens so we can develop new tools for surveillance and new ways to control an outbreak.

Canada is way ahead of the rest of the world when it comes to investigative and preventive food safety. There is no country in the world pursuing HACCP on the farm like Canada is determined and following the implementation of HACCP. The CFIA's food inspection programs are reviewed and well regarded by foreign countries that import Canadian products. However, the agency conducts self-evaluation and identified problems with the Agency's compliance activities. They examined 21 inspection files from establishments that had issued food recalls or had been prosecuted in the last two years. In 1999-2000, the Agency participated in 243 recalls and had 59 successful prosecutions. They found that in 16 cases, the same or similar problem persisted for many months and in some cases, years. The compliance actions taken were not sufficient to achieve the Agency's goal of timely correction of the compliance problem either because of the limitations in the legislation or a failure by the inspector to take more serious compliance action.

It has been noticed that Agency had not set expectations or measured performance to determine if its initiatives and activities have contributed to a more efficient and effective food inspection system. Their annual assessment of the performance information in the Agency's annual report has consistently noted that readers are not provided with the information necessary to understand the extent to which the Agency is achieving its objectives.

The Canadian Food Inspection Agency (CFIA) is the result of the amalgamation of food safety and inspection programs from three federal departments: Agriculture and Agri-Food Canada, Health Canada, and Fisheries and Oceans. It now has some 5,467 employees across the country and manages expenditures of $416 million. The Agency's main activities focus on inspecting the food supply, but it also conducts activities related to animal health and plant protection.

The Agency is not solely responsible for food safety. It shares this responsibility with other federal departments and provincial, territorial, and municipal authorities. Industry and consumers also play an important role. Health Canada is responsible for establishing policies and standards relating to the safety and nutritional quality of food. The Agency is responsible for delivering federal inspection programs that enforce these policies and standards.

The agency finds that a formal strategy for the implementation of the HACCP-based approach is needed. A plan for the transition period, including considering how to manage resources during the transition period needs to be developed. Further, insufficient information has been collected to allow the Agency to measure the success of implementing the HACCP-based approach in improving food safety. It could take many years to develop and implement the further redesign of the HACCP-based approach in the meat industry. This redesign would require industry to perform ante- and post-mortem detection with continuous government monitoring and oversight in the beef and pork industries. It could also take a long time to introduce a pathogen-reduction effort in these industries. This situation is in contrast with the important progress made in the poultry industry.

The Agency is lacking important information on the incidence of food-borne illness in humans and the prevalence of pathogens in the food supply. This is complicated by the fact that the Agency is not responsible for gathering some of the information. However, without this information, it is more difficult to manage risks to food safety and measure the success of Agency initiatives and its contribution to the safety of the food supply.

In Canada future course of action and initiative taken by CFIA has assured important strategic initiatives, which will contribute to the effective and efficient delivery of food inspection and safety activities.

Integrated Inspection System Setbacks: Integrated Inspection System has encountered setbacks that are to be improved. The Agency made a commitment to an Integrated Inspection System to improve the efficiency and effectiveness of food inspection activities by integrating them into two dimensions. First, it would integrate inspection activities across all food inspection programs to have a more uniform approach, that is, to treat similar risks to food safety in a similar manner regardless of which food inspection program they relate to. Second, it would develop an integrated "production to consumption" approach to food safety with producers, processors, provinces, and consumers. This project has received support from industry, which generally considers the IIS as a positive initiative.

Integrated Inspection System development: The Canadian Food Inspection Agency should revitalize and complete the development of the Integrated Inspection System. The CFIA is not in conflict with this notion and it has taken action to further enhance the efficiency and effectiveness of its food inspection system within legislative boundaries. The initiative has refocused on integration of inspection approaches in the area of import control systems and consistency of audit and verification protocols related to science-based inspection procedures.

Risk-Based Resourcing: Risk-Based Resourcing is a critical element in risk management decisions. The concept of risk and relative risk is a difficult and complex subject, and risk analysis is still evolving in Canada and at the international level. To be credible, risk analysis must be supported by a rigorous and systematic scientific approach. It requires that risks be identified and assessed based on relative risks, which means that risks across programs that are of equal severity receive a similar degree of attention and reflect an appropriate level of protection. Based on this analysis, the existing program design can be assessed to ensure that the program appropriately deals with the risks, and the appropriate level of resources needed to deliver the program can be determined.

Import Concerns: One area that concerns most is the inspection of imported commodities. Several of the Agency's internal reviews have identified the need for a more consistent, risk-based allocation of resources across these commodities imported from different countries in the form of raw materials, finished products and as food ingredients. The Agency has not conducted an analysis to demonstrate the adequacy of resourcing for imported commodities covered by the *Food and Drugs Act.* The need for risk-based resourcing is also required to regularise resourcing of food ingredients and raw materials.

Operational indecisiveness: Guidance is needed to assist operational decisions. Further guidance would be helpful when it is deciding how to allocate resources between competing program demands. For example, it would need guidance to determine whether a traditional inspection of a fish importer is of higher priority than a HACCP inspection of a fish processor. This guidance could be a priority listing or a series of criteria that outline what staff should consider in choosing among competing program demands. A parallel importance should be followed, as both are important in the view of food safety.

CFIA's Resourcing Capabilities: The Canadian Food Inspection Agency should assess and report the extent to which its food inspection programs are appropriately resourced based on relative risks. Further, the Agency should develop guidelines to assist staff in making operational decisions on competing program demands. The CFIA is undertaking a comprehensive resource review in conjunction with the Treasury Board Secretariat. The goal of the review is to ensure that the CFIA's activities, including its food inspection programs, are appropriately resourced. The resource review, which has been expected to be completed by April 2001, should assess all CFIA activities, resources and develop a projection of the resource requirements for the next five years. An effective work planning and quarterly reporting process involving both the program design and delivery staff of the CFIA will provide guidance on operational decisions and enhance reporting.

Strategic Approach Needed: The Agency needs a strategic approach to the Management of Imported Food Commodities. Managing safety is different for imported commodities than for commodities produced domestically. The Agency is expected to develop an overall strategic approach for imported commodities that would allow it to consistently manage the risks to food safety of imported commodities. There are concerns among local producers and consumers alike about the absence of a strategic approach for imported food commodities.

Limiting Inspection Factors: Current Canadian legislation is limiting to imports inspection. Imported commodities that are covered under trade and commerce legislation, such as meat or fish, can be stopped at points of entry and inspected. Imported commodities covered by the Food and Drugs Act cannot be inspected. They are declared at the point of entry, but may only be inspected on the importer's premises, unless they are subject to an import alert or other special control measures. These limitations in the legislation make it difficult to manage imported commodities. To deal with these limitations, Bill C-80, the *Canada Food Safety and Inspection Act,* was tabled in the House of Commons. This bill will allow the following:

- Licensing of all food importers;
- Inspection of all food products at points of entry;
- Designation of specific points of entry for certain commodities;
- Enhancement of inspectors' powers; and
- Implementation of electronic commerce.

For imported commodities, the Canadian Food Inspection Agency should develop an overall strategic approach to enhance consistency. Further, the federal government should address limitations in existing legislation. The CFIA is aware of this limitation and actions are being taken to develop an overall strategic approach to enhance and guide the integration of various import control systems and to improve the effectiveness and efficiency of control, monitoring, and enforcement actions.

In the spring of 1999, the Government of Canada introduced Bill C-80, the Canada Food Safety, and Inspection Act. This bill addressed the limitations in the existing legislation, which were identified by the audit. It is perceived that people's food safety takes a punishing body blow under Bill C-80. The consolidation and deregulation forces central to Bill C-80 do little to restore consumer confidence. This bill must be rethought and revisited, and include widespread national debate. The production of nutritional, healthy, ecologically and logically produced food is not centrally recognized as the cornerstone of Bill C-80. Bill C-80 will open the door further to the sale of a whole new generation of altered foods, including those that are genetically engineered. It also allows for the possible introduction of as-yet-undefined "novel" altered seed, feed chemical fertilizer and supplements in food production, and for their release into the environment. Furthermore, what is officially billed as the biggest government effort at modernizing and harmonizing food legislation in 130 years will maintain a system of selective and weak inspection that will rely even more on industry self-policing. These concerns should be removed.

Bureau for Food Safety and Consumer Protection: The Agency has recognized a need to change the focus in managing the sector. Following the organizational and program reviews, the Agency created the Bureau for Food Safety and Consumer Protection. The reviews concluded that with existing resources of about 160 positions, the Bureau, through its programs would place priority on activities related to recall investigations and emergency response, and address specific problems in the food industry on a risk priority basis. To deal with specific risk related problems, the Agency will undertake projects that may include inspection, sampling, education, and partnerships with industry, provinces, and territories. This new approach focuses on identifying specific risks and necessary industry controls to effectively manage the risks, rather than focussing mainly on establishment inspection. For example, the Agency has been working on projects with the sectors of ready-to-eat meat, sprouts, bottled water, and unpasteurized juice. This approach means that the Agency will no longer endeavour to undertake regularly scheduled inspections of all non-federally registered establishments covered under the previous program design. The Food Safety Investigations Program (FSIP) enforces the safety and nutritional quality provisions of the *Food and Drugs Act* (FDA). The Fair Labelling Practices Program (FLPP) - administers and enforces the non-health and safety food components of the FDA and the Consumer Packaging and Labelling

Act (CPLA). Activities include: investigating consumer and industry complaints; developing programs designed to encourage compliance with the provisions of the respective Acts; and developing overall consumer protection policies for the CFIA.

Assessment of overall risks: Assessment of overall risks in food production is needed. The new approach is intended to focus on identifying and prioritizing risks based on risk assessments by Health Canada, reviews of problems resulting in investigations and recalls, information obtained through international environmental scans, the experience and knowledge of staff. Without an overall assessment of risks and decisions on how much risk to accept, the Agency cannot determine the number of resources it needs to adequately deliver its programs.

HACCP Approach Needed: Approach Based on Hazard Analysis and Critical Control Points. The approach based on the principles of hazard analysis and critical control points (HACCP) for food processing has been designed as a cost-effective alternative to improving food safety. It is rapidly becoming the international standard for trade in value-added products. Implementing HACCP-based systems will likely become essential for food producers and processors to enhance their competitiveness and access in the domestic and global markets. For example, in 1996 the United States began, in stages, to require that meat-slaughter and meat-processing establishments adopt a HACCP-based system, which affects Canadian establishments exporting to the United States (US). In Canada, a growing number of food retailers will only accept food from suppliers that have a HACCP-based system. As well, the United Nation's Codex Alimentarius Commission strongly recommends the use of HACCP-based systems to improve food safety. As a result, HACCP principles are being applied throughout the food production continuum, including on-farm and at food retailers.

HACCP-based systems are widely believed to have several benefits. They are designed as tools that produce safer food and require industry to take more responsibility for the production of safe food. HACCP-based inspection programs can allow inspectors to focus on those areas that present the greatest risks to food safety and can help to improve efficiency in inspections. They can also allow some resources of the Agency to be allocated to other areas.

To implement a HACCP-based system, the processor must develop operational plans based on HACCP principles. It must then incorporate these plans into its operations; perform regular monitoring and verification activities to determine whether the plans are functioning adequately.

As the food industry adapts its operations to HACCP-based systems, the government should adapt enhance its approach to food inspection. In a traditional inspection program, government inspectors focus on the food-processing establishments, inspecting the processing conditions and the final product before distribution. A HACCP-based inspection program is designed to include two functions. First, a review verifies that the processor's operational plans respect the HACCP principles and meet the minimum requirements of the program. Second, regular audits check the adequacy of the establishment's activities in ensuring compliance with the operational plans. This demonstrates and provides the confidence to the regulators that the food manufacturing or handling organization is consistent in applying the product safety measures resulting in food products that meet customer and applicable regulatory requirements and aims to enhance food safety satisfaction through the effective application of the HACCP system including continual improvement, elimination of recurrence and conformity to regulatory requirements of CFIA/FSIS.

The Agency has further redesigned the poultry slaughter inspection program for establishments operating under the HACCP-based approach. This program requires industry to perform ante- and post-mortem detection activities. Agency inspectors then provide continuous monitoring and oversight of industry's detection activities. This program also includes a pathogen-reduction effort.

A formal strategy is needed for the implementation of the HACCP-based approach. Planning for the Food Safety Enhancement Program began in 1989. In 1991 a goal of full implementation of mandatory participation in the FSEP was set for 1996. As a result of many factors, including the creation of the Agency, this goal was not achieved, and a new strategy to guide implementation has not been developed. Over the last several years, the Agency has focussed its efforts on recognizing the HACCP plans of those meat establishments that export to the U.S. The Agency and industry were successful in meeting the implementation deadlines established by the U.S. However, at the present rate of recognition of HACCP plans, the transition to the FSEP will likely continue for some time.

The Agency had no plan for dealing with resource constraints that would be created during the transition period to the FSEP. We noted that the Agency had recognized the HACCP plans of some establishments several years ago, but it has not yet conducted HACCP audits because of a lack of resources. We also noted that some employees who had received HACCP training to recognize an establishment's HACCP plan were concerned that their training would be "stale" by the time they were available to complete audits. In the interim, inspectors continue to perform traditional inspection activities in these establishments, which requires them to be trained in both types of inspection activities.

The Agency has neither completed an analysis of the resources that could be freed from the implementation of the FSEP nor has it calculated the possible savings from the further redesign of the HACCP-based approach to include the beef and pork industries. It has estimated that about $4 million of resources currently allocated to the poultry program could be reallocated annually to areas of higher risk through the implementation of the MPIP. It also has not formally considered where any saved resources would be reallocated.

The Agency has not developed a means to measure the success of implementing the HACCP-based approach in order to achieve its goals of improving the efficiency and effectiveness of food inspection programs and improving food safety. It is believed that a formal strategy for guiding the implementation of FSEP and the further redesign of the HACCP-based approach is needed.

Pathogen-reduction Drive: There is no pathogen-reduction effort for the Canadian market. A pathogen-reduction effort involves laboratory testing to verify the effectiveness of the control measures that exist to control microbial hazards. Laboratory testing programs have been developed in the U.S. in response to concerns raised by the U.S. National Academy of Science that new methods be developed to better detect microbial hazards. The effort involves the setting of standards, guidelines or action levels for unacceptable prevalence rates of certain hazards in the food supply based on existing prevalence rates of microbial hazards.

Because of the U.S. requirements, all Canadian meat exporters to the U.S. must meet the U.S. standard for _Salmonella sp._, and the U.S. guideline for generic _E. coli_. In the event that the standard was not met, the establishment would not be eligible to export but would still be able to produce for the Canadian market because there is no similar pathogen-reduction effort in Canada.

Canada has not introduced a pathogen-reduction effort as part of the HACCP-based approach (FSEP) for beef, pork, poultry, and dairy except for processors involved in the MPIP pilot. The MPIP pathogen-reduction effort, based on the U.S. Pathogen Reduction Program, requires testing for _Salmonella sp._, and generic _E. Coli_. Based on the results of the national baseline survey, interim action levels for these microbial hazards have been set for establishments that participate in the MPIP.

To introduce a pathogen-reduction effort in Canada, the Agency would need national baseline surveys on the prevalence of pathogens. The Canadian Poultry and Egg Processors Council initiated such a survey for the poultry industry. This survey was completed with the assistance of the Agency, Health Canada and Agriculture and Agri-food Canada. The results of the survey were used to develop the MPIP pathogen-reduction effort. The Canadian Meat Council intends to undertake a national baseline survey for the beef and pork industries, pending the acceptance of a funding request to Agriculture and Agri-Food Canada.

Given the issues of food safety and value-for-money, it is believed that the Agency needs to involve the public and Parliament in a broad public debate on questions such as the following: Should participation in HACCP-based programs be mandatory? Should Canada be leading internationally in implementing the further redesign of the HACCP-based approach in the meat industry? Should a pathogen-reduction effort be launched for the Canadian market? Should a pathogen reduction necessity be conducted for milk and milk products?

The Canadian Food Inspection Agency should develop a more formal strategy for managing the implementation of the approach based on the principles of hazard analysis and critical control points. Further, the Agency should consider developing programs that require industry to perform ante- and post-mortem detection for the beef and pork industries, ensuring that national baseline surveys are available, and implementing a pathogen-reduction effort for the meat industry.

Problems exist in compliance activities: Program audit is the chief mechanism that the Agency uses to determine whether inspectors are delivering food inspection programs according to the Agency's standards. As such, it is an important means to assess whether they are taking sufficient and appropriate action to obtain compliance.

Non-Recurrence Policy is Vital: The Canadian Food Inspection Agency should identify and adopt management practices that reasonably assure the achievement of its policy of timely correction of non-compliance with no recurrence. The Agency should develop possible regulatory and legislative options to provide the necessary tools for dealing with non-compliance. The author does not recommend non-compliance to recurrence as it still remains a non-complying food safety issue but certain regulatory guidelines should be in place to curb recurrence of a safety lapse.

Basic Objectives Important: The meat hygiene program ensures that meat and poultry products leaving federally inspected establishments for inter provincial and export trade or being imported into Canada are safe and wholesome. It also monitors registered and non-registered establishments for labelling to avoid fraud and audits the delivery of a grading program based on objective standards of meat quality and retail yield to facilitate the marketing of meats from producer to consumer.

CFIA activities include:

- Registration and inspection of slaughter and processing
- Establishments of meat products;
- Inspection and grading of exports and meat products for interprovincial trade;
  inspection of import meat products;
- Process, formula, labelling policy and program development, registration and verification;
- Verifying that food advertising complies with requirements;
- Retail inspection including enforcing label regulations at retail; and residue testing.

Such importance should include for dairy, restaurant, catering and on board food supplies. Over five hundred federally registered meat and poultry processing companies are now operating or in the process of converting to a HACCP system. Many other commodity sectors, including processed fruit and vegetable, shell and processed eggs, hatcheries, milk; dairy creams, fermented milk products, butter, honey and maple syrup are also voluntarily implementing HACCP principles in their establishments.

Dealing with HACCP Criticism

The Hazard Analysis Critical Control Points/Pathogen Reduction inspection system has come under criticism from the regulated food industry, critics in various scientific fields, politicians, and the regulator community.

The first problem concerns the role of microbiological sampling and has been raised by the industry. It is a well-argued point concerning the value, logic, and the resulting outcome of it. The meat and poultry industry argues that microbiological sampling by the government is ineffective and not useful to processing operations. In at least one of these areas, a Federal District Court judge, who has ruled that the presence of _Salmonella sp_. does not in and of itself indicates a failed process as USDA-FSIS has asserted, has supported the industry.

In its waning days, the Clinton Administration proposed two new rules for ready-to-eat (RTE) products. One requires product testing by establishments of all RTE products and the other requires environmental testing in the establishments where RTE products are produced; environmental testing included both food-contact and non-food-contact surfaces. The Bush Administration put both rule-making initiatives on hold pending review but the new Secretary of Agriculture, Ms. Veneman, interceded and the rules have been published in the Federal Register for public comment. Industry argues logically that environmental sampling is unnecessary because RTE products have a lethality step in their processing that is designed to kill pathogens.

Industry also argues that HACCP is not science-based because requirements for acceptable pathogen levels were established using a national baseline sample that was subject to several sampling biases, including selection bias. The claim is made that baselines resulting from this biased sampling were then used to establish regulatory standards. USDA-FSIS argues in return that the baselines are simply baselines and the regulatory standards are based on scientific principles. The courts probably will ultimately settle this issue.

A trained risk analyst might point out that attempting to establish a standard dose-response curve for a microbial pathogen is futile. It is possible to quantify a dose-response within a range, but the range would be so wide as to be meaningless because of the wide variances in Lowest Observed Effect Level among ages and health statuses, races and ethnic groups, socio-economic status groups, *ad infinitum*.

The industry's challenge of HACCP on scientific grounds has some merit. Some of the problems with exposure assessments and mathematical models are outlined below.

Lack of necessary data - because many of these predictive tools require both input and validation data to ensure that the model reflects reality, this option may not be feasible. In many cases, laboratory costs, manpower utilization, time constraints, and political agenda will prohibit both businesses and government regulatory agencies from obtaining more than a one-time vertical slice sample.

Bacterial growth models may not reflect reality - it must be constantly borne in mind that, with microbial pathogens, the unit of infection is the single cell and, while the risk of infection from a single cell is exceedingly small, it is not zero. For example, ten individual vegetative *Campylobacter jejuni* cells have been shown to cause morbidity.

Bacterial dose-response levels are undefined - because bacterial levels are not constant, exposure by consumers can only be estimated. In order to estimate exposure, one must be able to estimate the probability that the pathogen is present in target foods, the initial level of the pathogen if it is present, and how this initial level varies as a result of food processing operations. The biggest challenge in bacterial dose-response comes from post processing circumstances where lack of controls during production to consumption may result unhealthy outcome.

Model inaccuracy - as shown in the risk analysis example, many models use the beta Poisson equation to model bacterial growth, but many growth patterns are more closely described by Gomperz's equation, while still others evade precise mathematical modeling.

Hazard analysis is not risk analysis - when establishments determine where potential biological, chemical, and physical hazards exist in their food processing operations, they are relying on historical data and not scientific validation. USDA-FSIS has recently been attempting to make the claim that absence of evidence is not acceptable as proof of absence of potential hazard. Especially in microbiological hazard, absence in per gram of a pathogen does not mean that it is absent in hundred grams signalling the way to increased numbers whenever suitable conditions develop from production to consumption.

Individual susceptibility is variable - individuals with healthy immune systems are seldom at risk for most food borne toxins. There is even with relative sensitivity to staphylococcal enterotoxin. However, susceptibility for most deficient immune person should be identified and categorised.

All of the points raised indicate that risk characterization is an uncertain process. It must be stated in terms of probabilities of pathogen presence, exposure odds, probable average dose-response, and so forth. We cannot categorically state that, because a particular ground beef lot contains 5,000 colony-forming units per millilitre (CFU/ml) of Coliform bacteria, there is a specific percentage of the population exposed to this lot that will become ill. In addition to all of the uncertainties posed by the nature of microbial pathogens, we must highlight preventive measures in the vagaries of food processing operations; home food preparation efficacy; home food safety practices; post-preparation handling;

retail establishments' responsibilities, distribution agents' responsibilities, where methods of handling, storing, and further processing need the same preventive care as in a manufacturing unit.

It is also stipulated that HACCP is only a preventive approach to hazards while its importance as a total food quality approach is short sighted. HACCP stands as a generic model in food safety; it should also incorporate food quality based on a comprehensive and fundamental rule in operating a food manufacturing and handling organization, aimed at continually improving quality performance over the long term by focusing on customers demand while addressing the needs of all stakeholders.

HACCP for Regulatory Analysis:

United States Food and Drug Administration (USFDA) and FSIS jointly proposed and introduced HACCP in 1996 to bring food safety to American people as well next-door neighbour consumers in Canada. In support of HACCP regulations, they also prepared regulatory analyses, which set the stage for a revolutionary expansion in federal jurisdiction over the food processing technology in the United States (US). Further to these changes, a considerable research work and feasibility studies were also conducted to analyse the economics of HACCP food safety system [190].

The review proceeds by taking HACCP principles, as applied to food products, and applying them to these regulatory analyses as products. The analytical principles set forth in Executive Order 12866 are described metaphorically as comprising a "generic HACCP plan." This plan includes the following areas in which "critical control points" may be located: The clear identification of the market failure, Basis for government intervention; An examination of the extent to which existing laws or regulations have caused or contributed to the problem that regulatory action is intended to correct; A comparative risk analysis used for both priority setting and as a real-world reality check on whether regulatory action is warranted; Non-efficiency concerns including incentives for innovation, consistency, predictability, flexibility, distributive impacts and equity; The fair analysis of a reasonable number of alternatives, including innovative approaches; and competent assessment of social benefits and costs.

Reviewing these analyses using the lens of HACCP, demonstrates that neither of them provided a credible prediction of the likely effects of the Seafood HACCP and Meat and Poultry HACCP rules. Both analyses exhibited extensive, material errors across multiple dimensions. Had they been food products regulated under a system of HACCP controls, both analyses would have been seized, recalled, and ordered destroyed.

Based on the problems noted, several hazards to quality regulatory analysis are identified. These hazards begin with the dubious competence of some of the analysts charged with producing regulatory analysis, for quality persons unskilled in the relevant analytic methods cannot produce products. Hazards extend to limitations and gaps in the relevant science, for the absence of scientific information invites the use of convenient but specious assumptions, defaults, and models. Finally, a host of conflicting objectives acts as a gauntlet of hazards, whether from program management, the agency's general counsel staff or political appointees.

Like in the application of HACCP to food, overcoming these hazards requires careful attention to identifying critical control points and the levels beyond which corrective action is necessary. Even then, safe quality is enhanced but not guaranteed. In the case of regulatory analysis, the HACCP system also lacks a set of credible enforcement tools. The depth of non-compliance with HACCP principles in regulatory analysis may be attributed to this fact.

Conclusion:
It is believed that USFDA have a good structure in place on which to build further food safety improvements. HACCP is implemented, surveillance and risk assessment are improving, and a substantially increased investment in research will continue to provide with more information that can be used to evaluate policies and programs.

Meeting food safety goals will require the efforts of both the public and private sectors. In addition, it will require a farm-to-table approach. For example, we know that consumers have a responsibility for food safety, but they need the right information to carry out that responsibility. That is why United States-FSIS and Canadian-CFIA have carried out an extensive information campaign to educate consumers in North America at risk of contracting Listeriosis about how to protect themselves and why these agencies are enthusiastic founding members of the Partnership for Food Safety Education and Improvements-77.

FSIS is continuing the HACCP-Based Models Project because the Agency believes that the project has been shown to improve food safety and other consumer protections and expects to publish a proposed rule. The new models capitalize on the food safety and other consumer protection gains garnered by the HIMP project thus far, while still meeting the demands of the inspection laws. Under the Models Project, FSIS is requiring improvements in the protections that are currently achieved under the traditional inspection. Data collected from this project show significant improvements in both food safety and other consumer protections.

For Canadian livestock and poultry producers who depend on the world market, the actions of importing countries, like Japan, the European Union, and the US, are crucial to their futures. HACCP is, or soon will be, an import requirement for animal products into these markets.

With HACCP awareness campaign, Canadian consumers too are becoming choosier. They're looking for quality products that are safe. They expect the federal government, the Canadian Food Inspection Agency, retailers, restaurateurs, food manufacturers, processors, and primary producers to provide it.

Canada's dairy, egg, poultry, and livestock producers share with food partners in industry, with governments and with consumers, the responsibility for ensuring that the food they produce is safe. Through the implementation of Canadian industry's codes of practice, GMP's concerning animal health products and other measures; food manufacturers in Canada are already doing a remarkable job of producing high-quality and safe food.

Despite increasing demands and pressures, the CFIA's achievements continued to be diverse and far-reaching. The sum of the CFIA's work contributed to the quality of life of Canadians, to a safe food supply, to the health of Canada's animal and plant resources. The CFIA's work also helped to foster Canada's international reputation as having a world-class food-safety and quarantine system.

The Hazard Analysis and Critical Control Point (HACCP) system has now become generally accepted as the key safety management system for the food industry worldwide. It reduces the incidence of food borne illness; reduces the regulatory burden on business; it is cost effective for the community, government and industry; introduces a preventative approach to food borne contamination; encourages a business environment that can respond quickly to new hazards; encourages businesses to take full responsibility for the safety of food they produce; it is consistent with international best practices; supports export initiatives for Canada to compete more effectively on world food markets; and facilitate trade through consistency with moves, by some primary industry sectors and other industry-driven initiatives, to rely on HACCP-based food safety programs to ensure food safety.

We in the food industry must remember some major points when starting a HACCP system. All employees, including management, must be trained to understand the overall working of this program.

A procedure must be worked out for every process performed. This could be translated to every recipe prepared in the kitchen and every recipe recombined and reconstituted in a food manufacturing plant. The end result is in a food product and a food service providing the safest food possible, which takes

Qamrul A. Khanson

Chapter: 09
HACCP – Worldwide Acceptance

Overview:

We have already discussed the original HACCP system, which was developed and originated at Pillsbury in the 1960's. HACCP was first conceived when Pillsbury-USA was asked to design and manufacture the first space foods for Mercury flights. As they moved onto Gemini with its more complex foods and longer flights, the problems were magnified. By the time the Apollo program landed on the moon, HACCP was developed. Within two years of that first moon landing HACCP was in commercial use in the manufacture of consumer foods at Pillsbury.

Pillsbury concluded, after extensive evaluation, that the only way they could succeed in having safe food would be to have control over the raw materials, the process, the environment and people, beginning as early in the system as possible. In using this approach they developed the Hazard Analysis Critical Control Points (HACCP) concept for food safety.

Canada, the European Economic Community (**EEC**), the United States, Gulf Cooperation Council (**GCC**), and other countries are being guided with regard to the HACCP approach by the deliberations taking place at the Food and Agriculture Organization (**FAO**) and the World Health Organization (**WHO**) of the United Nations and the pertinent Codex Alimentarius Committees. Canada's food trading partners are reaching out to harmonize the food safety system through their national agencies by applying HACCP process in the food manufacturing system. Canada's economy is the 8th largest in the world after United States, Japan, Germany, United Kingdom, France, China, and Italy. The United States of America being the next-door neighbour, super economic power and most advanced nation on the earth is naturally the largest trading partner of Canada. Japan is taking the second place, EU markets taking third place and the Asian markets taking the important fourth place. All of Canadian food trading partners take references from Codex Alimentarius Commission (CAC) for the food safety issues.

Let us highlight the few international approaches towards food safety agencies that have an impact on Canadian import and export of food products. Codex has initiated a working group to formalize a worldwide approach and application of HACCP principles. The concepts incorporated in the Canadian model, FSEP, are consistent with the Codex approach towards HACCP.

CODEX ALIMENTARIUS:

The Codex Alimentarius Commission was created in 1963 by FAO and WHO to develop food standards, guidelines, and related texts such as codes of practice under the Joint FAO/WHO Food Standards Programme. The main purposes of this Programme are protecting health of the consumers and ensuring fair trade practices in the food trade, and promoting coordination of all food standards work undertaken by international governmental and non-governmental organizations.

The Codex Alimentarius system presents a unique opportunity for all countries to join the international community in formulating and harmonizing food standards and ensuring their global implementation. It also allows them a role in the development of codes governing hygienic processing practices and recommendations relating to compliance with those standards.

The Codex achievement: The Codex Alimentarius Commission (CAC) has drawn world attention to the field of food quality and safety. The major points, which have come under the influence of CAC, are examination of the safety systems, back-up towards safety, responsiveness towards food safety and a supporting will to regularise global food safety systems. The points could be described as follows: -

❖ **A**ll-important aspects of food pertaining to the protection of consumer health and fair practices in the food trade have come under the Commission's scrutiny.

❖ **T**he Commission has encouraged food-related scientific and technological research as well as discussion.

❖ **I**n doing so, it has lifted the world community's awareness of food safety and related issues to unprecedented heights and has consequently become the single most important international reference point for developments associated with food standards.

❖ **A**n increasing number of consumers and most governments are becoming aware of food quality and safety issues and are realizing the need to be selective about the foods people eat.

❖ **I**t is now common for consumers to demand that their governments take legislative action to ensure that only safe food of acceptable quality is sold and that the risk of food-borne health hazards is minimized.

❖ The Codex Alimentarius Commission has helped significantly to put food as an entity on political agendas.

❖ The Codex Alimentarius Commission has been supported in its work by the now universally accepted maxim that people have the right to expect their food to be safe, of good quality and suitable for consumption.

❖ The positive effect of the Commission's work has also been enhanced by the declarations produced by international conferences and meetings, which have been influenced by the Commission's activities.

BROAD COMMUNITY INVOLVEMENT: The role of the Codex Alimentarius Commission has evolved with development of the Codex itself. The task of creating a food code is immense and, because of continuing research and product development, virtually endless. The finalization of food standards and their compilation into a code that is credible and authoritative requires extensive consultation as well as the collection and evaluation of information, followed up by confirmation of final results and sometimes objective compromise to satisfy differing sound, scientifically based views.

Creating standards that at once protect consumers, ensure fair practices in the sale of food and facilitate trade is a process that involves specialists in numerous food-related scientific disciplines, together with consumers' organizations, production and processing industries, food control administrators and traders. As more people become involved in the formulation of standards and as the Codex Alimentarius - including related codes and recommendations - covers further ground, so the Commission's activities are becoming better known and its influence strengthened and widened.

A Code of Scientifically Sound Standards: While the Codex Alimentarius as it stands is a remarkable achievement, it would be quite wrong to see it as the only product of the Codex Alimentarius Commission, although it is the most important. Resulting from the creation of the Codex, another major accomplishment has been to sensitize the global community to the danger of food hazards as well as to the importance of food quality and hence to the need for food standards. By providing an international focal point and forum for informed dialogue on issues relevant to food, the Codex Alimentarius Commission fulfils a crucial role. In support of its work on food standards and codes of practice, it generates reputable scientific texts, convenes numerous expert committees and consultations as well as international meetings attended by the best-informed individuals and organizations concerned with food and related fields. Countries have responded by introducing long-overdue food legislation and Codex-based standards and by establishing or strengthening food control agencies to monitor compliance with such regulations.

The Codex Alimentarius now has such a well-established reputation as an international reference that it has become customary for health authorities, government food control officials, manufacturers, scientists, and consumer advocates to ask first of all the directives of the Codex Alimentarius on food safety issues.

Today, there are 167 member countries including Canada. Canada's participation in Codex is coordinated through the Office of the Codex Contact Point for Canada, located in the Food Directorate, Health Products, and Food Branch of Health Canada.

The Codex Program in Canada is managed by an interdepartmental Committee consisting of senior officials from Health Canada, The Canadian Food Inspection Agency, The Pest Management Regulatory Agency, Foreign Affairs, International Trade and Agriculture and Agriculture and Agri-Food Canada.

Codex Role in Food Protection: Trade in food can be of great benefit to member countries of the United Nations. Food import increases the choice of products, allowing improvements in the nutritional and health status of the population. Food export stimulates the development of local industry and helps to upgrade food production facilities, standards and practices, which can lead to improvements in the standard of living. Under these conditions, trade makes a positive contribution to food security.

It is assumed that substantial economic losses result from unsafe food entering the international market, although they have not been systematically quantified worldwide. Such losses involve the costs of food spoilage and damage from contamination; the direct and indirect costs of illnesses caused by unsafe food, including health care treatment and losses in productivity resulting from morbidity, disability, and mortality; and the costs to the industry entailed in recall of products, court actions and recovery of product credibility.

Despite substantial progress in basic and applied science relating to food safety, contaminated food (including water) remains a major public health problem. Food borne diseases are very common in every country. They constitute one of the most important types of health problem. Furthermore, they are an important cause of reduced economic productivity[178 & 91]. In the United States alone, it has been reported that as many as 9 000 deaths and 6.5 million to 33 million illnesses occurring each year are food related[190]. For only seven specific pathogens, costs for lost productivity have been estimated to range between US$6 000 million and $9 000 million. The cost of Salmonellosis alone in the United States was estimated to be about US$1 000 million in 1987[183].

The observation of hygienic practices in food processing, transport and storage has gained more importance as the distance between producer and consumer has increased and consumers have become more dependent on processed and semi-prepared foods. A worldwide initiative on food safety is therefore becoming indispensable. While the public commonly shows concern about the safety of additives in food, the scientific evidence indicates that unhygienic practices represent more significant risks to human health.

THE CODEX ALIMENTARIUS INITIATIVE: Food laws and regulations existed in some form in most ancient cultures, as today it exists in modern societies, to address consumers' concerns. Historically speaking, regulations dealing with food production, manufacture and trade were chiefly related to the criterion of honesty in commerce. During the first half of the twentieth century it was scientifically validated that some substances in food can damage consumers' health. Contaminated or adulterated food moving into the international market can impair health in remote countries.

Consumer safety became a subject of international concern in the late 1950s and early 1960s. FAO and the World Health Organization (WHO) were requested to address this emerging issue in food trade. The Codex Alimentarius Commission (CAC) was established in 1962 as an executive organ of the Joint FAO/WHO Food Standards Programme, with the chief objective of protecting the health of consumers and ensuring fair practices in food trade. CAC is the only international forum that is able to bring together scientists, technical experts, government regulators, and international consumer and industry organizations.

With over 200 Codex standards, more than 2500 maximum limits for pesticide residues, 41 codes of practice and 25 guideline levels for contaminants adopted to date, CAC has proved to be one of the most successful programmes of the specialized agencies of the United Nations, contributing to international harmonization in the important area of food quality and safety[173]. Governments as part of their national food safety requirements use the final Codex texts. They are also used by commercial partners in specifying the grade and quality of consignments moving in international trade. During its more than 30 years of existence, CAC has never been indifferent to the changing demands of consumers and the needs of those who use international standards.

After adoption, Codex standards and other texts have been revisited when the necessity has arisen; in fact, many of them have been revised to take account of new scientific evidence or current food manufacturing techniques. CAC has adapted to emerging global challenges so that the international standards elaborated by the commission will remain pertinent and will always meet their purpose in the international trade of foods.

New Demands for Codex: Recent changes in the international environment arising from the conclusion of the Uruguay Round of multilateral trade negotiations have nearly redefined the role of Codex standards. These changes include the creation of the World Trade Organization (WTO) and the Agreement on the Application of Sanitary and Phytosanitary Measures (SPS Agreement) which all members of WTO are expected to observe. Under the SPS Agreement, which entered into force in January 1995, Codex standards, guidelines and recommendations have been granted the status of a reference point for international harmonization. They also serve as the basic texts to guide the resolution of trade disputes.

In 1991 the FAO/WHO Conference on Food Standards, Chemicals in Food and Food Trade adopted a number of recommendations, which set new directions for CAC-69. These have helped prepare the commission for its new role. Among the recommendations were:

- ❖ The use of a horizontal approach regarding food additives and possibly other areas;
- ❖ The strengthening of the work of general subject committees;
- ❖ Assurance of a sound scientific basis for standards;
- ❖ The use of explicit risk assessment methods by committees;
- ❖ Review of Codex elaboration and acceptance procedures;
- ❖ The establishment of a Codex committee to deal with import and export control problems is expected to eliminate constraints on this issue.
- ❖ Among the actions taken by CAC following these recommendations was the establishment of the Codex Committee on Food Import and Export Inspection and Certification Systems.

CODEX Committee on Food Hygiene: The CAC's subsidiary bodies undertake the principal work of developing standards. The Codex Committee on Food Hygiene is one of the most long-standing and active of the general subject committees. The recent work of the committee provides a good example of how CAC keeps its food standards and other texts relevant to current needs through the establishment of appropriate working principles. Hosted by the Government of the United States, the Codex Committee on Food Hygiene had convened 30 sessions by 1997.

Food hygiene means all conditions and measures necessary to ensure the safety and suitability of food at all stages of the food chain. The main task of the Codex Committee on Food Hygiene is to draft provisions on food hygiene that are relevant to all foods as well as provisions that are applied to specific food items or food groups. The basic texts on food hygiene developed by the committee are meant for use in preventing the spread of food borne pathogens and diseases. Considering both the health and economic consequences of unsafe food, governments should give greater attention to the prevention and control of food contamination at the national level.

A look at the more than 30-years history of the Codex Committee on Food Hygiene indicates that countries are paying increased attention to its work. Participation in its sessions has increased (see Figure). The thirtieth session, held in October 1997, saw a record attendance of 266 delegates representing 56 countries and 14 international scientific, technical, industry and consumer organizations.

Recent work of the committee: The Recommended International Code of Practice - General Principles of Food Hygiene is one of the most widely used Codex texts. It has been revised three times since its first adoption. The 1997 revised version has a new format and provisions based on the concept of risk assessment-187. The revised text sets out the objectives to be met throughout the food chain, from primary production to the final consumer, in order to ensure safety and suitability of food by applying a risk-based approach. One of the methods referred to in the text is the Hazard Analysis and Critical Control Point (HACCP) system. Guidelines for the application of HACCP-31 were initially adopted by CAC in 1993. The widest possible use of the basic text in all areas of food manufacturing implies the furthering of a horizontal approach and is expected to facilitate the efficient use of resources in key food safety and food control activities.

Another notable output of the Codex Committee on Food Hygiene is the Principles for the Establishment and Application of Microbiological Criteria for Foods (CAC/GL 21 - 1997), adopted by the twenty-second session of the Codex Alimentarius Commission-31. While adherence to good hygienic practices in conjunction with the use of the HACCP system is considered to be the best preventive system to ensure food safety, microbiological criteria may be used to examine foods of uncertain origin or when other means of verifying the efficiency of the HACCP system or good hygienic practices are not available. They can also be useful for determining whether processes are consistent with the General Principles of Food Hygiene. To avoid the possibility of microbiological criteria being applied in an arbitrary and non-scientific manner, this new text fully incorporates the idea of risk assessment and describes the principles to be applied in establishing microbiological criteria.

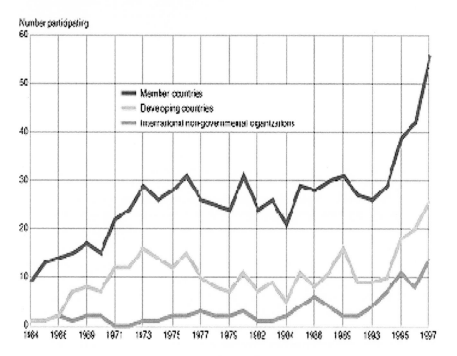

Fig: 09(1)-Participation in sessions of the Codex Committee on Food Hygiene-187 & 31.

Ongoing Work: Now that the text of the revised General Principles of Food Hygiene has been adopted by CAC, the Codex Committee on Food Hygiene will begin the work of revising the existing commodity-specific codes of practice to reflect the new philosophy in these texts: a preventive and risk-based approach.

In parallel, the HACCP system is being promoted in many areas. The Codex Committee on Food Hygiene, in cooperation with other Codex committees such as the Codex Committee on Food Inspection and Certification Systems, is also looking into the modality whereby countries should promote the use of HACCP or related systems nationally. The future work should take account of:

❖ The limited resources available in small businesses and the opportunity of recommending alternative approaches to the HACCP system;

❖ The status of the HACCP system as a possible component of more comprehensive quality control systems operated by food manufacturing companies is yet to be established.

Both issues are closely related to how government agencies should apply regulatory requirements to ensure compliance with food hygiene standards.

Another field of food hygiene of increasing importance regards fresh produce such as fruits and vegetables. As consumers' interest in foods perceived as healthy grows, so does the need to ensure the safety of fresh produce, which is often consumed raw or with minimal cooking.

The Codex Committee on Food Hygiene is also continuing its work on the general methodology of risk assessment for microbiological hazards. It has started elaborating the Principles and Guidelines for the Conduct of Microbiological Risk Assessment, which would provide guidance to CAC itself as well as to governments conducting microbiological risk assessment on their own. The principles are significant in that they attempt to identify the basic concepts of risk analysis, such as transparency, and to describe components and steps of microbiological risk assessment-33.

As shown above, the Codex Committee on Food Hygiene will incorporate further risk-based principles in the Codex texts addressing microbiological hazards for foods by building on the available scientific knowledge and data. This process will be pursued in close liaison with other bodies of CAC. To consolidate the scientific basis for its recommendations, the Codex Committee on Food Hygiene has requested that FAO and WHO consider the establishment of an expert group to conduct risk assessments on microbiological hazards. This recommendation has been endorsed by CAC. If approved by FAO and WHO, such a body will play a crucial part in the future work of the Codex Committee on Food

Hygiene. With the increasing input from scientific risk assessment, the committee is expected to offer further contributions to achieving CAC's objectives of protecting human health and facilitating food trade.

The Canadian Food Safety System:

Canada has a food safety system that is rigorous to protect consumers today, yet responsive to meet the challenges of tomorrow. Experts in nutrition, molecular biology, chemistry, toxicology, and environmental science base Canadian food safety system on evaluations. The system has the flexibility to keep pace with rapid changes in the production and processing of food, increased trade globalization, and shifting public expectations. It adheres to three fundamental principles.

Health Canada (**HC**) is responsible for establishing policies and standards related to the safety and nutritional quality of all food sold in Canada, and for carrying out food-borne disease surveillance for early detection and warning. Enhanced public health surveillance systems are in place at all times to provide immediate information on outbreaks of food-borne illnesses. The Canadian Food Inspection Agency (**CFIA**) enforces the policies and standards set by Health Canada. The creation of the CFIA in 1997 not only brought all federal inspection and enforcement together, it also clarified roles and responsibilities, tightening accountabilities and re-enforcing checks and balances right across the system. Strong communication links between the CFIA, provinces and territories, industry and consumers provide timely and accurate information. This information, together with statistical data on eating habits and food-borne illness outbreaks, for example, contributes to quick decision-making and response in the event of an emergency.

Health Canada, through the Food and Drugs Act (**C-FDA**), is the federal department that establishes standards for the safety and nutritional quality of food sold in Canada. It is also responsible for assessing the effectiveness of the Canadian Food Inspection Agency's (CFIA) food safety inspection activities.

The CFIA is responsible for the administration and enforcement of the following Acts: Administrative Monetary Penalties Act (**AMPA**), Canada Agricultural Products Act (**CAPA**), Canadian Food Inspection Agency Act (**CFIAA**), Feeds Act (**FA**), Fertilizers Act (**FERT.A**), Fish Inspection Act (**FIA**), Health of Animals Act (**HAA**), Meat Inspection Act (**MIA**), Plant Breeders' Rights Act (**PBRA**), Plant Protection Act (**PPA**), Seeds Act (**SA**), *the* Consumer Packaging and Labelling Act (**CPLA**) as it relates to food, and the enforcement of the Food and Drugs Act (**C-FDA**) as it relates to food.

The Food Safety Enhancement Program (FSEP) Manual has been prepared as an aid to the Canadian Food Inspection Agency's implementation teams, its inspection workforce, and to industry's management and employees. Its use is intended during the implementation phases of HACCP.

Due to copyrights constraints, a fully up-to-date and detailed information could be obtained from Web Site: http://www.inspection.gc.ca .

United States Food Safety System:

The United States Constitution prescribes the responsibilities of the government's three branches: executive, legislative and judicial, which all have roles that underpin the nation's food safety system. Congress, the legislative branch, enacts statutes designed to ensure the safety of the food supply. Congress also authorizes executive branch agencies to implement statutes, and they may do so by developing and enforcing regulations. When enforcement actions, regulations, or policies lead to disputes, the judicial branch is charged to render impartial decisions. General U.S. laws and statutes and Presidential Executive Orders establish procedures to ensure that regulations are developed in a transparent and interactive manner with the public. Characteristics of the U.S. food safety system include the separation of powers among these three branches, transparency, science-based decision-making and public participation.

Principal federal regulatory organizations responsible for providing consumer protection are the Department of Health and Human Services' (**DHHS**) Food and Drug Administration (**FDA**), the U.S. Department of Agriculture's (**USDA**) Food Safety and Inspection Service (**FSIS)** and Animal and Plant Health Inspection Service (**APHIS**), and the Environmental Protection Agency (**EPA**).

The Department of Treasury's Customs Service (**DTSC**) assists the regulatory authorities by checking and occasionally detaining imports based on guidance provided. Many agencies and offices have food safety missions within their research, education, prevention, surveillance, standard-setting, and/or outbreak response activities, including DHHS's Centers for Disease Control and Prevention (**CDC**) and National Institutes of Health (**NIH**); USDA's Agricultural Research Service (**ARS**); Cooperative State Research, Education, and Extension Service (**CSREES**); Agricultural Marketing Service (**AMS**); Economic Research Service (**ERS**); Grain Inspection, Packers and Stockyard Administration (**GIPSA**);

and the U.S. Codex office; and the Department of Commerce's National Marine Fisheries Service (**NMFS**).

The **F**DA is charged with protecting consumers against impure, unsafe, and fraudulently labelled food other than in areas regulated by FSIS. **F**SIS has the responsibility for ensuring that meat, poultry, and egg products are safe, wholesome, and accurately labelled. **E**PA's mission includes protecting public health and the environment from risks posed by pesticides and promoting safer means of pest management. No food or feed item may be marketed legally in the U.S. if it contains a food additive or drug residue not permitted by FDA or a pesticide residue without an EPA tolerance or if the residue is in excess of an established tolerance. **A**PHIS' primary role in the U.S. food safety network of agencies is to protect against plant and animal pests and diseases. FDA, APHIS, FSIS, and EPA also use existing food safety and environmental laws to regulate plants, animals, and foods that are the results of biotechnology.

Due to copyrights constraints, a fully up-to-date and detailed information could be obtained from Web Site: http://www.foodsafety.gov .

Food Standards Agency (FSA)-UK:

Canada sold nearly 6 percent of its Agricultural products to the European Union (EU), which falls as third largest importer of Canadian food products. An excellent food safety system in UK guarantees the requirement of Canadian imports from EU, which constitutes 13% imports of Agricultural products. UK being an important member of EU, the safety agency of UK and combined initiative of EU on food safety further guarantees the food supplies to Canada. UK is the 3rd largest investor in Canada. Trends in UK food investment in Canada (1996 - 2000) were $218 million increase from$2.82 billion to $3.04 billion. With such an important trade, a close knitted food safety relationship between CFIA and FSA is warranted.

The Food Standards Agency is an independent food safety watchdog set up by an Act of UK-Parliament in 2000 to protect the public's health and consumer interests in relation to food. FSA's aims are to reduce food borne illness by 20% by improving food safety right through the food chain, help people to eat more healthily, promote honest and informative labelling to help consumers, promote best practice within the food industry, improve the enforcement of food law, earn people's trust by what we do and how we do it.

Although the FSA is a Government agency, it works at 'arm's length' from Government because it doesn't report to a specific minister and is free to publish any advice it issues. A Board that has been appointed to act in the public interest and not to represent particular sectors leads the Agency. Board members have a wide range of relevant skills and experience. Our UK headquarters are in London, but the Agency also has national offices in Scotland, Wales, and Northern Ireland. The Meat Hygiene Service is an Executive Agency of the Food Standards Agency. FSA is accountable to Parliament through Health Ministers, and to the devolved administrations in Scotland, Wales, and Northern Ireland for its activities within their areas-81.

The FSA advocates the Hazard Analysis and Critical Control Point (HACCP) system of food safety management - one that is internationally recognised as the most effective way for food businesses to ensure consumer protection. The Agency believes that application of effective HACCP-based controls across the food chain will help reduce food borne disease, and is taking action to increase the awareness and application of HACCP in UK food businesses.

The Food Standards Agency acts as the national contact point for the UK in Codex. Much of the work of Codex is specialized and is therefore delegated to members of staff in FSA with the appropriate expertise. These internal Codex Committee Contact points take responsibility for specific Codex Committees and distribute all Codex papers relating to their committee/s to NCCC members, interested parties etc. Respond to Codex on standards and other texts in the step procedure. FSA represents the UK at the Codex Committee meeting.

Ministry of Agriculture, Forestry and Fisheries (MAFF) MAAF – Japan:

Canada sold nearly 9 percent of its Agricultural products to Japan in the year 2000. Grains and red meat were two major Canadian exports, representing 19 and 14 percent of total Agricultural shipments. Other exports included oilseeds and oilseed products (13 percent) and live animals (7 percent). Thus Japan becomes a single largest trading partner in food products. Canadian Agricultural imports from Asia amounted to a 6% level even this figure makes Japanese food safety system important to Canada. Ministry of Agriculture, Forestry and Fisheries (MAFF) manage the food safety systems in Japan. Agriculture, forestry and fisheries industries, as an important sector of Japan's economic structure, contribute outstandingly to the development of national economy and stabilization of national life through their role of providing stable supply of foods indispensable to our daily life.

MAFF is responsible not only for promoting the industries under its jurisdiction but also for regulating food safety. However, since a large percentage of its budget and subsidies are funnelled to the industries that it supervises, and since Diet members with close ties often stick their fingers into the pie, MAFF tends to devote more attention to the concerns of producers rather than those of consumers. Japan will have to adopt a new approach to guaranteeing food safety that will make it possible to trace the flow of food from the farm to the dinner table, and that includes a framework for disclosing information and for conducting scientific analyses of risk. Storing information on the flow of food from the harvest stage to kitchens in databases will make it easier to discover the cause of food poisoning outbreaks and other incidents involving food safety, and serve as a deterrent against improper behaviour and transgressions of standards and rules.

To guarantee the safety of its food supplies, Japan should not only enact food safety standards bill but also set up an independent agency to regulate food safety. While the creation of a new agency would fly in the face of the efforts to streamline government, any increase in personnel could be offset by eliminating positions at MAFF and the health ministry, which would have less work to do.

Farmland and forest also play the role of cleaning air and water, fostering water resources and conserving national land resources. Furthermore, nature and verdant scenic sights abundant in the rural communities is closely related to the national life as they provide mental tranquility for the people through communion between man and nature.

The circumstances surrounding the Agriculture, forestry and fisheries industries of Japan are severe, due to such factor as imbalance between supply and demand in Agricultural products (e.g. rice), delay in the management scale expansion in the so-called' land-extensive Agriculture' like rice cultivation, and the escalating pressure for opening up the market from various overseas countries.

In addition, in order to promote the harmonious development of economic society and stability of national life sound development of the Agriculture, forestry and fisheries industries and advancement of the welfare of the people engaged in these industries would be indispensable.

In order to assure healthy and abundant dietary life for the people, moreover, it is necessary to strive towards maintenance and reinforcement of the ability to attain self-sufficiency in food supplies at all times, maintaining, on the other hand, an appropriate combination of import and domestic production.

From these viewpoints, the Ministry comprehensively undertakes administration related to Agricultural, forestry and fisheries products, covering from production to consumption and also to rural development and promotion of the welfare of rural inhabitants with a view to achieving stable supply of food, sound development of the Agriculture, forestry and fisheries industries and upgrading of the welfare of rural inhabitants.

CQCCS – Japan: Center for Quality Control and Consumer Service (CQCCS) is Japanese response to Food Safety. In response to the higher consumer interest in food quality and so forth, it is a requirement that quality be improved and safety ensured in foods and wooden products. Corporations are actively acquiring ISO 9000 and 14000 series certification, the international standards for quality control and environmental protection, as well as introducing HACCP. However, there are many small and medium-size corporations in the food manufacturing industry, and they tend to delay adopting higher levels of quality control because of lack of funds and information. For such manufacturers, the centre provides various kinds of technical support by utilizing technical information and technical knowledge concerning manufacturing and quality control, which has been accumulated through past business activities.

In order to adjust international food standards (Codex standards) to Japan's actual conditions, the centre is collecting information regarding overseas manufacturing techniques and the actual status of distribution for Japan's essential foods. It is also conducting investigations into, and analysis of, the quality and labelling of foods and wooden materials concerned.

The centre also dispatches staff to the Codex Committee for Methods of Analysis and Sampling in order to adjust the analysis methods, which are the major component of international food standards, to Japan's actual conditions. At the request of consumers or manufacturers, the centre performs inspections on the quality or ingredients of Agricultural or forestry products they hand in. The centre also responds to requests to determine the causes of food related accidents, such as the evaluation of foreign compounds.

The centre has a contact point for corporate consultation for factories regarding quality control and other technical consultations. Depending on the type of consultation, the centre provides individualized technical guidance. For the proper and smooth guidance of quality control at factories, the centre creates high-level quality control technical standards for each product item.

GCC Food Safety Initiative:

The Gulf Cooperation Council (GCC) have taken strong initiative on food safety though different states have not yet harmonized a long awaited unification of Food Control and safety System. The GCC member nations are United Arab Emirates (UAE), Saudi Arabia, Kuwait, Bahrain, Oman, and Qatar. In the last two decades, the relative dependence on Agri-food imports has yielded the development of the infrastructure and import facilities in the region. GCC countries are multi-ethnic markets, resulting in a wide variety of food products offered on local market. The expatriate community throughout the GCC has influenced the food consumption in the region and the Agri-food product imports. As a result of nationals traveling to Europe and North America, GCC consumers have become more aware of quality, nutritious value, price and packaging, willing to pay extra for premium quality products, in addition to the integration of the Arab women in the social life, and their entrance to the workplaces.

UAE is the founding member of GCC and imposes stringent food safety regulations in all the individual Emirates. Nearly 85 percent of all foods that are sold in retail outlets are imported consumer ready products, while the remaining 15 percent is food that processed locally. The food safety system is enforced through municipal food inspectors belonging to food control section of different Emirates' municipalities. Abu Dhabi and Dubai are making the bulk of imports from Canada and are important centres for the food safety drive and HACCP implementation in UAE. In 2000, UAE was Canada's third largest export market for Agri-food products. According to Statistics Canada, approximately 70 percent of total Canadian Agri-food exports to UAE consisted of wheat and approximately 13 percent of barley in 2000. In the same year, Canada exported $3.7million worth of chickpeas (dried, shelled whether or not skinned) to U.A.E., which represent 4.8 percent of total Canadian Agri-food exports. Lentils (dried, shelled whether or not skinned) account for 2.3 percent of total Canadian Agri-food exports to U.A.E.

From 1998 to 2001, Canada's value-added Agri-food exports to U.A.E. decreased. According to Statistics Canada, Canadian cheese exports to U.A.E. were $836,016 in 2000 and $264,731 in 2001.

The most significant Canadian value-added products exported to U.A.E. were grain preparations, beverages, spirits, vinegar, and margarine and meat preparation. In 2000, U.A.E. was Alberta's third largest export market for Agri-food products. More than 95 percent of Alberta's Agri-food exports to U.A.E were wheat and barley. In 2000, Alberta's Agri-food exports to U.A.E. were $27 million, an increase of 80 percent over 1999.

Kingdom of Saudi Arabia being the largest member of GCC with a population of about 22 million and with a GDP estimated at US$ 173 billion in 2000 heavily depends on imported food products. Saudi Arabia leads the food safety regulatory drive with its head office in Riyadh. For Canada, Saudi Arabia is an attractive export market and, not surprisingly, it is also very competitive. Its vast oil, gas and mineral resources, modern infrastructure, and market economy provide considerable opportunities for Canadian food business.

Saudi Arabia allows imports of goods from other members of the Gulf Cooperation Council (GCC) under preferential tariffs and gives them a 10 percent price preference over non-GCC products for government procurement. Saudi Arabia's pre-shipment food inspection regime is designed to protect Saudi Arabian consumers from inferior foreign food products. It adds inspection costs to imported food products, may delay shipments to Saudi Arabia, and can increase exporter overhead. Canadian exports to the Kingdom added up to $324.4 million, with barley the least in the list. From 1996 to 1999, Alberta Agri-food exports to Saudi Arabia decreased substantially, dropping from $80 million in 1996 to $287,000 in 1999; because barley exports dwindled. In 2000, Alberta's Agri-food exports to the Kingdom were $15.2 million, which consisted of barley, prepared potatoes and oilseeds-[16]. Saudi Arabia is Canada's fifth largest export market for Agri-food products.

Canada's Agri-food exports to Saudi Arabia were $56 million in 2000, a substantial increase over 1999. In 2001, Canada's Agri-food exports to Saudi Arabia were $35 million. According to Statistics Canada, Canada's Agri-food exports of value-added products to Saudi Arabia were $7.2 million in 2000,which included dairy products, eggs, honey, sugar, preparations of grains (pasta), meat and edible meat offal, live animal and beverages. In 2001, Canada's value-added Agri-food exports to Saudi Arabia were $7.5 million, an increase of 4 percent from last year, consisted of: dairy products, grain preparations, meat and edible meat offal, live animals, cocoa preparations, caseins and albumins. According to Statistics Canada, almost 98 percent of Saudi meat imports from Canada were bovine and veal.

Kuwait is Canada's sixth largest export market for Agri-food products. Kuwait is also an important member of GCC. Canada's Agri-food products to Kuwait were $12.2 million in 2000, an increase of 37 percent over 1999. In 2001, Canada's Agri-food exports to Kuwait were $11.5 million and it is expected to reach $17 million by the end of the year. According to Statistics Canada, Canada Agri-food exports to Kuwait of value-added products were $11.4 million in 2000, which included: dairy products, eggs, honey, preparations of vegetable, preparations of grains (pasta), animal/vegetable fats (margarine), beverages, spirits, and cocoa preparations. In 2001, Canada's value-added exports for Agri-food products to Kuwait were approximately $11 million, which included: dairy products, eggs, honey, preparations of vegetables and grains, beverages, spirits, and vinegar. Milk, unsweetened cream, and prepared/ preserved potatoes were the most significant Canadian value-added exports for Agri-food products to Kuwait in 2001[16].

Kuwait is dependent of imports for than 90 percent if its food needs. Nearly 83 percent of Kuwaiti Agri-food needs are consumer-ready products. The balance of Kuwait food needs is ingredient imports for the local manufacturing industry, which includes wheat and feed grain, meat processing, dairy production, soft drinks bottling and dry pulse canning.

Bahrain, Oman and Qatar have almost the same food habits and retail system. The main difference between their distribution systems is the market shares of consumer cooperatives. In Qatar, consumer cooperatives, which are government owned, are the largest purchasers of goods and services in the country. Qatari co-ops have 40 percent of market share of all the food retail trade in the country. In Qatar, the distribution network includes importers, which supply the national market; wholesalers, which carry out the distribution of imported products either to retailers or directly to consumers through their own points of sale; middlemen who receive a commission and finally retailers. Such a distribution is gradually being oriented towards the creation of supermarkets and commercial centres. These GCC countries control their food safety through municipalities and look to Saudi Arabian Standards Organization (SASO) of Saudi Arabia. SASO coordinates with CAC for HACCP related issues in the kingdom and put efforts to integrate food safety issues with other GCC countries.

Oman food retail is quite similar to the ones on other Gulf countries. Supermarkets and self-service stores are available offering a wide selection of food products and complementary services. Oman has a small heterogeneous population (2.3 million),

25 percent of which live in the capital area (Muscat). About 25 percent of the population is expatriates (Westerners, Indians, Pakistanis, other Arabs).

Bahrain has a very small population (645,361); more than a half are expatriates. The GDP per capita reached $15,900 in 2000, which the second highest in the region. In addition to the strong purchase power, Bahraini consumers have become brand literate and are aware of quality attributes, due to the diversified and complex food distribution system, which is similar to Saudi Arabia. The best strategy for food exporters is to focus on importers and supermarkets. It is recommended to avoid wholesalers at the beginning, to focus on creating demand before entering the high volume market sector and to work pricing backwards from retail selling price to cost and freight label, taking into consideration retail profits, distributor margins, duties (mostly 5% for all food products), and successful price points vis-à-vis competition-78.

A series of food safety scares in recent years has heightened consumer awareness of the need for effective monitoring and enforcement of the existing food safety drive in Gulf Cooperation Council countries. While extensive legislative measures in different GCC countries regulate the safety and quality of food, evidence of deliberate avoidance of harmonized regulations is growing. The efforts are continual to harmonize the food safety regulations and procedures with in different emirates of United Arab Emirates (UAE). New analytical tools are needed to improve the effectiveness of monitoring and enforcement. However the infrastructure is already in place, the will to harmonize the food safety issues have gained momentum in recent years.

The European Food Safety Authority (EFSA):
Panels for EFSA have now been appointed, opening the way for the body to start work on streamlining safety within the European food and drinks industry. The EFSA will now take over the responsibility for the scientific assessment of food safety issues from the European Commission. This is a major milestone in European food safety. The Scientific Committee and panels are responsible for providing the scientific opinions of the Authority within their individual areas of competence. If and when appropriate, they can also organize hearings so that broader input can be obtained.

The EFSA stated that members of the Scientific Committee and panels have been appointed for a three-year term, which is renewable. In addition, EFSA will have its own scientific staff, and most of these will be recruited in late 2003 and 2004, following what the body says will be the imminent appointment of the deputy director (Head of Science). Together, these different scientific elements will give the Authority the flexibility that it needs; to answer the regular questions asked by the main stakeholders; to undertake the necessary strategic work and; to react to short term needs and emergencies.

The Scientific Committee, itself, is composed of the chairs of each of the eight panels plus a number of independent experts. These experts are not members of panels, but collectively possess the most appropriate balance of expertise to support the functioning of the committee. Although the panels primarily operate as independent entities, the EFSA says that the committee is responsible for the general coordination necessary to ensure the consistency of the scientific opinion procedure. In this respect, the adoption of working procedures and decisions on the harmonisation of working methods will be of particular importance. The committee will provide opinions on issues, which affect more than one panel, and on those, which do not fall within the competence of any of the panels.

The list of panels which has been created will include, amongst others: food additives, flavourings, processing aids and materials in contact with food; plant health, plant protection products and their residues; genetically modified organisms; contaminants in the food chain.

The EFSA says that the members of the panels are independent scientific experts who have been appointed as a result of a worldwide call for expressions of interest and an extensive evaluation exercise. During the course of time, the number, responsibilities, and membership of the panels may be adapted to take into account new developments relating to food safety.

In 1999, France established an Agency of Food Safety (Agence Francaise de securite sanitaire des aliments; **afssa**), and the European Commission also set up its Health and Consumer Protection Directorate-General In 2000, Britain inaugurated its Food Standards Agency.

Food Safety Issues In India:
The Directorate General of Health Services, Ministry of Health and Family Welfare (MOH&FW) has been designated as the nodal Ministry for liaison with the Codex Alimentarius Commission. It is also responsible for framing and implementation of the Prevention of Food Adulteration Act, 1954 and Rules, 1955, http://mohfw.nic.in/pfaact.pdf the statutory Act under which the quality and safety of food at the national level is regulated. The National Codex Contact Point (NCCP) as well as the National Codex

Committee (NCC), constituted by the Ministry of Health and Family Welfare for keeping liaison with the CAC, has been functioning since 1971.

A National Codex Resource Centre was set up in 2002 as the focal office for the work of Codex in India. It was set up under the FAO Project to Strengthen the National Codex Committee TCP/IND/ 0067 (A). All those with some responsibility or interest in food safety and quality and/or trade in food should consult the Training Manual prepared by "Strengthening the National Codex Committee - TCP/IND/0067(A)". It is directed to all relevant government agencies, autonomous bodies, and primary producers, food processing industry, traders in food (including import, export and domestic trade), research institutions, educational institutions, the hospitality industry and consumers and covers both the international food standards setting framework, achieving transparency through the consultative process, and the application of Codex norms to specific sectors. The Manual is available from the National Codex Resource Centre. Those interested to use the National Resource Centre may please contact the following address:

National Codex Resource Centre
Directorate General of Health Services
Ministry of Health and Family Welfare
Nirman Bhavan, New Delhi-110011
Fax: +91-11-3014968
Email: Codex-India@nb.nic.in

Conclusion: Consumers all over the western hemisphere as well as in Asian economies want their governments to pay closer attention to food safety and quality. That means more parameter, legislation, science based safety approach and harmonized controls which if ill defined or excessive can damage trade and well-being. Weighing up the costs and benefits of particular regulations, parallel to assessing risk, could help improve safety, while avoiding -protectionism.

Consumers are generally and traditionally everywhere in the world who have a commonality towards much less tolerance about food borne health risks than about risks from tobacco and alcohol. Smokers probably accept the risks they run from cigarettes, but eating food, particularly fresh food, is not supposed to be a risky venture, particularly in today's modern, hygiene conscious world. However, consumer confidence in the food industry has been badly shaken not once but many times due to different incidents and terrorist acts in Japan, USA, and Middle East. The scares caused by mad cow disease in UK and outbreaks of food-borne poisoning in United states, such as from *E. Coli* 0157 and *Listeria Sp.* There have been steep drops in demand for certain products as a result of these scares, and serious economic hardship has been the lot of some in the sectors concerned.

Nevertheless, governments are responding very well in developed countries. Canada, France, United Kingdom, and New Zealand have established food agencies with broad mandates for health, safety, and inspection responsibilities. Canada took a lead in establishing most conscious and scientifically orchestrated food safety system, which makes the Canadian food products the best and safest in the world. The United States has been announcing untiring initiatives continually to address the health risks of food consumption involving several federal agencies with related responsibilities. The authority of the US Department of Agriculture in this area has been enhanced and appreciated by North American public.

Since Canada is an ever looking food trading partner with developed and developing countries, with open immigration policy and diversified food production; Canadian food technologists, food regulatory agencies, educationists and students alike should keep in touch with other food trading countries' food safety agencies with a close eye on their HACCP based food safety drive. This will help screen, understand, and harmonize the drive to wards safe food consumption, imports, manufacturing, and distribution.

Chapter: 10
HACCP MANUAL

Overview:

HACCP manual entails systematic method of analyzing all chains of a production process, the identification of potential hazards and judgement of risks for the product quality and safety. That enables the companies in a chain to establish an adequate control of all possible risks. The manual contains a weighed and reasonable balance between preventive measures, monitoring and actual inspection and analysis of raw materials on the presence of risks that may yield problems in the consecutive chains of the food production and sales chain. Besides, food-manufacturing companies may use the different risk analyses of product streams that are published by FSIS, CFIA and other regulatory agencies as per the host countries concerned.

HACCP manuals should be food simple to understand and easy to implement very practical, yet comprehensive. It shall provide details of logical steps in food safety management of a particular food-manufacturing establishment. The manual must be the first easy-to-understand, a comprehensive safety document, an easy-to-follow guide to all HACCP techniques, processes, and procedures, tested in the application field, corresponding to local recommendations of HACCP generic model's guidelines, illustrated flowcharts, all diagrams complete with transparency checklists, and other valuable records.

A typical HACCP manual would include: Product Description, List of Product Ingredients and Incoming Materials, Process Flow Diagram, Plant Schematic, Hazards Identification, Biological Hazards, Chemical Hazards, Physical Hazards, Critical Control Points Determination, Process Flow Diagram with CCPs, Biological Hazards - Controlled at, Chemical Hazards - Controlled at, Physical Hazards - Controlled at, HACCP Plan, Relationship of the Various Forms Used in HACCP, and fulfilment of Prerequisite Programs.

There are different manuals tailor made for different regions or countries. The manufacturers shall follow the guidelines of the country where the manufacturing unit is located and at the same time products intended marketing jurisdictions should accommodate host countries requirements wherever applicable.

Because of Codex harmonizing involvement, seriousness of USDA to enforce HACCP, Canadians untiring effort to excel its application and G 8s given strength to support it, HACCP stands tall enough to ify international food safety systems. Food standards may vary with their numerical specifications, HACCP control points, control limits, corrective measures and system of verification principally remains the same for any given product. Canada's FSEP fits all requirements of science based HACCP system.

Those food manufacturers who are with ISO 9000 standards (Quality Assurance), it provides an excellent framework for the inclusion of the HACCP principles and an ongoing basis for continual improvement in food safety and quality. Monitoring, corrective actions, recording keeping and verification requirements are already contained within ISO 9001:2000. Adding hazard analysis and CCP's to the quality system is relatively simple and compatible for a comprehensive control. Many companies include too many CCP's in their HACCP system thereby making it cumbersome and unproductive. The key is to break up the important control issues from those that have no real impact. CCP's are those where the failure of the process would cause or contribute to the incidence of a hazard. Critical Limits are then customized for each CCP. These limits may be determined by regulatory and internal standards, which are used to establish that the HACCP system is working correctly. Meeting regulatory limits is mandatory exceeding regulatory limits brings excellence.

Many overlook important CCPs in a HACCP system. Let us take the example of training and education of the food workers and their responsibilities in Food Safety at every Processing Step. The Food factory staff shall be trained and be made responsible for as many as half of the Control Measures and Monitoring Procedures identified in a HACCP system.

In dairy industry, supervisory staff identifying the CCPs, HACCP Coordinator or manager establishes its affirmation and CCLs. The HACCP manual is designed in such a way that it would fulfill all the requirements of a compatible and comprehensive HACCP system.

Logic Sequence of HACCP Implementation:

The following sequence of 12 steps is the approach for the development of a HACCP program and should be considered by any HACCP team.

1. Assemble HACCP team

2. Describe product

3. Identify intended use

4. Construct process Flow Diagram and Plant Schematic

5. On-site verification of Flow Diagram and Plant Schematic

6. List hazards associated with each step - (principle 1)

7. Apply HACCP decision tree to determine CCP - (principle 2)

8. Establish critical limits - (principle 3)

9. Establish monitoring procedures - (principle 4)

10. Establish deviation procedures - (principle 5)

11. Establish verification procedures - (principle 6)

12. Establish record keeping/documentation for principles one through six (principle 7)

ASSEMBLE HACCP TEAM:

Prior to proceeding to the HACCP team selection, it is extremely important to get full commitment from the management of the factory at all levels to the HACCP initiative. Without a firm commitment, the HACCP plan may be more difficult to implement.

The first step in the application of HACCP is to assemble a team having the knowledge and expertise to develop a HACCP plan. The team should be multi-disciplinary and could include representatives from: production, sanitation, quality assurance, food microbiology, food chemistry, and food engineering and inspection staff.

The team should also include personnel who are directly involved in the daily processing activities as they are more familiar with the variability and limitations of the operations. Their representation will foster a sense of ownership among those who will have to implement the plan. The HACCP team may require independent outside expertise (e.g. an expert in public health risks associated with the product/process). However, a plan, which is developed, totally by outside sources may lack support by the plant personnel.

When selecting the team, focus on:

- Those who will be involved in hazard identification;
- Those who will be involved in CCPs determination;
- Those who will monitor critical control points;
- Those who verify operations at critical control points;
- Those who will examine samples and perform verification procedures.

Selected personnel should have a basic understanding of:

- The technology/equipment used on the processing lines;
- The practical aspects of food operations;

- The flow and technology of processes;
- Applied aspects of food microbiology;
- HACCP principles and techniques.

HOW TO SELECT A GENERIC MODEL:

A complete description of each food product must be done by the HACCP team to assist in the identification of possible hazards that may be inherent either in the ingredients or in the packaging materials used in the formulation of the product. It is important that the team is familiar with the product properties, destination and usage. It is important, for example, to take into consideration whether sensitive segments of the population may consume the product in the form in which it leaves the processing plant.

IDENTIFY INTENDED USE:

The intended use of the product should be based upon its normal use by end users or consumers. The HACCP team must specify where the product will be sold, as well as the target group, especially if it happens to be a sensitive portion of the population (i.e. senior citizen homes, hospitals, baby food). The intended use of the product should be described in PDF 01.

Process Flow Diagram:

A process Flow Diagram, using Product Flow Diagram PFD 03 must be constructed following interviews, observations of operations, and other sources of information such as blueprints. The process Flow Diagram will identify the important process steps (from receiving to final shipping) used in the production of the specific product being assessed. There has to be enough details to be useful in hazard identification, however not so many as to overburden the plan with less important points.

Plant Schematic:

A Plant Schematic, using Product Plant Schematic Form PPS 04 must be developed to show product flow and employee traffic patterns within the plant, for that specific product. The diagram should include the flow of all ingredients and packaging materials from the moment they are received at the plant, through storage, preparation, processing, packaging, finished product holding, and shipping. The personnel flow should indicate employee movement through the plant, including change rooms, washrooms and lunchrooms. The location of hand wash facilities and footbaths (if applicable) should also be noted. This plan should aid in the identification of any areas of potential cross contamination within the establishment.

PRODUCT DESCRIPTION FORM: PDF 01
Product Name: Yoghurt

Product Name	Yoghurt
Product Characteristic	PH 4.30 – 4.50
Product End Usage	Finished Product for Consumption
Packaging	Plastic cups with Aluminium foil Heat Sealed
Product Shelf life	Fifteen Days from the date of production
Product Marketing Area	GTA
Product Labelling Instruction	Keep refrigerated between 2°C – 4°C
Product Marketing Control	Keep refrigerated between 2°C – 4°C

PRODUCT INGREDIENT FORM: PIF 02

Product Name: Yoghurt

Dairy Solid Ingredients	Dairy Liquid Ingredients	Non-Dairy Ingredients
Spray Dried Whole Milk Powder (P+B)	Bulk Starter (CH-1) (B+V)	Water, Stabilizer
Spray Dried Butter Milk Powder(P+B)		
Packaging Material	**Flavouring**	**Colorant**
Food Grade Plastic Cups 500 g (P+B)	Nil	Nil
Food Grade Aluminium Foils (Lids)		

ON-SITE VERIFICATION OF FLOW DIAGRAM AND PLANT SCHEMATIC:

Once the Process Flow Diagram and Plant Schematic have been drafted, they must be verified by an on-site inspection for accuracy and completeness. This will ensure that all the major process steps have been identified. It will also validate the assumptions made with respect to the movement of product and employees in the food premise.

IDENTIFICATION OF HAZARDS - HACCP Principle 1

Hazard analysis is the first HACCP principle. As the name HACCP implies, hazard analysis is one of the most important steps. A wrong hazard analysis would inevitably lead to the development of an inadequate HACCP plan. Hazard analysis requires technical expertise and scientific background in various domains to properly identify all potential hazards.

Preparation for the Hazard Identification and Analysis:

The preceding sections describe the various steps required to prepare for the application of the HACCP principles. They explain the importance of having a multidisciplinary HACCP team with much combined knowledge and experience with the product and process under review. They further outline the format for the basic information required on the specific product characteristics and inputs, as well as the specific operational steps and the layout of the process under review. The HACCP team is almost ready now to apply HACCP principle 1. However, before starting the hazard identification and analysis, some background work in the way of a brief literature review should be carried out. This literature search will provide the team with an up-date and scientific review of general information related to the control of food safety hazards related to the products and processes under study.

PROCESS FLOW DIAGRAM
Yoghurt (SET TYPE) PFD 03

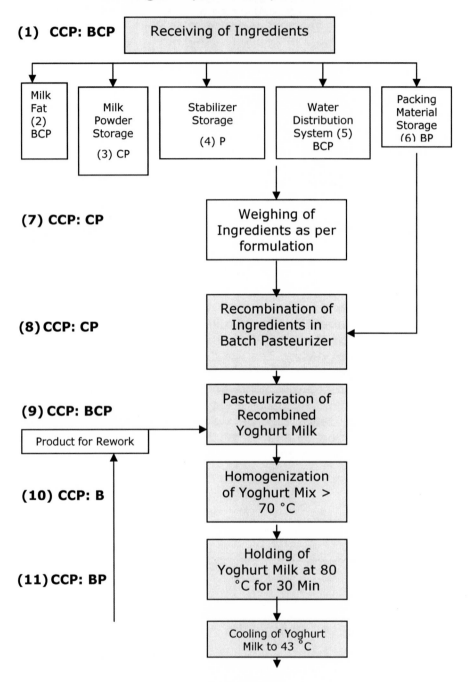

(1) CCP: BCP Receiving of Ingredients

| Milk Fat (2) BCP | Milk Powder Storage (3) CP | Stabilizer Storage (4) P | Water Distribution System (5) BCP | Packing Material Storage (6) BP |

(7) CCP: CP — Weighing of Ingredients as per formulation

(8) CCP: CP — Recombination of Ingredients in Batch Pasteurizer

(9) CCP: BCP — Pasteurization of Recombined Yoghurt Milk

Product for Rework

(10) CCP: B — Homogenization of Yoghurt Mix > 70 °C

(11) CCP: BP — Holding of Yoghurt Milk at 80 °C for 30 Min

Cooling of Yoghurt Milk to 43 °C

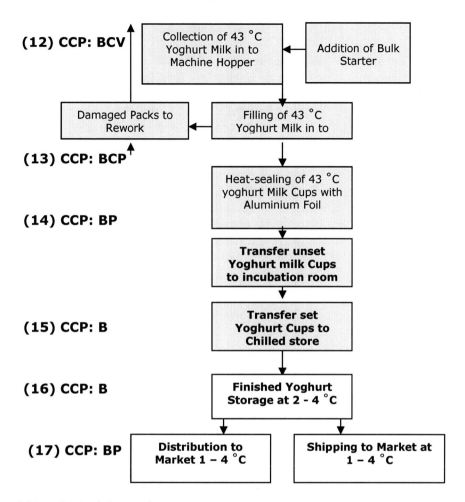

(12) CCP: BCV

Collection of 43 °C Yoghurt Milk in to Machine Hopper

Addition of Bulk Starter

Damaged Packs to Rework

Filling of 43 °C Yoghurt Milk in to

(13) CCP: BCP

Heat-sealing of 43 °C yoghurt Milk Cups with Aluminium Foil

(14) CCP: BP

Transfer unset Yoghurt milk Cups to incubation room

(15) CCP: B

Transfer set Yoghurt Cups to Chilled store

(16) CCP: B

Finished Yoghurt Storage at 2 - 4 °C

(17) CCP: BP

Distribution to Market 1 – 4 °C

Shipping to Market at 1 – 4 °C

CCP= Critical Control Point
C   = Chemical
B   = Bacteriological
P   = Physical
V   = Viral (Bacteriophage) if desired

Note: The total number of Critical Control Points mentioned here is plant specific and could vary from plant to plant. The declaration of CCPs would depend on chances of particular contaminants.

In this section, guidance will be given on what kind of information can be most useful and where it can be found. That way, the time spent on this activity can be minimized and its preparatory effect can be maximized. Examples and references for this necessary background information are described.

The information required can be obtained from the following sources:

a. **Reference Database for Hazard Identification.** A reference database is available to industry and inspection staff to assist in the hazard identification. For a commodity type (e.g. dairy products), the user can access usual incoming materials and process steps. For each of the above, the database will list hazards that should be given consideration by the HACCP Team. The intent of the database is to facilitate hazard identification and augment uniformity in this exercise. It must be understood that the reference database is a guide only and that the HACCP Team is responsible to ensure that additional hazards that may be specific to a food premise will be considered in the hazard identification and evaluation process.

b. **Reference Texts.** Depending on the experience and knowledge of the team, review of texts on HACCP, food microbiology, food chemistry, food processing and plant sanitation may be useful.

Examples of texts of this kind are:

IAMFES, Procedures to Implement the HACCP System, 1991, Ames, Iowa 50010-6666, U.S.A.

ICMSF, HACCP in Microbiological Safety and Quality, 1989, Blackwell Scientific Publications, Boston Mass., U.S.A.

NRC, Committee on Food Protection, An Evaluation of the Role of Microbiological Criteria for Foods and Food Ingredients, 1985, National Academy Press, Washington, D.C., U.S.A.

ICMSF, Microrganisms in Foods 1 - Their Significance and Methods of Enumeration, 1978, University of Toronto Press, Toronto ON.

Gould, W.A., CGMP's/Food Plant Sanitation, 1990, CTI Publications Inc., Baltimore Md., U.S.A.

Marriott, N.G., Principles of Food Plant Sanitation, 1989, Van Nostrand Rheinhold, New York, N.Y., U.S.A.

Texts with more specific information on particular food products and food processes are of course available, depending on the product being considered. However, the best places to obtain access to these texts would be for example, library, community colleges or universities.

c. Health and Welfare Canada Reports on Food Safety Related Illnesses, Recalls and Complaints. The Food Directorate in Ottawa publishes epidemiological information on reported food-borne disease in Canada. An example of one of the reports published is;

Todd, E.C.D., Food-borne Disease in Canada - A 10 Year Summary 1975-1984, 1991, HPB, Health and Welfare Canada, Ottawa, Ont.

The Bureau of Field Operations, Health Protection Branch in Ottawa, compiles the food recall and complaint information. This information is on computer and can be accessed by food product type. This is critical information because it can point to hazards that need to be controlled. One can learn from the mistakes of others.

d. **Company's complaints file.** This file should be thoroughly examined. The causes of the complaints should be reviewed to assist in the hazard identification.

e. **Scientific Research and Review Papers.** These papers are published in the many food journals from around the world. Again, community college or university libraries can help search their library indexes, as well as international data network systems, for pertinent information on specific food products, ingredients, processes and packages. Abstracts can be reviewed and the papers obtained, if appropriate.

This collection of basic data and information by the HACCP team is very important. However, because this preparation for hazard analysis can be very time-consuming, it must be focused on the identification of the following for the product under review:

- The likelihood of occurrence of the various hazards
- Locations where mishandling occurs
- Frequently identified vehicles of transmission, and
- Some contributing factors such as those listed below (examples only)

Table: SOURCES OF CONTAMINANTS IN THE FOOD CHAIN

RAW MATERIALS	In the production of **dairy foods**, raw milk could be a potential source of contamination. E.g. *Mycobacterium tuberculosis*, *Salmonella sp.*, *S. aureus*, *E. coli*, *Campylobacter* sp., *Yersinia* sp., *Streptococcus pyogenes*, *L. monocytogenes*,
	In the production of **Meat and Poultry products**, raw material from meat and poultry source could carry potential microbial hazards. E.g. *Salmonella sp.*, *Campylobacter sp.*, *C. botulinum*, *C. perfringens*, *Yersinia entericolitica*, *E. coli*, *S. aureus*, *L. monocytogenes*, etc. EGGS by: *Salmonella sp.*, *S. aureus*, *L. monocytogenes*,
	In the processing of **Fruits & Vegetables** raw materials could be potentially contaminated by *C. botulinum*, *Salmonella* sp., *L. monocytogenes*, Yeast, molds...
PROCESSING TECHNOLOGY	Processing of raw materials to destroy microrganisms necessary to make them safe for human consumption and for a desired shelf life is of paramount importance in the food industry.
CROSS CONTAMINATION	Cross contamination of finished product from raw food or contaminated objects via raw product (common contacts), workers' hands, equipment and utensils pose a threat to product safety.
PACKAGING	Aseptic packaging plays a vital role in food safety
PERSONNEL	Nasal carriers of *S. aureus*, persons infected with hepatitis A, or Norwalk virus, or being a carrier of *Shigella*, uncovered wounds or cuts being infected with *Streptococcus* or *E. coli* carry potential risks to food products
PLANT DESIGN	Plant Schematic would affect the safety of the product after its heat treatment
FLOW LINE	Raw Material should never be in touch of final food products
CIP INSTALLATION	Improper cleaning or sanitation during food operations are dangerous
WATER ACTIVITY	Final water activity of the food products determine its safety
PRODUCT NATURE	Product needing special pH must conform to its specification e.g. Yoghurt, Ripened Cheeses etc.
STORAGE	Contamination during storage such as condensation, cross contamination, alteration in storage temperatures,

	backflow of water in equipment or container, contamination by leaking or overflowing sewage systems create Food safety issues
MARKETING	Outdoor sales in the market shall be covered with food products storage temperature recommendations.
RENOVATION	Recycling of the food product shall be cautious. The products returned from the market shall not be recycled.

How to Conduct a Hazard Analysis:

A hazard analysis must be conducted for each existing product/process type and for each new product. In addition, the hazard analysis done for a product or process type must be reviewed and validated if any of the following changes are made in: raw material, product formulation, preparation, processing, packaging, distribution and intended use of the product.

Hazards may vary from one establishment to another because of differences in:

- Sources of ingredients
- Formulations
- Equipment and layout
- Preparation/processing methods
- Duration of process/storage, and
- Experience/knowledge/attitude of personnel

For more simplicity, the Hazard Analysis procedure has been broken down into the five (5) following steps. Applying them in a logical sequential manner will help to avoid any omissions.

Step 1: Review Incoming Material:

a. In order to complete this step, use the product description form (**PDF 01**) and the list of product ingredients and incoming materials (**PIF 02**).

b. Review the product description form (**PDF 01**) and determine how this information could influence your interpretation during the analysis of the process. The end product is ready to eat thus process involved must assure safety for the consumer. For the purpose a process of heat and holding could be determined and set.

c. For each incoming material (ingredient or packaging material), write B, C, or P directly on **PIF 02** (as per example provided), to indicate if a biological, chemical or physical hazard exists using previously described sources of information. Each time a hazard is identified on **PIF 02**, fully describe that hazard on Product Biological Hazards **PBH 05** for biological hazards, on Product Chemical Hazards **PCH 06** for chemical hazards and on Product Physical Hazards **PPH 07** for physical hazards. The information should be as specific as possible when describing the hazards (e.g. instead of using "bacteria in incoming ingredient" write "*Escherichia coli* in incoming milk").

PBH 05

Product Biological Hazards

Biological Hazards	Controlled At
Date _____	Approved by:_____

PCH 06

Product Chemical Hazards

Chemical Hazards	Controlled At
Date _____	Approved by:_____

PPH 07

Product Physical Hazards

Physical Hazards	Controlled At
Date _____	Approved by:_____

PHP:08

Product HACCP Plan

Process Stage	CCP Number	Hazard ID	CCL	Monitoring Procedure	Deviation Procedure	Verification Procedure	HACCP Records

Date _____ Approved by:_____

d. In order to facilitate the identification of hazards, answer the following questions for each incoming material:

i. Could pathogenic microrganisms, toxins, chemicals or physical objects possibly be present on/in this material? If so, note the hazard on the appropriate forms.

ii. Are any returned/reworked products used as ingredients? If yes, is there a hazard linked to that practice?

iii. Could any ingredients, if used in amounts lower than recommended or if left out, result in a hazard due to microbial vegetative or sporulated cells outgrowth? If yes, note this on the biological hazards form.

iv. Does the amount and type of acid ingredients and resulting pH of the final product affect growth/survival of microrganisms?

v. Does the type of humectants and the aw (water activity) of final product affect microbial growth? Do they affect the survival of pathogens? (Parasites, bacteria, fungi,).

vi. Should adequate refrigeration be maintained for products during transit or in holding?

Step 2: <u>Evaluate Operations for Hazards</u>

The objective of this step is to identify all potential hazards related to each processing step, the product flow and the employee's traffic pattern. This is accomplished by:

1. Reviewing Process Flow Diagram Form and by:

    a. Assigning a number to each processing step on the production flow diagram horizontally as per example provided (**PFD 03**), from receiving to shipping.

    b. Examining each step on the process flow diagram and determining if a hazard exists for that step (biological, chemical or physical) using previously described sources of information such as the reference database.

    c. Writing "B" for biological, "C" for chemical and "P" for physical, beside each step on the flow diagram as per example (**PFD 03**), where such hazard has been identified.

    d. Fully describing hazards identified on the flow diagram on the pre-printed hazard analysis forms (Forms 5, 6 and 7). The hazards should be related to the process. For example, if a biological hazard is identified at a "storage" step, a letter "B" will be placed close to the "storage" step on the process flow diagram. Then "bacterial growth during storage of ingredient XYZ" will be written on Form 5 (biological hazard).

2. Reviewing Plant Schematic and Employees' Traffic Pattern: (niches), splashing, etc.

Step 3: <u>Observe Actual Operating Practices</u>

The HACCP team must be very familiar with every detail of the operation under investigation. Any identified hazard must be recorded on the appropriate forms. The observer shall:

a. Observe the operation long enough to be confident that it is the usual process/practices.

b. Observe the employees. Could raw or contaminated product cross-contaminate workers' hands, gloves or equipment used for finished/post

The following questions should be answered for each processing step:

a. Could contaminants reach the product during this processing step? Consider workers' hands, contaminated equipment/material, cross-contamination from raw materials, leaking valves/plates, dead ends (niches), splashing, etc.

b. Could any microorganisms of concern multiply during this processing step to the point where it becomes a hazard? Consider temperature, duration, is there a kill step (process which destroys all microorganisms) during the process? If so, focus attention on the areas after this processing step in relation to potential cross contamination.

Step 4: Take Measurements

It may be necessary to take measurements of important processing parameters to confirm actual operating conditions.

Before measuring, make sure all devices are accurate and correctly calibrated.

For example, some of the measurements that may be done, depending on the product/process type is:

a. Measure product temperatures. Consider the heat processing and the cooling/chilling. Take measurements at the coldest point of the product when heat processing is evaluated and at the warmest point of the product when cooling/chilling (frequently the centre of the largest piece) is evaluated.

b. Measure time/temperature for cooking, pasteurization, canning (appertization), cooling (rates), storing, thawing, reconstituting,

c. Measure the dimension of the containers used to hold foods being cooled and depth of the food mass.

d. Measure pressure, headspace, venting procedure, adequacy of container closure, initial temperatures, and any other factors critical to the successful delivery of a scheduled process.

e. Measure pH of the product during processing and also the pH of the finished product. Measure pH at room temperature whenever possible.

f. Measure water activity (a_w) of the product. Run duplicate samples whenever possible (because of variations). Make corrections for ambient temperatures according to the chart.

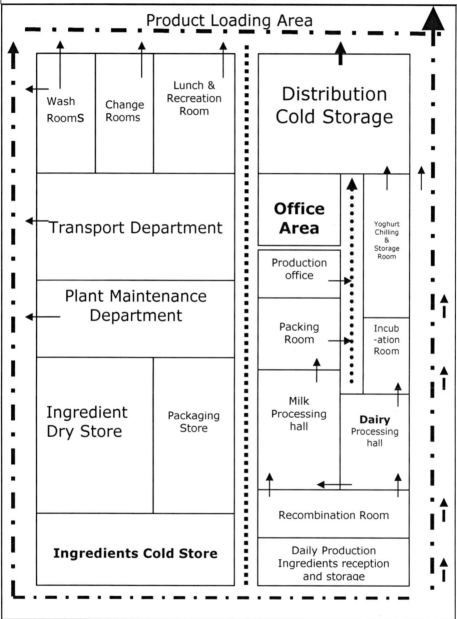

PLANT SCHEMATIC
PPS: 04
PRODUCT NAME: YOGHURT

Product Loading Area

Wash RoomS

Change Rooms

Lunch & Recreation Room

Distribution Cold Storage

Transport Department

Office Area

Yoghurt Chilling & Storage Room

Production office

Plant Maintenance Department

Packing Room

Incub-ation Room

Milk Processing hall

Dairy Processing hall

Ingredient Dry Store

Packaging Store

Recombination Room

Ingredients Cold Store

Daily Production Ingredients reception and storage

PCCPD: 09

CCP Determination

Product Name:

CCP IDENTIFICATION	HAZARDS	CONTROL LIMITS	PARAMETER ACHIEVED	VERIFICATION PROCEDURE

Date _____ Approved by:_____

g. Sample collections, inoculated-pack studies, and microbial challenge studies could be necessary when information on hazards is not otherwise available, or for new products; or for assessing the expected shelf life.

Step 5: <u>Analyze the Measurements</u>

A qualified individual (with proper scientific background) analyzes the measurement in order to correctly interpret the data collected. During the review and interpretation of the data, identified hazards will be fully described on the Forms 5, 6 and 7.

For example:

a. Plot time/temperature measurements on a computer printout or on graph paper. Interpret controlled data vs. optimal growth temperatures of microrganisms and temperature ranges at which they can multiply.

b. Estimate and evaluate probable cooling rate. Interpret cooling rates and compare the measured temperatures with temperature ranges within which bacteria of concern multiply rapidly vs. temperature at which growth begins, slows and ceases (see reference material). Determine whether covers are used on containers to cool down foods (may delay the cooling but may also prevent contamination...) or if containers are stacked against each other. An evaluation of its impact must be done.

c. Compare a_w and pH values to ranges at which pathogens multiply or are eliminated.

d. Evaluate the shelf stability of products.

Once those five (5) steps have been completed, the HACCP team should have an extensive list of potential hazards on PBH-5 (biological hazards), PCH-6 (chemical hazards) and PPH-7 (physical hazards). The team is now ready to proceed to the determination of critical control points.

<u>DETERMINE CCPs - HACCP PRINCIPLE 2</u>

The determination of critical control points (CCPs) is the second HACCP principle. A CCP is defined as any point; step or procedure at which control can be applied and a food safety hazard can be prevented, eliminated or reduced to an acceptable level.

1. Introduction to CCP Determination

The determination of critical control points (CCPs) is based upon the assessment of severity and likely occurrence of hazards and upon what can be done to eliminate, prevent or reduce the hazards at a process step.

The selection of CCPs is made on the basis of:

a. Identified hazards and likely occurrence with relation to what constitutes unacceptable contamination;

b. operations to which the product is subjected to during processing and preparation, and;

c. Intended use of the product.

A separate critical control point does not have to be designated for each hazard.

However, actions must be taken to ensure elimination, prevention of all identified hazards.

Examples of CCPs may include: cooking/pasteurization, chilling, and formulation control.

1. Cooking / Pasteurization

Incoming raw foods often contain pathogens; therefore, inspection for condition at time of receiving may be a critical control point depending on the origin and anticipated use of the products. One or more steps during processing (e.g., Pasteurization / cooking) may eliminate or greatly reduce the other biological hazards. Cooking or Pasteurization would therefore be a CCP. If there is no heat process then the food should be obtained from a safe source or the raw material should be inspected. Heat processing inactivates certain pathogens and spoilage microrganisms.

2. Chilling

Cooling may be a CCP for some products. Rapid lowering of the temperature of pasteurized foods is an important consideration. Pasteurization of food products do not sterilize the food or totally eliminate all bacteria but only reduce the bacterial load to a certain level depending on the process time and the temperature. Spores surviving these processes will grow if there is improper cooling or inadequate refrigeration during the storage of non-shelf stable product. This bacterial growth and germination of sporulating bacteria may represent a health hazard.

3. Formulation Control

Formulation control may be a CCP. Some ingredients affecting the pH or the water activity (a_w) levels of the food mixture will prevent bacterial growth. Acidifier will prevent growth or kill microorganisms if used in sufficient amounts to lower the pH. Ingredients substitution (ex. peanuts) could cause allergic reactions if not declared on the label.

Curing salts create a selective environment for microbial growth, and nitrites in sufficient concentration will prevent the outgrowth of heat-injured spores. Therefore, a sufficiently high concentration of salts and nitrites in food products must be specified as a CCP and monitored to ensure safety.

Certain temperatures, salt concentrations and pH are used to create conditions that select for and promote the multiplication of fermenting micro-organisms. Control of these conditions and/or the addition of starter cultures or cultures from a previous batch (back slopping) are essential for the safe production of fermented food products e.g. yoghurt, sour cream, cheese etc.

If the processing procedures are changed and as a result are different from those originally assessed as safe, the hazard analysis must be repeated and the CCPs redefined if necessary.

In highly microbiological sensitive areas (e.g. packaging of ready-to-eat products), particular handling / hygiene practices may be necessary to be identified as CCP.

ESTABLISH CRITICAL CONTROL LIMITIS - HACCP PRINCIPLE 3

At each critical control point (CCP), critical limits are established.
Critical limits are defined as criteria, which separate acceptability from unacceptability. These parameters, if maintained within boundaries, will confirm the safety of the product.

The critical limits will meet government regulations, company standards or other scientific data. Critical limits may exceed a regulatory requirement.

One or more critical limits are set to control the identified hazard. Critical limits may be set for factors such as temperature, time (minimum time exposure), physical product dimensions, water activity, moisture level, etc.

Once the critical limits are established, they will be written on PCCPD: 09 together with the description of the process step, the CCP number and hazard description.

Critical Limits - Examples
1. An acidified beverage that requires a hot fill and hold as the process may have acid addition as the CCP. If insufficient acid is added or if the temperature of the hot fill is insufficient, the product would be under processed with

potential for the growth of pathogenic spore-forming bacteria. The critical limits in this case would be pH and fill temperature.

2. Kebobs are cooked in a continuous oven. More than one critical limit is set to control the hazard of heat-resistant pathogen survival. The critical limits could be; minimum internal temperature of the Kebob; oven temperature; time in the oven determined by the belt speed in rpm; Kebob thickness.

3. In a ready-to-eat operation, the final packaging has been identified as a CCP. The hazard to be controlled is the contamination of the meat due to inadequate working techniques. The critical limit in this case would be that the working techniques are in accordance with the documented work procedures (e.g. Product contact utensils and gloves are sanitized at prescribed frequencies).

These examples illustrate that CCPs may be controlled by more than one critical limit.

ESTABLISH APPROPRIATE MONITORING PROCEDURES - HACCP PRINCIPLE 4

Monitoring is the act of conducting a planned sequence of observations or measurements of control parameters to assess whether a CCP is under control.

At each CCP, the monitoring requirements and the means to ensure that the CCP remains within the critical limits are specified. Monitoring procedures generally relate to on-line processes and are rapid type tests, visual, monitoring of documentation (for example, product certification) or any other appropriate procedures. The frequency of testing, who is responsible for carrying out the testing, and the testing procedures must also be specified. The monitoring specifications could be written on a newly created Form 10 for each CCP.

Monitoring tracks the system's operation and allows for action to be taken in the event of a loss of control or if there is a trend toward the loss of control. It provides information to an establishment on a timely basis, allowing for decisions to be made on the acceptability of the lot at a particular stage in the process. Monitoring procedures performed in the establishment during operation will result in written documentation that will serve as an accurate record of the operating conditions.

If any one of the critical limits is out of control as determined by the monitoring procedures, the CCP will be out of control. Lack of control at a CCP is defined as being a critical defect or a deviation. Deviations will result in the production of a hazardous or unsafe product. Therefore, adequate and effective monitoring procedures are essential due to the serious consequences arising from deviations. Most monitoring procedures for CCPs must be rapid because they relate to on-line processes and there is not sufficient time for lengthy analytical testing. Physical and chemical measurements or visual observations are preferred because they may be done rapidly and can indicate control of the process. All monitoring equipment must be properly calibrated for accuracy. Examples of some physical and chemical measurements taken to monitor the critical limits are: temperature, time, pH, and moisture level and water activity.

There are many ways to monitor critical control points. Monitoring can be done on a continuous or batch basis. The reliability of continuous monitoring (100 %) is preferred where feasible. The established monitoring frequency must be sufficient to substantiate that the hazard is under control. Responsibility for monitoring is clearly identified and individuals monitoring the CCPs must be trained in the testing procedure and must fully understand the purpose and importance of monitoring. The individual must have ready access to the monitoring activity and must be unbiased in monitoring and reporting. Finally, the individual must accurately report the monitoring activity.

All operational records and documents that are associated with CCP monitoring must be properly filled in and signed by the person doing the monitoring and verified/signed by a responsible official of the company.

Monitoring Procedures - Examples

1. The scheduled final thermal process for pasteurized fluid milk in a pasteurizer is continuously monitored by the recorder-controller. The recorder-controller makes a permanent record of the process time and temperature. The pasteurizer operator is to ensure proper functioning of the thermal process and its record.

2. No deviation from documented work techniques has been identified as the critical limit for the evisceration step in a slaughter process. The foreman monitors working techniques 2 / hour and fills out the appropriate record.

ESTABLISH CORRECTIVE PROCEDURES - HACCP PRINCIPLE 5

A deviation is defined as failure to meet the specified critical limits. Deviation procedures are pre-determined and documented set of corrective actions that are implemented when a deviation occurs.

All deviations must be corrected by taking appropriate corrective action(s) to control the non-compliant product and to correct the cause of non-compliance. The corrective action(s) taken must be recorded and filed. A deviation procedure must describe the acceptable corrective action(s) for a deviation. The diversity of possible deviations at each CCP means that more than one corrective action may be necessary at each CCP. The corrective action(s) must correct the cause of the deviation and must control the actual or potential hazard resulting from the deviation. Product control includes proper identification and handling of the affected lots. The deviation procedures at each CCP are written on prescribed Form.

Corrective actions are prescribed and formalized so that employees responsible for critical control point monitoring understand and are able to perform the appropriate corrective action(s) in the event of a deviation.

When a deviation occurs, it will most likely be noticed during the routine monitoring of a CCP. A deviation results when the pre-determined critical limit for a CCP is out of compliance. If the proper corrective action is not taken the deviation may result in an unacceptable health risk.

Deviation Procedures - Examples

1. The scheduled thermal process for canned spaghetti is not met due to a loss in steam pressure during retorting. The operator notices the deviation before the end of the process time and she refers to the written deviation procedure. The deviation procedure states that the operator should add on the required additional processing time. Additional minutes are added on. This is only part of the corrective action. The deviation procedure also states that the action must be recorded and the affected lots held until a process authority has authorized and signed off for the release of the product. After the process cycle is finished, the lot is tagged and is moved to the detention area. The corrective action taken has corrected the problem and has controlled the affected product.

   During the next shift, the scheduled thermal process for a different batch of canned spaghetti is not met due to another loss in steam pressure. The operator notices the deviation after the end of the process cycle and he refers to the written deviation procedure. The deviation procedure for canned spaghetti states that product is to be tagged and moved to the detention area. The deviation procedure also states that the action must be recorded and the affected lots held until a process authority as to disposition of the product does a full evaluation. After the process cycle is finished, the lot is tagged and is moved to the detention area. The corrective action taken has corrected the problem and has controlled the affected product.

This illustrates that there could be more than one-way to handle a similar deviation. It also illustrates that the deviation procedure will address the various actions that are acceptable.

2. Antibiotics in incoming raw milk are detected by a rapid screening test. The detected level exceeds the established critical limits. The milk receiver refers to the deviation procedure. The deviation procedure states that the milk is to remain in the truck and not be unloaded. The procedure also describes the follow-up action. The milk receiver phones the provincial inspector who will follow up with the milk shippers. All corrective actions are recorded.

3. Cooked sausages are being sliced with equipment that had not been cleaned at the specified frequency. The foreman notices that the slicer has excessive product build-up and he believes that the sausages are being subjected to excessive bacterial contamination. The deviation procedure states that the foreman must hold all products produced since the last recorded clean-up. The product under hold is subjected to microbiological laboratory testing and is not released until the laboratory results are received. The deviation procedure also states that the employee responsible for equipment cleaning is questioned as to the reason for the deviation from specified procedure and is retrained as necessary.

ESTABLISH VERIFICATION PROCEDURES - HACCP PRINCIPLE 6

Verification activities are methods, procedures and tests that are used to determine if the HACCP plan for that establishment is valid and is operating properly.

Verification activities are generally involved and may include analytical testing. In carrying out the verification activities, the establishment may find that some hazards were overlooked or they may discover new or unexpected hazards. In this case, the plan needs to be modified appropriately. The verification procedures at each CCP are written on prescribed Form. Both the establishment and the Canadian Food Inspection Agency will have a role in verifying HACCP plan compliance and they will carry out activities to verify that the HACCP plan is operating properly. Verification activities differ from monitoring activities. Results from verification activities are not intended to make decisions on the acceptability of lots of product. Verification activities involve for example, analytical testing or auditing of the monitoring procedures, product sampling, audits of monitoring and verification records, plant inspection audits, environmental sampling or any other appropriate activities.

Verification Procedures - Examples

1. Checking each incoming lot does the monitoring of the acceptability of peanuts for Aflatoxins. The certificate of guarantee from the manufacture is examined by the raw material receiver to ensure the peanuts meet the critical limits set (Aflatoxins free). As well, every load is visually examined for mould presence.

    Verification of the monitoring activity involves an audit of the supplier's Aflatoxins-free claim by having the peanut analyzed at a private laboratory. A private laboratory for Aflatoxin levels tests a sample of peanuts from every tenth load.

2. The pasteurizer operator does the monitoring of whole egg pasteurization time/temperature for each lot. The pasteurization verification activities are numerous. An example of one verification activity is the microbiological testing of finished product to ensure that the pasteurization is adequate. Another verification activity is the monthly pasteurization thermometer check to validate the accuracy of the indicating thermometers.

3. The monitoring by the foreman of the cleanliness of equipment and utensils in the post-cooking area is done on an hourly basis. The quality control personnel verify the monitoring activity through unexpected audits. The quality control personnel swab the product contact surfaces and do the microbiological testing to determine the microbiological cleanliness of the area.

ESTABLISH DOCUMENTATION / RECORD KEEPING - HACCP PRINCIPLE 7

The HACCP documentations or records are defined as the in-plant record keeping that is done at each CCP and that contain the information required to ensure that the HACCP plan is followed.

Documentations are essential in determining the compliance of the establishment in following the agreed-upon HACCP plan. The HACCP records differ from the records that are kept to ensure compliance to the pre-requisite program requirements. The required HACCP records to be kept at each CCP are written on a separate prescribed Form.

Monitoring results are documented together with any deviations and corrective action taken. Failure to document the control of a CCP would be a critical departure from the HACCP plan. Verification activities are also to be recorded. Records must specify who recorded the information and must indicate who reviewed and signed off the information.

A record may be in any form (processing chart, written record, computerized record) and shows the historical record of the process, the monitoring, the deviations and the corrective actions (including disposition of product) that occurred at the identified CCP. The information contained in the records is used to establish the product's processing profile that would be used if there were any subsequent problems. Accurate records allow for trace back of the actual manufacturing conditions, which will aid in troubleshooting if a problem arises. The importance of records to the HACCP program must be emphasized. The records are an important tool that an inspector will have to ensure that the establishment is following the agreed upon HACCP plan. It will be imperative that the establishment maintain up-to-date, properly filed, and accurate records.

Record Keeping - Examples

1. Pasteurization charts record the time and temperature processing data. The records will show if a drop in temperature occurred and the frequency pen will indicate if a proper flow diversion occurred. The records register additional information such as; indicating thermometer temperature, lot size, operator, date, and product.

2. The retort processing records show a loss in steam during the cooking cycle and the temperature dropped below the temperature specified in the scheduled process. The records must acknowledge that this was a process deviation, and the file must show any process calculations that were done

by the process authority to determine the safety of the product. The file must also show what action was taken with the product.

3. Cooked salami is being sliced with equipment that had not been cleaned at the specified time period. The records must show that a deviation occurred and must indicate the corrective action taken.

Chapter: 11
HACCP-DOCUMENTATION

Overview:

HACCP system documentation can be defined as a documented system to run or manage a food manufacturing and distribution business. It covers all aspects of the company's food manufacturing and dispensing operations. Companies that possess a quality system or HACCP system or a combination of both have documented their systems in writing in the form of manuals, procedures, format, records, and instructions. All members of the company strive to produce a standard, consistent, safe and healthy product or product service that follows these documents.

The food regulators worldwide have shifted their concern from end product testing to monitoring throughout the chain of primary production of raw material to the end product, which is finally consumed. Application of Hazard Analysis and Critical Control Points (HACCP) at every level of food chain from primary cultivation, raising, harvest, grading, transportation, distribution, handling at distribution centres, storage, recombining, processing, packing, to retail outlets till finally consumed by consumers that provides assurance of safety of the food to the punter.

HACCP system can be designed through a safety software system to ensure that HACCP is easy for Food Manufacturers, Food Packaging, Hotel, Catering, Food Safety, and Training Consultancy businesses. The HACCP software system could cover the entire process of HACCP from planning, writing to implementation of the HACCP Plan.

Whatever software for HACCP is used, it must include the requirements of local food inspection agency. In Canada FSEP for HACCP is the standard and CFIA is responsible to implement HACCP accordingly. For Canadian food manufacturers it is important to have uniformity with FSEP. However, consultants who have vast experience in the field may design the HACCP soft wares to meet the international guidelines set out by the World Health Organisation (WHO) and Codex Alimentarius. Which are equally good but for Canadian conditions, FSEP is specific and important for the unified approach to Canadian food safety.

HACCP Documents:

The HACCP Documents can be defined as a record, reference literature, factory specific or generic guidelines, referral point for food safety information of a food manufacturing unit where Hazard

Analysis Critical Control Points (HACCP) process has been validated by a local regulatory agency or accredited by registered agency recognised by the regulating government agency or being implemented for accreditation whether by local, state, federal, foreign or international agencies.

Based on the FAO/WHO Codex Alimentarius, the HACCP procedures identify specific hazards at various points of the production process and set out preventive measures for their control. HACCP programs can be adapted to changes occurring in equipment design, processing procedures or technological developments.

The HACCP lists the points that must be analysed: Raw material and Packaging material; Production equipment, including probes; Production environment; Production personnel; Ingredients preparation; Recombination system, Homogenization system, Deodorization system, heat treatments (Sterilization, Pasteurization); Additives validation, Fermentation process; transfers of products; Microbial Cultures, Finished products; Hygiene, Sanitation and general cleanliness.

The process specifically deals with the quantitative and qualitative evaluation of risks based on the consequences of the possible harm to human health and the probability of their occurrence. Probability can be measured by reference to company documentation, literature, and statistical data. Control of the HACCP analysis procedures must be carried out after every modification in process or changes in official regulations. All documents pertaining to the monitoring of the HACCP system must be kept in the firm's documentation together with working instructions, records, and procedures of the quality system (ISO 9000); HACCP documents are internal documents and must be controlled. However, documents are generic in HACCP but may vary from product to product and plant to plant. Some of the documents most commonly used are as follows:

- ❖ Product Description Form
- ❖ Incoming Product Ingredients Form
- ❖ Incoming Packaging Material Form
- ❖ Process Flow Diagram
- ❖ Plant Schematic
- ❖ Biological Hazards Identification Form,
- ❖ Chemical Hazards Identification
- ❖ Physical Hazards Identification
- ❖ Critical Control Points (CCPs)
- ❖ Process Flow Diagram with CCPs
- ❖ Identified Biological Hazards - Controlled at
- ❖ Identified Chemical Hazards - Controlled at

❖ Identified Physical Hazards - Controlled at
❖ Hazards not Controlled by Operator
❖ HACCP Plan
❖ HACCP Plans for new product line
❖ Relationship of the Various Forms Used in HACCP
❖ Prerequisite Program Requirements
❖ HACCP Manual
❖ HACCP Plant Audit Checklist
❖ Plant Monitoring Records
❖ Laboratory Records
❖ HACCP Audit Records
❖ HACCP Management Review Records
❖ Corrective Action Required (CAR) Records

The HACCP Manual:

1. Cover Pages:

Cover page of any document or literatures identifies the content of that document. The HACCP Manual outlines the prerequisite Good Manufacturing Practices (GMPs), HACCP program, and seven principles of Hazard Analysis and Critical Control Points (HACCP) protocol for product safety. It is simply a tool that will organize you, point out what information you need to gather from suppliers to production and provide you with a format to keep that information on file for easy and logical retrieval.

1 - 1. Title of the Manual: - HACCP Food Safety Manual is the normally mentioned title, which refers to the all food safety related detailed information. The title of the manual encompasses all the list of contents reflecting the title. The title of manual may also indicate version of the HACCP user's manual, which does not pretend to be complete, or without errors but a continual improvement remains a part of the process. Because of product/process additions/deductions, the HACCP manual may still be found to develop quite rapidly, the program may not in every detail correspond to what the manual says it should do. Therefore, constructive criticism, suggestions, ideas and audit reports for the manual should be welcome by the HACCP team, as well as reports of other disorders of the program.

1 - 2. Plant Name and Address: - The registered name of the plant and the address where communication can be conducted. It will be an ideal way to mention complete street address, post box no., and telephone no., fax no., E-mail address and Web site if any.

1 - 3. Purpose Statement: — A statement detailing the purpose of the manual (e.g., This manual lists the products manufactured in this establishment and provides a full description of the hazards, preventive measures, corrective actions, and verifications used in the safe manufacture of food products at this establishment). To reduce the incidence of food borne illness due to microbial and other contaminations to the greatest extent possible, an effective food safety system that will drive future progress for years to come is a purposeful intent.

1 - 4.Commitment Statement: — A statement committing the management to initiate and perform the program detailed in this manual (e.g., The owners of this establishment by signature agree to accept and perform the duties described in the HACCP manual and further to empower the employees of the establishment to carry out the procedures described in the manual). The key methods for addressing microbial contamination and preventing food borne illness are through surveillance, education, research, risk assessment, outbreak containment, and improved inspections and compliance. A commitment statement can spearhead this by the establishment's administration.

1 - 5.Signatures of officials: – The signatures of the company's officials associated with the business and food safety management signify a commitment to the program. With this commitment we see the opportunity to start connecting the early-care issue to having a quality and safe food being manufactured. Much of the increase in support to comprehensive food safety activity will come from officials and down the line of involvement, which are seeing the variable steps and procedures with food safety issues.

1 - 6.Date program will be initiated: - It means that the existing gaps and those certain segments of the food safety issues clearly lagging behind are eliminated. Instituting a mid-course correction to its HACCP program is to focus on those products that present the highest risk to consumers. Before initiation the efforts will intensify its focus on processing steps/stages whose activities present the highest safety risk.

1 - 7.Revisions in the HACCP Manual: - It will include changes and additions that are implemented in the main copy, simultaneously in duplicate copies and followed by authorized signatures.

2. HACCP Team:

HACCP Team works together to provide food plant staff with necessary training and resources to produce safer food products in a food factory. The team uses innovative and effective techniques in their HACCP training activities.

The first step involves identifying the individuals who will serve as lead HACCP persons for the establishment. According to the author's judgement and Hazard Analysis and Critical Control Point (HACCP) system's regulation, the individual who is developing the HACCP plan must have successfully completed a course of instruction in the application of the seven HACCP principles to food product processing. Therefore, the second step is to make sure the individuals complete the required training. Proposed team members can obtain a list of introductory HACCP courses from the CFIA office in Canada.

After the completion of the HACCP training, the individuals should have a working knowledge of the process required to develop and implement a HACCP program. They should also have a HACCP reference book and handouts from the training course that should help them move forward. The HACCP trained individual should then identify the people that he/she needs on the HACCP team. It is prudent to select the HACCP staff according the food segment. For dairy plant operations, a HACCP team should include technologists, operators, and laboratory technicians from the dairy field. So is the perception for other food segments.

The HACCP manual should include the following details of the team in order to facilitate identification and confidence among the members of the Management, HACCP team, Audit Team and Regulatory authorities.

- ❖ HACCP Coordinator's name
- ❖ Credentials of Coordinator
- ❖ Team members and titles

3. List of Products Covered in each Plan: This document is to clarify its policy with regard to HACCP requirements for products like meat and poultry establishments producing either multiple products that fall within a single processing category or single product that pass through multiple processing categories. The same could be applied for other products with similar ingredients and processing steps but different flavours or rheology. HACCP is a flexible system that enables establishments to develop and implement control systems customized to the nature and volume of their production. HACCP plans for products that fall into the multiple processing categories could be exemplified as follows:

Slaughter--all species, Raw product—ground, Raw product--not ground, Thermally processed--commercially sterile, Not heat-treated--shelf stable, Heat-treated--shelf stable, Fully cooked--not shelf stable, Heat-treated but not fully cooked--not shelf stable, and Product with secondary inhibitors--not shelf stable-108.

A single HACCP plan may encompass multiple products within a single processing category identified in this paragraph, if the food safety hazards, critical control points (CCP's), critical limits, and procedures required to be identified and performed are essentially the same, provided that any required features of the plan that are unique to a specific product are clearly delineated in the plan and are observed in practice. Many meat and poultry establishments, especially processing establishments, manufacture numerous products that have most of their processing steps in common. Allowing a single HACCP plan for such products is intended to simplify and improve both compliance and inspection.

For example, an establishment producing both ready-to-eat corned beef and ready-to-eat roast beef could develop and implement a single HACCP plan for both products. The HACCP plan would identify the common CCP's and critical limits (cooking and cooling product in accordance with time/temperature combinations predetermined by the establishment), as well as any processing differences (the corned beef would undergo a curing step). In this example, compliance with HACCP requirements is simplified, and it is probably more efficient and cost-effective to develop and implement a single HACCP plan for the two products than to produce two separate plans.

In another example, the production of fruit yoghurt involves almost the same ingredients, processing, culturing and mixing of fruit preparations with yoghurt to fill in the packaging, or filling fruits and stirred yoghurt from separate filling nozzles making an attractive layer allowing consumers to mix it at the time of consumption. The only difference is in the types of fruit preparations e.g. strawberry, raspberry, cherry, apricot, kiwi, etc. The whole plan will be the same but the difference in fruit pronto/preparation and hazards involved from that particular fruit preparation could be different and must be identified.

Inspection is also improved and simplified because CFIA/FSIS inspection personnel can more efficiently and effectively review a single, unified HACCP plan.

Meat and poultry establishments may develop a single HACCP plan for a single product that passes through multiple processing categories. It is likely that such HACCP plans would be developed and implemented, for the most part, by establishments that both slaughter meat or poultry. For example, there are numerous establishments that slaughter, grind, and package meat for retail sale. There also are numerous establishments that slaughter, cut up, and package poultry for retail sale. Many of these and similar establishments probably will choose to develop and implement a single HACCP. Plan covering both slaughter and processing; developing and implementing a single HACCP plan for a closely related product often would be more efficient and cost effective than producing two plans (one for slaughter and one for processing).

Seafood processors also should be aware that HACCP regulation covers the processing and importing of Fish and Fishery Products. The products coming under fisheries products could include fresh or saltwater fish, crustaceans, all molluscs, alligators, frogs, aquatic turtles, jellyfish, sea cucumbers, sea urchins, other aquatic animal life except mammals and birds, and the roe from these animals, if intended for human consumption. A fishery product includes fish or shellfish as the characterizing ingredient.

Exempted are the harvesting or transporting the involved products without otherwise processing, retail operations and practices such as heading, eviscerating, or freezing intended solely to prepare [involved products] for holding on board a harvest vessel. Note, harvesters, and transporters can be influenced indirectly through processors' product and shipping specifications as it relates to their HACCP Plans.

CFIA lists generic models for many food products to cover as many processes and products as possible to facilitate the development of plant specific HACCP plans. Some categories of the products are as follows: -

Meat and Poultry Meat Products: Products available are Beef Slaughter -- slaughter operations for all red meat species, (except hog), Boneless Beef -- red meat boning operations, Cooked Sausage -- cooked, cured, ready-to-eat meat products e.g., wieners, bologna, Meat spread (Cretons) -- cooked, pasteurized meat products requiring refrigeration for preservation e.g., head cheese, Cretons.

Fermented Smoked Sausage: Dry fermented meat products sausages e.g., salami and some types of pepperoni, Assembled Meat Product (Pizza) -- multi commodity food products with or without meat e.g. pizza, submarines, sandwiches, Dried Meat (Beef Jerky) -- non-fermented dried cured meat products e.g., beef jerky Cooked/Sliced Ham -- cooked, sliced meat packaged after heat treatment e.g., luncheon meats.

Ready to Eat Poultry Products: (Fully Cooked Chicken Wings) -- cooked, ready-to-eat poultry products e.g., chicken wings, drumsticks Ready to Cook Poultry Products: (Chicken Breast Fillets) -- raw or partially cooked, may be cured e.g., seasoned or breaded breasts, fingers, Chinese Style Dried Sausage -- cured, dried/ sausages (not ready to eat) Mechanically Separated Meat (Chicken) -- mechanically separated or deboned meat products Poultry slaughter (Chilled Ready to Cook Whole Chicken) -- poultry slaughter operations e.g., turkey, Cornish hens, fowl Hog slaughter -- hog slaughter operations Ready to Cook Poultry Products (Seasoned Formed, Breaded Chicken Burger) -- poultry products such as burgers, nuggets.

Prosciutto (Salted Ham) -- Cured hind leg of pork, prepared in accordance with a variety of traditions Fresh/Frozen Stored Products (Meat, Non-meat, Food, Non-food)

Eggs and Processed Eggs: Products included are: Generic Models for Egg and Generic Models for Egg and Processed Egg are not available at this time. This list will be amended as they do become available.

Processed Products: (fruits, vegetables, honey, and maple): Low acid canned food -- canned vegetables, meats, and milk products. Acidified -- includes pickles, pork tongue in vinegar.

Frozen Vegetables: Frozen fruits and vegetables Aseptic Fruit Juice -- aseptically packaged fruit and most vegetable juices Pasteurized Honey -- honey operations that pasteurize and package Maple Syrup (Packer) -- maple product operations that heat treat and package.

Dairy Products: Unsalted Butter -- butter products e.g., salted, unsalted, light, dairy spreads and blends Ice Cream -- frozen dairy products e.g., light ice cream, ice milk, frozen yoghurt Soft serve ice cream -- frozen dairy product mixes e.g. includes soft serve yoghurt, milk shake mix. UHT milk -- ultra-high temperature treated milk products which are aseptically packaged and do not require refrigeration for preservation e.g., UHT cream, UHT milk.

However, the listed generic models do not cover all product types and/or processes. Some models or parts of models may serve as examples for other related operations. The HACCP coordinator/team may want to select a model from the list above that best represents the process under review.

Please note that these generic models are normally developed through pilot projects or expert committees to be used as examples or guidelines for various processes/product Generic models are designed as a reference to generate a spe plan out of it wherever applicable. They must be adapted to refle the specific conditions of a given plant operation.

4. <u>HACCP Plan:</u>

HACCP plan is a nucleus of HACCP system and contains Critical Control Point (CCP), Significant Hazard(s) in that point, Critical Limits for each Preventive Measure; it could be mentioned in numerical figure or mentioned in combination of procedural method, Monitoring; by what measurable means, How it is going to be measured or only observed, what is the frequency of monitoring and who will be responsible for collecting data, Corrective actions; to be taken or deviational procedure reference, Records of the whole activity maintained, referenced and it is verified by an auditor or designated person that corrective actions have been taken, they are effective and documented. For each process category following details are to be provided.

5. <u>Steps In Each Process Category:</u>

1. <u>Product Description:</u>

Describe fully the product and the method of its distribution. This ensures that the manufactured food products or commercial supply of food like dairy, meat, poultry, and egg products are judged correctly with respect to its natural characteristics corresponding to safety and wholesomeness. Processors are required to identify product and process information in the form of a product description for each type of product. The product description must identify those product attributes and characteristics that are important in ensuring a safe and acceptable edible food item.

Name of the Product: First of all the name of the product signifies initial identification which most of the consumers as well as processors are aware. Product name (common name) or group of product names (the grouping of like products is acceptable as long as all hazards are addressed) indicate the nature and characteristics of juice. For example orange juice clearly indicates the juice from orange fruits while citrus juice, which may contain a combination of different citrus juices may reflect a combined characteristic of different citrus juices.

Product Usage: Product description could refer to the food items which will be used as ingredients in the manufacture of another product or it may refer to the product which is ready to consume until expires as per written period of shelf life at a recommended

In either case product specification describes the ~~ucts~~, which will be labelled by the manufacturer. For ~~n~~ Concentrate Orange Juice (FCOJ) will reflect its the manufacturing of natural orange juice with ~~...~~ent. In another example; Frozen Cream 69% will ~~...ribed~~ as a milk fat source which could be used as an ~~ingredient~~ for the for the production of Table Cream, Recombined Milk, Coffee Cream etc.

Ingredient: For a product which is to be used as an ingredient a complete description of each food product must be done by the HACCP team to assist in the identification of possible hazards that may be inherent either in the ingredients or in the packaging materials used in the formulation of the product. It is important that the team is familiar with the product properties, destination, and usage. It is important, for example, to take into consideration whether sensitive segments of the population may consume the product in the form in which it leaves the processing plant. Let us take the example of a loaf, which may further be used to produce another product. A loaf may contain ingredients like unbleached enriched flour, stone ground wheat flour, canola oil, yeast, salt, dextrose, sugar, vinegar, calcium propionate, balding powder, potassium sorbate, citric acid, and cystine hydrochloride. Beside these ingredients, it is possible that Soya margarine and gluten could also be present which are not indicated on the label. Such presence of ingredients in the absence of a declaration on label causes allergic reactions and health problems to sensitive consumers.

List the product ingredients and incoming materials (including raw materials, product ingredients, processing aids, and packaging materials), which are used during the manufacturing process. This exhaustive listing is required to properly identify all potential hazards that could apply.

List of product materials for further processing to manufacture products like Liquid Ingredients, Dry Milk Ingredients, Flavouring, Stabilizers, Emulsifiers, and Packaging Materials etc shall be listed separately in another form. That form could be called "List of Product Ingredients and Incoming Materials".

Ready to Eat Product: For a product, which is being manufactured, its important end product characteristics require to ensure its safety could be aw, pH, preservatives, protein%, fat%, minerals %, moisture%, specific gravity, Aerobic Plate Count (APC), Total Coliform Count (TCC), and Yeast & Mould Count (YMC) etc.

All these characteristics of a particular food product indicate what type of storage temperature, shelf life, probable deterioration, possible risk the product may pose if it does not reach consumer in wholesome condition. In fact most of the critical points could be identified at this juncture, which will play a significant role in its safety during transition to ultimate consumer.

The end product mode of usage is another indication, which will require certain points to be taken care before its manufacture. A food manufacturer must list how it is to be used (i.e. ready-to-eat, for further processing, heated prior to consumption). Let us take the example of Flavoured Milk. Every one knows that such milk is consumed directly by children who are susceptible to any contaminants than the adults. Thus the flavoured milk in question shall be with zero defects otherwise a risk to health will exist. At the same time milk in bulk containers when supplied to restaurants or hotels for cooking, not for direct consumption then the leniency in total count may be tolerated. Because the milk will be given further heat treatment, which will minimise the microbial count. Therefore, the regulatory parameters may not differ but individual customer parameters may differ according to end product usage.

Product Packaging: Type of packing is to be described in a way, which clearly indicates the safety of product and its storage condition. Type of package, including packaging material and packaging conditions (i.e. modified atmosphere) are of significant importance as it affect the shelf life of the product. An aseptic pack differs from the non-aseptic pack. A pasteurized milk pack will differ from the long life milk pack.

Product Shelf Life: In the product description, the shelf life, recommended storage temperature and in some cases humidity are mentioned because these factors have a direct impact in the deterioration of food products especially by prompting the growth of microorganism under temperatures above 4 °C and humidity above 40%. Humidity plays an important role where products are dry and with very less water activity. Higher humidity would adversely affect products like milk powders, nuts, and bread. Higher humidity levels instigate the growth of fungus, which spoils most of the dried foods. Let us understand the scientific basis for establishing the 4 °C standard as this seems to be an adequate temperature to control rapid growth of all pathogenic microorganisms and is consistent with the requirements to enhance shelf life of all chilled products by keeping the food beyond the danger zone.

However, establishing a 45 °F (7°C) temperature to control rapid growth of *Salmonella* *enteritidis* microorganisms sounds appropriate and it is consistent with the USDA's Food Safety Inspection Service requirement that shell eggs packed for consumer use be stored and transported at an ambient temperature that does not exceed 45 °F (7 °C). However, a general guideline for other food product storage in shelves of supermarkets and groceries could be below 40 °F (4.5 °C) and above 34 °F (1 C). This is advisable for products like fresh pasteurized milk, milk drinks, fruit yoghurts, plain yoghurt, and chilled custards.

Market Segment:

The market and segment where the product will be sold is another step in product description. (I.e. retail, institutions, further processing). It will indicate if product will be used as an ingredient to complete the production of a product, it may not be subjected to further processing. The best example is whipped cream being used as cake topping. In this case whipped cream shall be fit for direct consumption. Similarly processed minced meat could be used as an ingredient for Indian Samosas, which will be deeply fried in oil beyond 99 °C. Thus processed minced meat will be further subjected to heat treatment, which will eliminate any chances of microbial contaminants due to manual handling. However, any ingredient or ready to eat product shall conform to laid parameters.

Product Labelling: Labelling instructions are indications to customers, consumers, and regulatory agencies. The labels enhance the information in detail about the product and its composition. Sensitive consumers identify the suitability of the products for their consumption by reading the ingredients list for allergens.

Certain products are very sensitive to storage temperatures. For example eggs may contain harmful bacteria, which are known to cause serious illness, especially in children, the elderly, and persons with weakened immune systems. For consumer's protection: keep eggs refrigerated; cook eggs until yolk is firm; and cook foods containing eggs thoroughly before eating. Such instruction on the label could save illness. Such statements are non-threatening, simple, and educational in a way that can be easily understood by consumers.

Guidance through labelling on storage temperatures could minimise the growth of pathogenic bacteria as well as spoilage organisms. Such guidance could prompt housewife and other manufacturers to take more precaution on safe refrigeration temperatures, specific cooking instructions, and post-preparation handling and storage procedures. Educating and advising end users and consumers through proper labelling messages; handling instructions, usage instructions, allergen content, compositional and nutritional information help advance the cause of food safety.

Product Distribution Control: Specific distribution control like shipping condition is another step in describing the safety of food products. Anhydrous milk fat is a product that can keep very well under ambient temperatures. Because it contains 0.3% moisture and 99.7% milk fat which will not allow any microbial activity. However, storage under direct sunlight will instigate oxidation of milkfat, which will reduce its shelf life and edible quality. An instruction "Store away from direct sunlight" is the criteria of shipping and storage conditions. Similarly "Frozen Milkfat for Recombination (FMR)" will have a recommendation for −0.4 °F (−18 °C) storage requirements though composition of both the product remains identical.

2. Identify Intended Use:

Identify the consumer and the intended use of the food. The intended use of the product should be based upon its normal use by end users or consumers. The HACCP team must specify where the product will be sold, as well as the target group, especially if it happens to be a sensitive portion of the population (i.e. senior citizen homes, hospitals, baby food). The intended use of the product should be described in PRODUCT DESCRIPTION FORM: PDF 01

If the product is labelled as sugar free then it is for the consumption of those consumers who are sugar intolerant. The Lacteeze milk is for the consumer who has lactose intolerance. Similarly, the product could be identified as an ingredient, or ready to eat product or a combination thereof. The raw milk sold in the farms may be intended for further processing, a note "boil it before a direct consumption" is a helpful guideline. The unpasteurized juices in Canada would carry a warning sign of "Unpasteurized Juice" though it remained intended for direct consumption. Many examples could be drawn to the point of making a difference.

3. Process Flow Diagram:

Provide a flow diagram for each step in the process. Guidance by using Fig. 13(01)- Form 3 Process Flow Diagram and Fig: 11(01) Process Flow Diagram Example should be obtained as a reference; it must be constructed following interviews, observations of operations, and other sources of information such as blueprints. The process Flow Diagram will identify the important process steps (from receiving to final shipping) used in the production of the specific product being assessed. There has to be enough details to be useful in hazard identification, however not so many as to overburden the plan with less important points.

In the most common configuration, the process flow diagram of a manufacturing unit is equipped to indicate each and every step of the process. A simple visual approach to map the different stages in a process and to identify areas for improvement is a prelude to a successful HACCP system. A Process Flow Diagram is a paper-based tool, which represents a series of activities as a diagram. Improvement teams with little formal training can use it. In HACCP process it to identify weaknesses in the process and Critical Control Points in existing process arrangements and to highlight improvement points.

Develop Product Concept: Based on the product requirements and specifications, multiple product concepts are developed that can potentially satisfy those requirements.

Fig: 11(01) - <u>Process Flow Diagram Example</u>

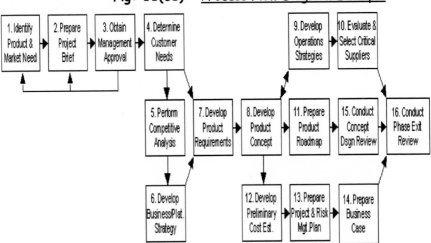

Brainstorming and other creativity techniques are used to generate a range of concept alternatives for improvements in the process. These concepts are analyzed with respect to the product safety requirements as well as the existing technology portfolio, company capabilities, and business strategy in order to select the most promising architecture. The architecture is refined and the best aspects of other concepts are synthesized into the concept.

Tasks

1. Brainstorm and develop top-level product or system concepts to satisfy product quality and requirements.

2. Analyze, evaluate and select a preferred product concept considering product requirements, company technology and capabilities, development risks, regulatory aspects and business strategy.

3. Partition the system into subsystems or modules (and derive subsystem requirements

4. Brainstorm and develop subsystem concepts to satisfy lower-level requirements.

5. Analyze, evaluate and select subsystem concepts considering customer's requirements, regulatory requirements, improved technology and capabilities, development risks, and business strategy.

6. Identify need for risk-reduction development or investigation and launch effort.

7. Document the concept.

Inputs

1. Product requirements document

Outputs/Deliverables

1. Product concept
2. Layout drawing
3. Identified CCPs
4. Establishment of CCLs
5. Preventive procedure
6. Concept selection matrix
7. Improvement in techniques

Personnel Involved

1. Quality Assurance Manager
2. Food Plant Manager
3. Design Engineers
4. Manufacturing Engineer
5. Test Engineer
6. Production @ Quality Supervisors
7. Plant Operators
8. Internal HACCP Auditors

4. Plant Schematic:

Provide a plant schematic for each step in the process. A Plant Schematic, using form 4 must be developed to show product flow and employee traffic patterns within the plant, for that specific product. The diagram should include the flow of all ingredients and packaging materials from the moment they are received at the plant, through storage, preparation, processing, packaging, finished product holding, and shipping. The personnel flow should indicate employee movement through the plant, including change rooms, washrooms, and lunchrooms. The location of hand wash facilities and footbaths (if applicable) should also be noted. This plan should aid in the identification of any areas of potential cross contamination within the establishment. All sections that apply must be provided.

Many of the modern days dairy operations are directed from a centralized, computerized control room situated either side of the building or centrally located. The facility may be staffed twenty-four hours a day with a minimum crew of two at all times, who generally work twelve-hour shifts. The drawing of plant schematic plan reflects the task of risk assessment, which should not be limited to a few specialists. In some situations, it may be appropriate to conduct and formally document very detailed schematic risk assessments that require input from several technical experts. Food Managers use the information provided by plant schematic diagram to assess, to complete the risk management and communication components of the HACCP analysis, and ultimately to make decisions.

The need for standardized specifications for a food plant installations and construction has long been recognized. Much of the blame of bottlenecks and safety issues can be attached to the lack of uniformity in conceptual models used to define a production plant control system. A state of the art plant schematic design accommodating Food Safety, Cycle Time Reduction and Human Safety holds significant promise for food processors, particularly in a production environment where manufacturing flexibility is causing even those with continuous processes to rethink the benefits of an efficient and model plant schematic plan. Reductions in troubleshooting time, paperwork, and simplified recipe changes, rapid changeover, and greater flexibility in mix making are among the benefits realized attributed to a proper schematic plan. Cycle Time Reduction is one of the benefits, which is identifying and implementing more efficient ways to do things. Reducing cycle time requires eliminating or reducing non-value-added activity, which is defined as any activity that does not add value to the product but may endanger food safety. Examples of non-value- added activity in which cycle time can be reduced or eliminated include repair due to defects, machine set-up, and schedule delays due to lack of preventive maintenance attributed to wrong plant design and congestion in the manufacturing hall. Reducing cycle time will have a significant impact on a company's rapid productivity and HACCP implementation.

Once the Process Flow Diagram and Plant Schematic have been drafted, they must be verified by an on-site inspection for accuracy and completeness. This will ensure that all the major process steps have been identified. It will also validate the assumptions made with respect to the movement of product and employees in the food premise.

HACCP is a preventative control program for the food industry. HACCP incorporates safety into the food production process by verifying each step in the process. Anticipating and preventing hazards during processing rather than relying on the final inspection and testing of the finished product is the corner stone, which help ensure food safety. On site verification of flow diagram and plant schematic verifies envisioned plan in to a reality, which paves the identification of many CCPs, which may deceive human brain.

A fine example of such a deception could be drawn from a process where a stainless steel elbow loop is used for a changeover between the three milk incubation tanks. The changeover elbow shall be cleaned each time and sanitized each time to eliminate chances of microbial contamination from atmosphere, human hands, and spill over and milk solids. In a plant schematic diagram such a CCP may not be visible unless recognized and listed in the product flow diagram. By visiting the plant, visualising each critical and practical step in the

process one can list this minor step and eliminate major contamination factor either by modifying the connection in to the CIP type or laying down the procedure of sanitation each time it is dismantled.

Flow Diagram for Production of Pasteurized Skim Milk and Cream

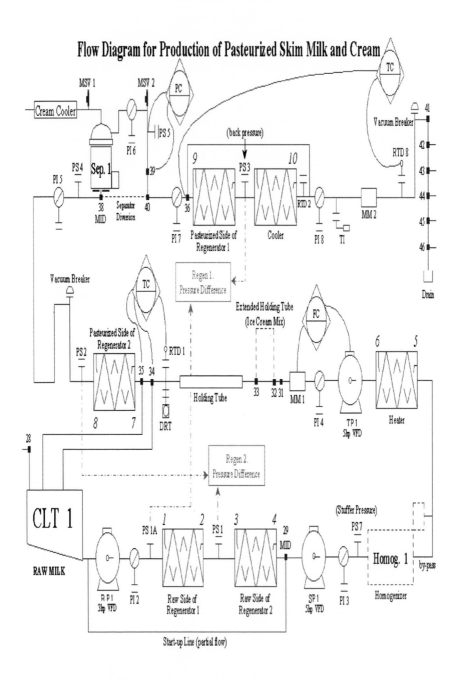

Fig: (11) 02 - Courtesy: Michigan State University Dairy Plant

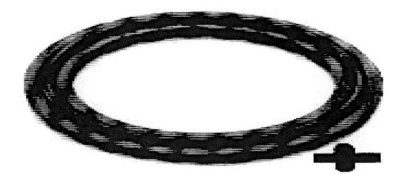

STANDARD CLAMP GASKET

Fig: (11) 03 - <u>Sound Gaskets Eliminate on Line Microbial Risks</u>

Sometimes, a standard clamp gasket in a pipe union may have a minor leak, which may go un-noticed by human eyes. One can mark such joints with rigid fixtures, which will not allow movement to prevent milk leakage and its solidification. Such leakage if un-noticed could provide a breeding media for Enterobacteriaceae bacteria. A multiple continual monitoring on day-to-day basis may help detect an early stage contamination. This may not be listed as a separate CCP but should be a part of SSOP.

5. Identified Hazards:

List hazards associated with each step - (principle 1). The primary purpose of this identification is to develop practical guidelines on risk prevention for chemical, microbiological, and physical hazards in food. In order to do this the process of identification will compare and review the approaches used in several generic model recent risk assessments. The findings will address issues such as "How the outcome should be expressed", "is it understandable"? "Characterization and effect of uncertainty" "quality assurance of the risk assessment, including validation of the estimated risk", "sensitivity analysis" "characterization of the adverse effects expected" "investigation of mitigation strategies" as these are key factors in the risk characterization. Based on currently available scientific knowledge and information, the HACCP process will formulate practical guidelines for the elimination conduct of risk hazards of foods in the process.

Hazard analysis requires multidisciplinary HACCP team with much combined knowledge and experience with the product and process under review, as it is the first HACCP principle and an important step. As hazard analysis is one of the most important steps it outlines the format for the basic information required on the specific product characteristics and inputs, as well as the specific operational steps and the layout of the process under review. A wrong hazard analysis would inevitably lead to the development of an inadequate HACCP plan. Hazard analysis requires technical expertise and scientific background in various domains to properly identify all potential hazards. Before starting the hazard identification and analysis, some background work in the way of a brief literature review should be carried out. This literature search will provide the team with an up-date and scientific review of general information related to the control of food safety hazards related to the products and processes under study.

Texts can be referred for more specific information on particular food products and food processes-119 & 142. Other references can also be availed from CFIA office-86.

List the identified hazards:
For a commodity type (e.g. meat products), the user can access usual incoming materials and process steps. For each of the above, the database will list hazards that should be given consideration by the HACCP Team. A Reference Database for Hazard Identification from CFIA is available to industry and inspection staff to assist in the hazard identification. The database lists are only for guidance and HACCP team investigating and listing hazards is responsible to ensure that additional hazards that may be specific to a food premise will be considered in the hazard identification, listing and evaluation process.

Before switching to the next stage, HACCP team should ask a question and brainstorm that where can a breakdown in the system cause customers to become ill from eating the food we manufacture? At what point in the flow of food through my establishment—from receiving and storing to preparing and serving—could something go wrong? The answers to these questions will aid the team in developing an effective food safety plan that helps to ensure the food being manufactured and distributed for consumption is safe.

State the significance of each hazard:
A microbial hazard will require adequate heat treatment as has been the practice known to humans that thermal treatment of food products is to render them free of pathogenic microorganisms and it has been practiced for more than five thousand years. However, a method by which to quantify the microbial destruction that takes place during a thermal treatment and that significance has to be stated in time and temperature combination. The amount of heat delivered by a food process is dependent on both the way in which the product is heated and its physical nature. The negative impact

of identified hazard should be stated and clearly understood in the worst-case scenario and no risk taken in elimination process.

For each incoming material; ingredient or packaging material, write B, C, or P directly on Form 2 to indicate if a Biological, Chemical or Physical hazard exists using previously described sources of information. Each time a hazard is identified on Form 2, fully describe that hazard on Form 5 for biological hazards, on Form 6 for chemical hazards and on Form 7 for physical hazards. The information should be as specific as possible when describing the hazards e.g. instead of using "bacteria in incoming ingredient" write "_Escherichia coli_ in incoming milk powder."

In order to facilitate the identification and significance of hazards, find a solution to the following questions for each incoming material: Could pathogenic microrganisms, toxins, chemicals or physical objects possibly be present on/in this material? If so, note the hazard on the appropriate forms. Are any returned/reworked products used as ingredients? If yes, is there a hazard linked to that practice? Could any ingredients, if used in amounts lower than recommended or if left out, result in a hazard due to microbial vegetative or sporulated cells outgrowth? If yes, note this on the biological hazards form. Does the amount and type of acid ingredients and resulting pH of the final product affect growth/survival of microorganisms? Does the type of humectants and a_w (water activity) of final product affect microbial growth? Do they affect the survival of pathogens? (Parasites, bacteria, fungi,). Should adequate refrigeration be maintained for products during transit or in holding?

Justify the significance: The distinctions between precautionary principle and actual risk need clarification and understanding. When human health is impacted by a hazard, zero tolerance remains the limit. In order to have a successful food safety plan, one must focus on having an infrastructure in place to embrace the program so it doesn't erode over time. A good management system will understand the significance of each hazard and would ensure an effective food safety plan, now and for the longer term. Retraining staff and verifying that food safety procedures are in place will help ensure the food you serve is safe. It will also demonstrate commitment to proper food safety procedures.

A frightening array of food-related hazards that can poison the most sumptuous feasts like Sea cucumbers plumped up with formaldehyde, Pork laced with clenbuteral, an asthma medication farmers use to make the meat lean. Moldy rice coated with carcinogenic chemicals to make it look fresh. Such hazards may look imaginary but a selector of ingredients or a consumer must ask such questions because it will have significant impact on human health.

In a manufacturing unit, an important factor is the significance of each step and its association with possible hazards. Identify all potential hazards related to each processing step, the product flow, and the employee's traffic pattern. This is accomplished by reviewing Process Flow Diagram Form and by assigning a number to each processing step on the production flow diagram horizontally as per example provided (Form 3), from receiving to shipping.

Examining each step on the process flow diagram and determining if a hazard exists for that step (biological, chemical or physical) using previously described sources of information such as the reference database. Writing "B" for biological, "C" for chemical and "P" for physical beside each step on the flow diagram as per example, where such hazard has been identified. Fully describing hazards identified on the flow diagram on the pre-printed hazard analysis forms (Forms 5, 6 and 7). The hazards should be related to the process. For example, if a biological hazard is identified at a "storage" step, a letter "B" will be placed close to the "storage" step on the process flow diagram. Then "bacterial growth during storage of ingredient XYZ" will be written on Form 5 (biological hazard).

Reviewing Plant Schematic and Employees' Traffic Pattern: Review product flow and employees' traffic pattern (Form 4), and identify all hazards in the same manner. To help in determining if a hazard exists; the following questions should be answered for each processing step:

Could contaminants reach the product during this processing step? Consider workers' hands, contaminated equipment/material, cross-contamination from raw materials, leaking valves/plates, dead ends (niches), splashing, etc. Could any microorganisms of concern multiply during this processing step to the point where it becomes a hazard? Consider temperature and duration.

Beside the literary information on the significance of hazards in manufacturing place, The HACCP team must be very familiar with every detail of the operation under investigation. Any identified hazard must be recorded on the appropriate forms. The observer shall observe the operation long enough to be confident that it is the usual process/practices. Observe the employees. Could raw or contaminated product cross-contaminate workers' hands, gloves, or equipment used for finished/post process product? Observe hygienic practices and note the hazards. Is there a kill step (process which destroys all microorganisms) during the process? If so, focus attention on the areas after this processing step in relation to potential cross contamination.

Describe preventive measures: The regulation defines critical limit as "the maximum or minimum value to which a physical, biological, or chemical hazard must be controlled at a Critical Control Point to prevent, eliminate, or reduce to an acceptable level the occurrence of the identified food safety hazard." Critical limits are expressed as numbers or specific parameters based on visual observation, such as: 140 °C for 3 seconds. It may be necessary to take measurements of important processing parameters to confirm actual operating conditions. Before measuring, make sure all devices are accurate and correctly calibrated.

For example, some of the measurements that may be done, depending on the product/process type is: Measure product temperatures. Consider the heat processing and the cooling/chilling. Take measurements at the coldest point of the product when heat processing is evaluated and at the warmest point of the product when cooling/chilling (frequently the centre of the largest piece) is evaluated. Measure time/temperature for cooking, pasteurization, canning (appertization), cooling (rates), storing, thawing, reconstituting, Measure the dimension of the containers used to hold foods being cooled and depth of the food mass. Measure the pressure, headspace, venting procedure, adequacy of container closure, initial temperatures and any other factor critical to the successful delivery of a scheduled process. Measure pH of the product during the processing and also measure the pH of the finished products. Measure pH at room temperature whenever possible and measure the water activity (a_w) of the product. Run duplicate samples whenever possible (because of variations). Make corrections for ambient temperatures according to the chart. Sample collections, inoculated-pack studies, and microbial challenge studies could be necessary when information on hazards is not otherwise available, or for new products or for assessing the expected shelf life.

Analyze the Measurements:
A qualified individual from the HACCP team analyzes the measurements in order to correctly interpret the data collected. During the review and interpretation of the data, identified hazards will be fully described on the same Forms 5, 6 and 7. For the purpose of a reference let us take few examples from the process:

1. Plot time/temperature measurements on a computer printout or on graph paper. This measurement is automatically recorded in modern Pasteurizers, UHT sterilizers, packaging machine sterilizing and heat seal devices. The record paper generated from the process is commonly known as thermograph.

2. Interpret controlled data Vs optimal growth temperatures of Microrganisms and temperature ranges at which they can multiply. For this the best example could be of fermented dairy products where culture bacteria are required to grow at 42 °C. Given the characteristics of _Lactobacillus bulgaricus_ and _Streptococcus thermophilus,_ this is the best suited temperature. Any interpretation of data would help formulate critical factor involved which optimum temperature and hour of incubation.

3. Estimate and evaluate probable cooling rate. Interpret cooling rates and compare the measured temperatures with temperature ranges within which bacteria of concern multiply rapidly Vs temperature at which growth begins, slows, and ceases (see reference material). Determine whether covers are used on containers to cool down foods (may delay the cooling but may also prevent contamination...) or if containers are stacked against each other. An evaluation of its impact must be done. The yoghurt containers after incubation require gradual cooling to bring down the temperature up to 4 °C and pH 4.20.

4. Compare a_w and pH values to ranges at which pathogens multiply or are eliminated. These two parameters are very critical to control the growth of microorganism. It differs from product to product that is where critical factors are measured to analyse and maintain safety. Lower pH values will help retard the growth of most of the Enterobacteriaceae microorganism while helping the growth of acidophiles and fungus. Lower water activity help reduce the microbial multiplication.

5. Evaluate the shelf stability of products. Shelf life of any product depends on its nature, process applied, end product microbial parameters, packaging material as well as regulatory requirements.

Upon completion of these five points, the HACCP team should have an extensive list of potential hazards on Forms 5 (biological hazards), 6 (chemical hazards) and 7 (physical hazards). The team is now ready to proceed to the determination of critical control points.

6. Determining the CCPs:
Apply HACCP decision tree to determine CCP - (principle 2). Think of a control point as a potential weak link in a chain. The

determination of critical control points (CCPs) is the second HACCP principle. CFIA defines a CCP as any point; step or procedure at which control can be applied and a food safety hazard can be prevented, eliminated, or reduced to an acceptable level. Control points are pertinent to all organizations.

During the stages of HACCP process development, some control points require more time and energy than others. The determination of critical control points (CCPs) is based upon the assessment of severity and likely occurrence of hazards and upon what can be done to eliminate, prevent, or reduce the hazards at a process step. The selection of CCPs is made on the basis of: Identified hazards and likely occurrence in relation to what constitutes unacceptable contamination Operations to which the product is subjected to during processing and preparation, and Intended use of the product.

The bottom line is this: The earlier the critical control points are incorporated into the HACCP process, the less they will cost (money & market reputation) to implement and the more short- and long-term value an organization will derive from the whole process. A separate critical control point does not have to be designated for each hazard. However, actions must be taken to ensure elimination, prevention, or reduction of all identified hazards.

Examples of CCPs may include: thermal treatment, chilling, and ingredients formulation control etc.

Thermal Treatment: Procured raw ingredients normally contain pathogens, impurities, and sometimes deviating from laid parameters. Therefore, inspection for condition at time of receiving may be a critical control point depending on the origin and anticipated use of the products. One or more steps during processing (e.g., Pasteurization, Cooking) may eliminate or greatly reduce the biological hazards. Pasteurization and Cooking would therefore be a CCP. If the food item is for direct consumption then the food must be accompanied by health certificate assuring the safety and quality. In case of doubt, raw material should be inspected and tested for the required parameters. If there is no heat process, then the food should be obtained from a safe source or the raw material should be inspected. Pasteurization inactivates all of the commonly known pathogens and reduces most of spoilage microorganisms.

Physical Treatment: If milk supplied from a tanker contains lumps of milkfat, a filter and homogenization will eliminate the concern. In third world countries, milk is adulterated with starch.

An inspection for solids in milk could be a CCP. Water supply containing foreign particle may be treated with filtration process of right size to eliminate coarser scale particles. Therefore, inspection for condition at time of receiving may be a critical control point.

Chemical Screening: At the time of receiving in reception dock pH, milkfat, alcohol test, clot on boiling (COB) test and other investigative tests are conducted to identify the risks involved. Therefore, inspection for condition at a time of receiving may be a critical control point.

Chilling: Time and temperature relationships are critical to the growth and spread of microbial contamination, contributing to sensory-quality and safety loss in foods. Every food-service manager and food technologist is aware of this fact, and of how difficult it can be to make all food-service employees use safe food handling and storage practices in an attempt to prevent quality loss and possible food-borne illnesses. Consider the consequences if prepared foods are contaminated by the following organisms and are cooled as slowly as Table: 11(01) - Bacteria Growth Rate Chart indicates.

Cooling may be a CCP for some products. Rapid lowering of the temperature of pasteurized foods is an important consideration. Pasteurization of food products do not sterilize the food or totally eliminate all bacteria but only reduce the bacterial load to a certain level depending on the process time and the temperature. Spores surviving these processes will grow if there is improper cooling or inadequate refrigeration during the storage of non-shelf stable product. This bacterial growth and germination of sporulating bacteria may represent a health hazard.

A HACCP program, through the use of documentation, will identify hazards at every processing step where loss of control could result in a food safety risk. Lack of timely chilling of food products leads to the multiplication of Mesophiles, which grow, between 77 °F - 95 °F (25 °C – 35 °C). For most bacteria, the growth range from minimum to maximum is about 86 °F (30°C) e.g., from 111.2 °F – 57.2 °F (44°C down to 14°C). Regardless of the type of bacteria, growth gradually increases from the minimum to the optimum temperature and decreases very sharply from the optimum to the maximum temperature, allowing many pathogens and spoilage bacteria to multiply. So it is CCP especially when raw milk is received from the farms and the stage after thermal treatment during pasteurization.

Table: 11(01) - Bacteria Growth Rate Chart-14

Organisms	Temperature	Generation Time
Escherichia coli	98.6°F/37°C	17 min. in broth 12.5 min. in milk
Salmonella typhi	98.6°F/37°C	23.5 min. in broth
Staphylococcus aureus	98.6°F/37°C	27-30 min. in broth
Streptococcus lactis	98.6°F/37°C	48 min. in broth 26 min. in milk

The air blast chiller provides critical temperature control during conventional food preparation. The blast chiller is more efficient in cooling foods than the standard storage refrigerator. In the Frozen Meat Burger Processing, a quick freezing is a critical point to be noted.

The following microbiological data in Table: 11(02) - Standard Plate Counts for Sliced Turkey and Gravy are the result of an unstructured test analyzing the effect of cooling time on the condition of sliced turkey and gravy prepared in a high school kitchen.

Table: 11(02) - Standard Plate Counts Sliced Turkey and Gravy-14

Time Following Chilling	Chill Processing Refrigerator	Holding Refrigerator
Initial	3,000	4,000
Day 3	8,000	151,000
Day 7	400	5,700
Day 10	4,500	30,000
Day 14	13,000	40,000

The growth factor in this case is clearly the temperature alterations, which effectively encourages the microbial population, which may include the pathogen if not screened. Immediate chilling of food products thwarts the transitional growth of microorganisms. The lag phase factor is favourably affected if food products are chilled to 39.2 °F (4 °C). As soon as food products are subjected to danger zone temperatures, microbial growth becomes a critical factor, which is evident in the Table: 11 (02) - Standard Plate Counts Sliced Turkey and Gravy.

Formulation Control: The more successful companies in product development start applying total quality management and HACCP at the very beginning, when a product idea is first discussed. R&D people need to be aware of what ingredients require HACCP programs. Formulation control may be considered a CCP. Some ingredients affecting the pH or the water activity (aw) levels of the food mixture will prevent bacterial growth. Acidifier will prevent growth or kill microorganisms if used in sufficient amounts to lower the pH. Ingredients substitution (ex. peanuts) could cause allergic reactions if not declared on the label.

Curing salts create a selective environment for microbial growth, and nitrites in sufficient concentration will prevent the outgrowth of heat-injured spores. Therefore, a sufficiently high concentration of salts and nitrites in food products must be specified as a CCP and monitored to ensure safety. Certain temperatures, salt concentrations, and pH are used to create conditions that select for and promote the multiplication of fermenting microorganisms. Control of these conditions and/or the addition of starter cultures or cultures from a previous batch (back slopping) are essential for the safe production of fermented food products.

Addition of certain additives like organic citric acid in orange juice to prevent early oxidative changes, lowering pH and meeting the regulatory maximum limit of it could be considered as a CCP.

Skimmed milk designed for specific people who need to be fed with minimum dairy fat shall be milk that contains not more than 0.3% milk fat. Here the composition of milk especially the fat% is a CCP.

Rheology of candies is important to quality but it may not be important to safety issues. When designing an aerated confection, which can include candies as light as a malted milk ball or as dense as a nougat centre, formulators should carefully select an ingredient with a minimum of ten percent protein, to create the proper foaming properties. Both non-fat dry milk, with 34% protein and whey protein concentrate 34 (WPC 34), contain sufficient protein levels to achieve the desired effect. WPC 34, for example, helps create a protein network within the foam to help stabilize the candy's final structure—or prevent the air bubbles in the aerated confection from collapsing. Stability factor is the CCP, which is to be listed and controlled.

If the processing procedures are changed and as a result, are different from those originally assessed as safe, the hazard analysis must be repeated and the CCPs redefined if necessary.

7. Decision Tree:

Apply HACCP decision tree to determine CCP - (principle 2) Critical Control Points (CCPs) will be determined using the HACCP decision tree (Form 8). A Codex Alimentarius working group on HACCP in June 1991 first developed the decision tree. Through its use in various pilot projects and workshops, the decision tree has been modified based on the comments/suggestions made by inspection staff and industry representatives. The first column on Form 8 is designed to identify the incoming materials, as delivered or the process steps where hazard(s) have been identified.

In the second column, you will identify which category of hazard (biological, chemical, or physical with a "B", "C", or "P" notation) is related to those particular incoming materials/ process steps and describe very concisely the identified hazard(s). When the identified hazard has been determined it should be fully controlled by the prerequisite program(s), write the abbreviation "prereq. Prog." for prerequisite program(s) in that column and proceed to next identified hazard. This determination is based on (1) the thorough assessment of the documented prerequisite program(s) and, (2) the on-site verification of these program(s). If the identified hazard is not fully controlled by a prerequisite program, then proceed to Question 1 (Q1) in the next column.

To decide if a step in a process is a CCP, a series of questions are asked about the product at that particular stage of production. These questions are illustrated in a Decision Tree. These questions are intended for processes in which processing of food is clarified. A CCP could net be controlled by the operator and the supplier will be required to guarantee the control of that CCP in the product. An example can be given from the presence of antibiotics in raw milk. This decision tree is an excellent tool for identifying CCP=s in operations where foods are fully cooked or sterilized; however, it should not be used for foods that are to be purchased raw. There are certain considerations when one is using a decision tree.

The decision tree is used after the hazard analysis of a food plant has been completed. The decision tree is used to find answer to probable aspects of risk control at the steps where a "significant hazard" has been identified. These are hazards that may reasonably be expected to occur. Non-significant hazards (i.e., of low risk and unlikely to occur) have been excluded. A process, which does not have a significant hazard, does not need a HACCP plan. Each step which is a CCP must agree with the definition: a point, step, or procedure at which control can be applied and a food safety hazard can be prevented, eliminated, or reduced to acceptable levels. A subsequent step in the process under control may be more effective for controlling a hazard and may be the preferred CCP. More than one step in a process may be involved in controlling a hazard. More than one hazard may be controlled by a specific preventative measure.

Decision Tree

Question 01: In case of a hazard detection what measures would be used by the operator to eradicate the hazard.

Question 02: What intensity of hazard could influence its level of control measure? What control measures would be taken to pacify the demand of HACCP?

Question 03: Would it be possible to eliminate the hazards completely.

Question 04: Why the procedure to pre-empt the identified hazard not present in the HACCP Manual

Question 05: Would it be sufficient to apply corrective procedure to eradicate identified hazard.

Having now established the critical control points (CCPs), the next step is report CCPs on Form 10 and documents the parameters that will be monitored and controlled on this form.

HACCP principles 3-7 will lead to the development of a HACCP plan that will be described on Form 10. The critical limits, monitoring procedures, deviation procedures, verification procedures and record keeping will be described in an establishment's HACCP plan. This HACCP plan will provide the written guidelines that will be followed in an establishment

8. Identify Critical Control Limits (CCL):

Establish critical limits - (principle 3). CFIA defines Critical Control Limits (CCL) as criteria, which separate acceptability from unacceptability. These parameters, if maintained within boundaries, will confirm the safety of the product. The critical limits will meet government regulations, company standards, or other scientific data. Critical limits may exceed a regulatory requirement. The U.S. seafood HACCP regulation defines critical limits in the following way: 21 CFR 123.3(c) Critical limit means the maximum or minimum value to which a physical, biological, or chemical parameter must be controlled at a critical control point to prevent, eliminate, or reduce to an acceptable level the occurrence of the identified food safety hazard-[61].

The third step in the HACCP process is to establish preventive measures with critical limits for each control point. One or more critical limits are set to control the identified hazard. Critical limits may be set for factors such as temperature, time (minimum time exposure), physical product dimensions, water activity, moisture level, etc. HACCP allows a great deal of flexibility in the manner in which you can go about this, as long as you monitor the critical limits. As an internal HACCP auditor and member of HACCP team, one is responsible for evaluating the preventive measures and critical limits to make sure that they are adequate, and that they are being properly observed.

Once the critical limits are established, they will be written on Form 10 together with the description of the process step, the CCP number and hazard description.

Critical Limits - examples an acidified beverage that requires a hot fills and holds as the process may have acid addition as the CCP. If insufficient acid is added or if the temperature of the hot fill is insufficient, the product would be under processed with potential for the growth of pathogenic spore-forming bacteria. The critical limits in this case would be pH and fill temperature.

Beef patties are cooked in a continuous oven. More than one critical limit is set to control the hazard of heat-resistant pathogen survival. The critical limits could be; minimum internal temperature of the patty; oven temperature; time in the oven determined by the belt speed in rpm; patty thickness.

In a ready-to-eat operation, the final packaging has been identified as a CCP. The hazard to be controlled is the contamination of the meat due to inadequate working techniques. The critical limit in this case would be that the working techniques are in accordance with the documented work procedures (e.g., utensils and gloves sanitized at prescribed frequencies).

These examples illustrate that CCPs may be controlled by more than one critical limit.

9. Describe Monitoring Procedures and Frequencies

Establish monitoring procedures - (principle 4). Having now established the critical control points (CCPs), the next step is report CCPs on Form 10 and documents the parameters that will be monitored and controlled on this form. HACCP principles 3-7 will lead to the development of a HACCP plan that will be described on Form 10. The critical limits, monitoring procedures, will be described in an establishment's HACCP plan. This HACCP plan will provide the written guidelines that will be followed in an establishment.

Monitoring is the act of conducting a planned sequence of observations or measurements of control parameters to assess whether a CCP is under control. For each processing step where "metal detection" is identified as a significant hazard on the HACCP Plan Form, describe monitoring procedures, monitoring equipment and its operational adjustment that will ensure that the critical limits are consistently met. To fully describe monitoring program one should find solution to few of the questions, which are detrimental to elimination of hazards: What is the hazard, which is being monitored? How it is being monitored? What is the interval of monitoring or there is a need to monitor continuously, which has been designated to perform the monitoring? A record specific to identified individual unit is to be maintained and reference given in the HACCP manual. The monitoring specifications are written on Form 10 for each CCP.

If equipment is used, the equipment itself performs monitoring. A check should be made at least once per day to ensure that the device is operating or is in place. The equipment operator, a production supervisor, and a member of the quality control staff, a member of the maintenance or engineering staff, or any other person who has an understanding of the operation of the equipment, may perform this.

The equipment operator, a production supervisor, and a member of the quality control staff, a member of the maintenance or engineering staff, or any other person, who has a thorough understanding of the proper condition of the equipment, may perform monitoring. In assigning responsibility for this monitoring function; one should consider the complexity of the equipment and the level of understanding necessary to evaluate its condition.

It is important to keep in mind that the feature of the process that one monitors and the method of monitoring should enable to determine whether the CCL is being met. At each CCP, the monitoring requirements and the means to ensure that the CCP remains within the critical limits are specified. Monitoring procedures generally relate to on-line processes and are rapid type tests, visual, monitoring of documentation (for example, product certification) or any other appropriate procedures. The monitoring process should directly measure the feature for which you have established a CCL.

Monitoring tracks the system's operation and allows for action to be taken in the event of a loss of control or if there is a trend toward the loss of control. It provides information to an establishment on a timely basis, allowing for decisions to be made on the acceptability of the lot at a particular stage in the process. Monitoring procedures performed in the establishment during operation will result in written documentation that will serve as an accurate record of the operating conditions.

If any one of the critical limits is out of control as determined by the monitoring procedures, the CCP will be out of control. Lack of control at a CCP is defined as being a critical defect or a deviation. Deviations will result in the production of a hazardous or unsafe product. Therefore, adequate and effective monitoring procedures are essential due to the serious consequences arising from deviations. Most monitoring procedures for CCPs must be rapid because they relate to on-line processes and there is not sufficient time for lengthy analytical testing. Physical and chemical measurements or visual observations are preferred because they may be done rapidly and can indicate control of the process. All monitoring equipment must be properly calibrated for accuracy. Examples of some physical and chemical measurements taken to monitor the critical limits are: temperature, time, pH, and moisture level and water activity.

There are many ways to monitor critical control points. Monitoring can be done on a continuous or batch basis. The reliability of continuous monitoring (100 %) is preferred where feasible. The established monitoring frequency must be sufficient to substantiate that the hazard is under control. Responsibility for monitoring is clearly identified and individuals monitoring the CCPs must be trained in the testing procedure and must fully understand the purpose and importance of monitoring. The individual must have ready access to the monitoring activity and must be unbiased in monitoring and reporting. Finally, the individual must accurately report the monitoring activity.

All operational records and documents that are associated with CCP monitoring must be properly filled in and signed by the person doing the monitoring and verified/signed by a responsible official of the company. A reference of the records should be mentioned in the HACCP manual.

Monitoring Procedures examples can be taken from the scheduled thermal process for a canned meat product in a steam-still retort is continuously monitored by the recorder-controller. The recorder-controller makes a permanent record of the process time and temperature. The retort operator to ensure proper delivery of the thermal process checks this record.

10. Describe Corrective Actions to be taken:

Establish deviation procedures - (principle 5) Describe corrective action to be taken in case of a non-performance of prescribed procedure resulting in nonconformity of the standard. In one example, for each processing step where "metal inclusion" is identified as a significant hazard on the HACCP Plan Form, describe the procedures that one will use when monitoring indicates that the CCL has not been met. These procedures should ensure that unsafe product does not go to palletizing section, correct the problem that caused the CCL deviation and consequently non-detected package does not reach to sales and consumer. It is to be remembered that deviations from operating limits do not need to result in formal corrective actions. The frequency of such incidence may lead to a chronic situation, which should be formally corrected.

Let us take sceneric situations when it is found that package has not been detected by the monitoring system and it may or may not contain the metal. It cannot be found unless the pack is opened which will make the product unsolvable, in some cases if metal is not found that product could still be safe to move on for consumption. Alternatively, many options could be taken by an incharge, one could take decision to destroy, divert to a non-food use, rework, or hold and evaluate any product in which the metal detector has detected metal fragments and later may divert to rework.

Attempt to locate and correct the source of the fragments found in product by the metal detector or separated from the product stream by the magnets, screens, or other devices. Take one of the following actions when product is processed without a properly functioning metal detector or separation device: Destroy the product; Hold the product until it can be run through a metal detector; Hold the product until an inspection of the processing equipment that could contribute metal fragments can be completed to determine whether there are any broken or missing parts; Divert the product to a use in which it will be run through a metal detector (e.g. divert fish fillets to a breading operation that is equipped with a metal detector); Divert the product to a non-food use.

Take one of the following corrective actions to regain control over the operation after a CCL deviation: Stop production; If necessary, adjust or modify the equipment to reduce the risk of recurrence; Take one of the following actions to the product involved in the critical limit deviation: Destroy the product; Run the product through a metal detector; Divert the product to a use in which it will be run through a metal detector (e.g. divert fish fillets to a breading operation that is equipped with a metal detector); Divert the product to a non-food use.

Describe Plant Specific Deviation Procedures:
HACCP principles 3-7 will lead to the development of a HACCP plan that will be described on Form 10. Deviation procedures will be described in an establishment's HACCP plan. This HACCP plan will provide the written guidelines that will be followed in an establishment.

A deviation is defined as failure to meet the specified critical limits. Deviation procedures are pre-determined and documented set of corrective actions that are implemented when a deviation occurs. This procedure establishes a method, procedure, and the controls to effectively and efficiently deviate from approved procedural documentation. This procedure provides the capability and authority for an operator, supervisor or managing personnel to officially record deviations to test documentation in order to expedite a processing completion, maintain safety control of the affected product, and to satisfy the HACCP process requirements.

All deviations must be corrected by taking appropriate corrective actions to control the non-compliant product and to correct the cause of non-compliance. The corrective actions taken must be recorded and filed. A deviation procedure must describe the acceptable corrective actions for a deviation. The diversity of possible deviations at each CCP means that more than one corrective action may be necessary at each CCP. The corrective actions must correct the cause of the deviation and must control the actual or potential hazard resulting from the deviation. Product control includes proper identification and handling of the affected lots. The deviation procedures at each CCP are written on Form 10.

Corrective actions are prescribed and formalized so that employees responsible for critical control point monitoring understand and are able to perform the appropriate corrective actions in the event of a deviation.

When a deviation occurs, it will most likely be noticed during the routine monitoring of a CCP. A deviation results when the pre-determined critical limit for a CCP is out of compliance. If the proper corrective action is not taken the deviation may result in an unacceptable health risk.

Deviation Procedures - Examples
The scheduled thermal process for Aseptic Long Life Flavoured Milk is not met due to a loss in steam pressure during the processing. The operator notices the deviation in control panel before the end of the production cycle, which is followed by the restart of plant sterilization phase. However, due to lack of steam plant cannot reach the temperature and circle goes on with out end. The operator refers to the written deviation procedure. The deviation procedure states that the operator should shut the product feed line, run the plant with water, take corrective action on steam supply and put the plant back on CIP mode with Alkali cleaning followed by plant sterilization. Segregate the packed product from the time of steam failure for a 10 days product observation. After the process cycle is finished, the lot is tagged and is moved to the detention and observation area. The deviation procedure also states that the action must be recorded and the affected lots held until a process authority has authorized and signed off for the release or destruction of the product after the observation period. The corrective action taken has corrected the problem with steam and has controlled the plant to satisfactory operation.

In a spaghetti factory, the scheduled thermal process for a batch of canned spaghetti is not met due to loss in steam pressure. The operator notices the deviation after the end of the process cycle and he refers to the written deviation procedure. The deviation procedure for canned spaghetti states that product is to be tagged and moved to the detention area. The deviation procedure also states that the action must be recorded and the affected lots held until a process authority as to disposition of the product does a full evaluation. After the process cycle is finished, the lot is tagged and is moved to the detention area. The corrective action taken has corrected the problem and has controlled the affected product.

This illustrates that there could be more than one-way to handle a thermal deviation for the different product. It also illustrates that the deviation procedure will address the various actions that are acceptable.

Antibiotics in incoming raw milk are detected by a rapid screening test. The detected level exceeds the established critical limits. The milk receiver refers to the deviation procedure. The deviation procedure states that the milk is to remain in the truck and not be unloaded. The procedure also describes the follow-up action. The milk receiver phones the provincial inspector who will follow up with the milk shippers. All corrective actions are recorded.

Cooked sausages are being sliced with equipment that had not been cleaned at the specified frequency. The foreman notices that the slicers have excessive product build-up and he believes that the sausages are being subjected to excessive bacterial contamination. The deviation procedure states that the foreman must hold all products produced since the last recorded clean up. The product under hold is subjected to microbiological laboratory testing and is not released until the laboratory results are received. The deviation procedure also states that the employee responsible for equipment cleaning is questioned as to the reason for the deviation from specified procedure and is retrained as necessary.

11. Describe the Verification Procedures to be used:
Verification activities are methods, procedures and tests that are used to determine if the HACCP plan for that establishment is valid and is operating properly. Establish verification procedures - (principle 6). In other words, those activities, other than monitoring, that determine the validity of the HACCP plan and that the system is operating according to the plan.

Principle 6 emphasises establishment of verification procedures explaining in simple language the definitional value of this principle and stating how verification impacts the success of HACCP process as a whole. The procedure is to be established to verify that the HACCP system is working correctly. The HACCP team needs to verify that the HACCP system is working the way it is expected to work. In carrying out the verification activities, the establishment may find that some hazards were overlooked or they may discover new or unexpected hazards. In this case, the plan needs to be modified appropriately. The verification procedures at each CCP are written on Form 10.

There are different types of verifications that must take place within this principle. First, there are verification activities for CCPs to determine the personnel responsible and frequency to verify the results of those performing monitoring activities. Supervisory or quality control personnel several times per shift would typically complete this. Second, there must be a verification that the entire HACCP Plan is performing as expected and written. This is critical to complete following the initial implementation of the plan and at least annually thereafter. An outside consultant who can be unbiased during the review often performs this task. Third, there must be a plan validation completed upon implementation and annually thereafter. The validation process is defined as the scientific and technical process for determining that the CCP and Critical Limits are adequate and sufficient to control likely hazards. An independent expert external to the organization also frequently completes this step.

Verification may include: Reviewing the HACCP plan; Reviewing the CCP records; Reviewing and determining the adequacy of corrective actions taken when a deviation occurs; Reviewing the critical limits; Reviewing other records pertaining to the HACCP plan or system; Direct observation or measurement at a CCP; Sample collection and analysis to determine the product meets all safety standards; may include analytical testing, On-site observations and Record review. Verification Procedures must not omit Ongoing checks, Review of deviations, Product dispositions, Instrument calibration, Annual audits, Prior shipment review, Confirmation that CCPs are kept under control and Unscheduled reassessments when conditions change or problems persist.

In the United States, establishments are responsible for verifications, the Food safety and the Inspection Service (FSIS) which is the agency with in USDA responsible for the verification of food safety, wholesomeness, accurate labelling of meat poultry and egg products have a regulatory role in compliance.

Similarly in Canada, both the establishment and the Canadian Food Inspection Agency will have a role in verifying HACCP plan compliance and they will carry out activities to verify that the HACCP plan is operating properly. Verification activities differ from monitoring activities. Results from verification activities are not intended to make decisions on the acceptability of lots of product. Verification activities involve for example, analytical testing or auditing of the monitoring procedures, product sampling, audits of monitoring and verification records, plant inspection audits, environmental sampling or any other appropriate activities.

Verification Procedures - Examples

Checking each incoming lot does the monitoring of the acceptability of peanuts for Aflatoxin. The manufacturer provides the certificate of guarantee and it is further examined by importer or purchaser that the peanuts are Aflatoxin free and meets other CCL requirements. As well, every load is visually examined for mould presence.

Verification of the monitoring activity involves an audit of the supplier's Aflatoxin-free claim by having the peanut analyzed at a private laboratory. A private laboratory for Aflatoxin levels tests a sample of peanuts from every tenth load.

The monitoring of whole egg pasteurization time/temperature is done for each lot by the pasteurize operator. The pasteurization verification activities are numerous. An example of one verification activity is the microbiological testing of finished product to ensure that the pasteurization is adequate. Another verification activity is the monthly pasteurization thermometer check to validate the accuracy of the indicating thermometers.

The monitoring by the Leadsman (Foreman) of the cleanliness of equipment and utensils in the post-cooking area is done on an hourly basis. The quality control personnel verify the monitoring activity through unexpected audits. The quality control personnel swab the product contact surfaces and do the microbiological testing to determine the microbiological cleanliness of the area.

Verification procedures will be described in an establishment's HACCP plan. This HACCP plan will provide the written guidelines that will be followed in an establishment.

12. Establish Record Keeping:

Describe the record-keeping system to be used. Record keeping will be described in an establishment's HACCP plan. This HACCP plan will provide the written guidelines that will be followed in an establishment. The HACCP records are defined as the in plant record keeping that is done at each CCP and that contain the information required to ensure that the HACCP plan is followed.

Records are essential in determining the compliance of the establishment in following the agreed-upon HACCP plan. The HACCP records differ from the records that are kept to ensure compliance to the pre-requisite program requirements. The required HACCP records to be kept at each CCP are written on Form 10.

There are several types of records that must be maintained. First is the written Hazard Analysis along with supporting documentation. Secondly, the written HACCP Plan, which includes the decision-making, documents regarding critical control points and critical limits. Third, the production records relating to the monitoring of the critical control points. These forms should also include columns for documenting verifications and corrective actions, unless you elect to record these on another form. The fourth and last type of records involves the pre-shipment approval record. This record must include verification that the critical control points have been properly monitored and met to release the product for shipment. The timing of this document is extremely critical to assure completion before the shipment of product. Without this step, product may be considered adulterated and subject to recall.

Individuals with record-keeping responsibilities need to be well trained. Complete records must include specified information such as the date, time, product, lot, monitoring data, and signature. Information must be recorded in ink. Records cannot be recorded in pencil, nor should white out or complete erasure be evident. Erroneous information should be lined out with initials and the correct information recorded.

Monitoring results are documented together with any deviations and corrective action taken. Failure to document the control of a CCP would be a critical departure from the HACCP plan. Corrective actions should be documented at the time they occur. Records must also be timely. Production records should be completed throughout the day at the time of processing. These cannot be completed at the end of the shift from memory. Inspection personnel will need to exercise good judgment in this area because some part of the corrective action may be documented sooner than others. Corrective actions should not be documented until they are performed, but when they are performed they should be documented within a reasonable amount of time. In the United States, Regulation 417.5 requires that each entry on a record maintained under the HACCP plan shall be made at the time the specific event occurs. So is the recommendation in Canada. It will be imperative that the establishment maintain up-to-date, properly filed, and accurate records.

Verification activities are also to be recorded. Records must specify who recorded the information and must indicate who reviewed and signed off the information.

A record may be in any form (processing chart, written record, computerized record) and shows the historical record of the process, the monitoring, the deviations, and the corrective actions (including disposition of product) that occurred at the identified CCP. The information contained in the records is used to establish the product's processing profile that would be used if there were any subsequent problems. Accurate records allow for trace back of the actual manufacturing conditions, which will aid in troubleshooting if a problem arises. The importance of records to the HACCP program must be emphasized. The records are an important tool that an inspector will have to ensure that the establishment is following the agreed upon HACCP plan. It will be imperative that the establishment maintain up-to-date, properly filed, and accurate records.

Food plants may be required to retain documentation related to outdated, replaced parts of the HACCP plan or hazard analysis for a period of time. The establishment should consider that they might still have product in commerce represented by the portion of the plan that was modified, and it would be a good business practice to keep that "old" portion of the plan until that product has left the market. The regulatory retention requirements are for the records generated by the HACCP plan. Records have to be maintained for specific periods of time. In the United States, slaughtered and refrigerated product records have to be retained for a period of one year. Frozen product records have to be retained for a period of two years. Records may be stored off site after six months; however they must be available to US-FSIS within 24 hours of request. Electronic records are permissible. Such records should be designed with adequate security measures and be routinely backed up.

Under certain application, a processing authority is used to evaluate a process, under such circumstances also scientific data supporting his/her decisions be available as part of the HACCP documentation e.g., Critical limit not met for time and temperature for cooked beef in a catering situation due to power failure. It is expected that the data to be available.

There is new technology available to ease the burden of record keeping. Microsoft ® Windows® 95, Windows 98, NT or higher systems could use programs to process HACCP data. Many systems have remote units to input CCP monitoring information. This information resides in a central computer, which maintains the information and alerts the user in the event of a deviation. Data collected may be entered into the computer on the forms that were created in HACCP module. Special features to assist in data entry include a pop-up calendar for the date field, a clock for the time field, and a flashing red or yellow light if a number is outside critical control limits or quality limits. The forms with data may be printed out. These systems are moderately priced and offer many benefits to organize your record keeping system. They also simplify the process of pre-shipment approvals. The number of records that can be entered into record module of HACCP could be limited by the storage space on the computer-65.

During the regulatory inspection or external audits Inspection personnel on all shifts should have access to the records in a reasonable amount of time. If there are questions concerning the availability of records, these should be addressed through the chain of command. Record-keeping responsibilities involve the organization of the record-keeping system. Records need to be maintained in an organized fashion and be available for review on request. It is helpful to have a centralized location to maintain the records.

It is advised that all of your HACCP Plan and related records be designated as Controlled Documents. Monitoring records should be designated as "Confidential Commercial Data". These steps will limit access to the documents through the Freedom of Information Act. Accordingly, the company must treat the documents as such to afford this protection. Companies should not make the documents available for public review.

Record Keeping - Examples

Pasteurization charts record the time and temperature processing data. The records will show if a drop in temperature occurred and the frequency pen will indicate if a proper flow diversion occurred. The records register additional information such as indicating thermometer temperature, lot size, operator, date, and product.

The retort processing records show a loss in steam during the cook cycle and the temperature dropped below the temperature specified in the scheduled process. The records must acknowledge that this was a process deviation, and the file must show any process calculations that were done by the process authority to determine the safety of the product. The file must also show what action was taken with the product.

Cooked salami is being sliced with equipment that had not been cleaned at the specified time period. The foreman notices that the slicer has excessive product build-up and he believes that the salami is being subjected to excessive bacterial contamination. The records must show that a deviation occurred and must indicate the corrective action taken. The lot number, lot size, hold tag number, laboratory testing results, and disposition of the sliced salami are recorded. The records also indicate that the employee responsible for the clean-up was notified as to the unsatisfactory nature of the area at that time.

If the HACCP plan includes the management review meetings once in a month to assess the HACCP management and its impact on food quality and safety, then the matter on the agenda, attending management representatives and HACCP team members names, corrective actions taken and verified, Non conformity reports, decisions and any amendments pertaining to HACCP process must be made available in the form of a report/record.

Employee Training Records: As HACCP pioneer Dr. Howard Bauman stated: "HACCP is a cooperative program and should involve everyone from the CEO to the newest employee in the plant. Everyone should be receiving training in the HACCP concept so that it is fully understood. Personnel used to train plant employees must have an extensive knowledge of the program. An overall trust must be developed in the company, since under the HACCP system people on the line have a responsibility to monitor CCPs and take corrective action if a problem occurs."

Effective implementation is absolutely imperative for the HACCP Plan. Implementation involves a significant commitment to employee training and continuing involvement and direction from the HACCP Team. GMPs are the basic principles of operations in a HACCP system where a food processor should follow to produce a consistent, quality food product. Specific GMP guidelines exist for specific Canadian products: soft drinks, dairy products, dried dairy products, bottled waters, nuts and principal nut products, low acid and acidified low acid canned foods, processing and aseptic packaging, processed eggs, and fermented meats.

HACCP systems rely on a trained teamwork to support the process and the system. Prerequisite programs required in HACCP are essentially GMPs and follow on requirements in the manufacturing places are mostly generic. However, the specific requirements for each unit will differ due to variability with food, preservation, packaging, and many other products related specifications. It is a legal requirement that staff involved in a food environment are adequately trained and /or supervised commensurate with their work activity. The responsibility for training and supervision of staff lies clearly with the proprietor of every food business.

The Canadian Food Inspection Agency (CFIA) approach to HACCP / FSEP is consistent with internationally accepted standards including those supported by Codex Alimentarius. CFIA recommends that any provider that is considering the development of a HACCP / FSEP course should acquire the CFIA Food Safety Enhancement

Program Implementation Manuals Volumes I, II, III and IV as well as the Reference Database for Hazard Identification and the appropriate generic models. The implementation manuals provide detailed descriptions of the Food Safety Enhancement Program (FSEP) as well as recommendations concerning the process and format for HACCP system development, and the use and application of generic HACCP models. Please refer Chapters 07-08-09 & 10 for further details.

The part of HACCP team responsibility is to demonstrate and impart adequate training with in self and to food manufacturing employees of the factory. One can use modules to track competency or outcomes-based training provided to entire workforce. For any training program for the staff, maintain the following records:

- ❑ Lay down specification of competency requirements for each employee.
- ❑ Maintain details of all Training programs and course modules, with outcomes per module.
- ❑ Maintain records of incurred cost and attendance at all internal and external training.
- ❑ Skill assessment tests records to be maintained.
- ❑ Certification of HACCP renewals to be done in time.
- ❑ Maintain records of current and past employee training.
- ❑ Always maintain prerequisite criteria for employees to work
- ❑ HACCP and quality related systems.
- ❑ New food production hires should have criteria of selection.
- ❑ On-the-job training should be segmented to train people with specific skills and variable segments of a manufacturing unit.
- ❑ Training plans for the year should be in place to advance the
Commitment and pre-empt shortcomings.
- ❑ Special courses requirements to be envisaged

Many types of courses may be offered according to the targeted population. The main courses are:

1. HACCP/FSEP Orientation for Executive Managers -- Duration: 2 to 4 hours
2. Courses for HACCP Coordinators -- Duration: 2 or + days according to needs
3. Courses for Production Staff working at CCPs -- Duration: 1 or + days according to needs

Checklists are developed for each of the three types of courses. They could be used by the providers of HACCP / FSEP courses as a self-evaluation tool or by people looking for training on HACCP / FSEP, regarding the evaluation of the different courses available in order to choose the one(s) most appropriate to their needs. Furthermore, the participants of HACCP / FSEP courses could use these checklists to evaluate a course after attending it or, if applicable, to recommend the course to other staff for their establishment or their commodity sector.

It is important to note that the checklists were developed as guidelines to evaluate if courses follow the HACCP approach as described in CFIA's FSEP Implementation Manuals. Course format, content and duration may vary from one provider to the other.

Courses for HACCP Coordinators:

The objective of these courses is to train the HACCP Coordinators in order for them to have the necessary knowledge and skills to assume their roles and responsibilities under HACCP / FSEP. This includes training on the HACCP system (i.e. prerequisite programs & HACCP plans) development, implementation, and maintenance in a specific food establishment as well as audit principles and internal audit. The courses should explain the prerequisite programs content and evaluation as well as the plant specific HACCP plan(s) development according to CFIA guidelines, with or without generic models. Practical exercises should be included in the courses. Take note that some providers could choose to offer courses covering specific parts of the program, i.e. one course on the prerequisite programs and another course on the development of a HACCP plan.

HACCP Internal Auditor Training: The objective of this training course is to enable participants to understand, develop, and implement an in-house HACCP audit programme.

The training with computerized HACCP module systems could enhance its application. This HACCP training module could enable to schedule and record all internal audits needed to verify that your system has been implemented and that is effective. It helps to set up an audit schedule for all user-defined elements of the food safety system, automatically tracks audits due and reminds you when not completed by the scheduled date, enter results each time an audit is conducted, generate and print audit findings and one could generate Corrective Actions for audit deficiencies.

CFIA developed for each of the three types of courses. They could be used by the providers of HACCP / FSEP courses as a self-evaluation tool or by people looking for training on HACCP / FSEP, regarding the evaluation of the different courses available in order to choose the ones most appropriate to their needs. It is important to note that the checklists were developed as guidelines to evaluate if courses follow the HACCP approach as described in CFIA's FSEP Implementation Manuals. Course format, content and duration may vary from one provider to the other. Checklists for recommended HACCP Course Content please see Appendix-1

Assistance and Support: In order to encourage the implementation of in-plant HACCP system, the Canadian Food Inspection Agency has established Area and Regional Food Safety Enhancement Program Teams. People needing more information on the program are encouraged to contact members of these teams. A list of the main resource persons in each area is included in Appendix 2. Another source of information, for their members, can be the National Industry Associations. A list of these national associations is included in **Appendix 3**. Please refer to the CFIA's Internet address-107.

Additional Reference Material: Depending on the commodity area, there are a number of reference documents and manuals, which may be used. In particular, the proposed Good Manufacturing Procedures (GMP) Regulations from Health Canada are pertinent to prerequisite programs. For more information, please consult your local Canadian Food Inspection Agency Area and/or Regional Food Safety Enhancement Program Team member, or the applicable National Industry Association-107.

13. Machine maintenance Record:
To qualify for HACCP accreditation one will need to incorporate machine maintenance & safety record, stringent temperature controls, calibration records; machines, equipments, related to monitoring, testing and evaluating safety parameters. Such documents into the production processes provide proof of your standards of operation. Preventive maintenance—avoiding trouble before it starts—is a major job in safety related issues.

The most common problem with machine maintenance in authors experience is machine safety guards. All the food-packaging machines need guarding and guard switches. If a risk assessment, which is an essential part of machinery design, shows that a machine carries a risk of food safety and human injury, then the hazard must be eliminated or contained. Because of the conflicting demands of cost effectiveness, speed and efficiency, on the one hand, and of safety on the other, many machine designers opt for a guard interlocking system, which gives freer access, where this will contain or eliminate the risk posed by the machine.

Broadly speaking, there are two basic types of electrical safety interlocking systems: power interlocking, where the power source of the hazard is directly interrupted before the opening of a guard; and control interlocking, where the power source of the hazard is interrupted by the switching of a circuit which controls the power switching device. Safety interlock switches, which are designed without a guard-locking feature, do not restrict access. The guard can be opened at any time, but as soon as it is opened the switch isolates the power to the hazard via the contactor control circuit. If the hazard always ceases immediately, the requirements are satisfied because the operator cannot reach the parts while they are dangerous.

The guards not only provide safety to humans but also minimises physical and chemical contaminants. Let us take the example of a cup-filling machine where cups are being filled with fruit yoghurt. If the upper guard or the side guards are not there to protect falling debris, insects, water, or CIP spill over then very purpose of food safety will be lost. Thus for each food packaging machine and recombination equipments, products physical safety guards shall be maintained and recorded in a general maintenance form.

People see guarding as a limitation to interaction with a machine. This is wrong. This is how arms and fingers are chopped off. People need to realize that guarding, as with any other safety rules, are there for their benefit, protection and product safety.

Food, Pharmaceutical and medical packaging engineers can benefit from improved machinery performance by asking their equipment manufacturers to incorporate a detailed food safety and hygiene guides into their packaging machinery. They can also benefit from improved machinery performance by asking their equipment manufacturers to incorporate pre-packaged, ready-to-install linear guides into their packaging machinery. Off-the-shelf linear guides optimize functionality and throughput and minimize downtime, cost, and contamination. They provide guidance for critical movement in applications from product insertion into containers, bottles, boxes, and cartons to folding, assembly, and sealing.

Accessories are available for linear motion products to maximize uptime. Bellows, or way covers, protect critical bearing components from contamination such as cardboard dust, which is found in many packaging applications. Another way to maximize uptime is to ensure that bearings are properly lubricated to avoid failure resulting from oxidation or wear. Maintenance-free, self-lubricating linear guides ensure proper lubrication and minimize cost by reducing or eliminating the need for expensive lube systems or manual maintenance.

Standard Operating Procedures (SOPs) are descriptions of particular tasks undertaken in a food processing operation. Similarly a specific SOP will address the maintenance of machine from operational and hygienic perspective. Both of the tasks are important to the safety of products; long machine failures may result in the spoilage of culture added milk for yoghurt, improper hygiene maintenance program could lead to microbial hazards. To safeguard the interest of food and human health, the basic purpose and frequency of doing a task, who will do the task, a description of the procedure to be performed that includes all the steps involved, and the corrective actions to be taken if the task is performed incorrectly shall be referenced in HACCP manual.

Referring to machine and plant related hygiene maintenance, these should describe procedures during operations that include equipment and utensils cleaning, sanitizing, disinfecting during production, at breaks, at midshift and between shifts, pre-operation sanitization or sterilization and final CIPs.

Temperature Measuring Devices are very important where microbial control is a safety factor. Few food borne illness outbreaks associated with inadequate cooking of eggs and hamburger patties have shown that it is very important to be able to accurately determine the temperatures associated with these products as well. A bimetal bayonet style thermometer with a dial face scale with a range of -18 to 105°C (0 to 220°F) may be used for certain applications in food temperature measurement. The scale must be in 1°C (2°F) increments. The dial face should be a minimum of about 1 inch in diameter and is usually available in larger sizes. The stem length should be a minimum of 127 mm (5 inches) and may need to be much longer to measure thicker foods. Specific measurement and maintenance instructions from the manufacturer of the instrument should be followed.

Thermistor has Advantages in high output and fast response at a very low cost. Disadvantages include nonlinearity and a limited upper temperature range, typically 300°C (572°F). Thermocouple device relies on the voltage generated by the junction of two dissimilar metals. The advantages are a relatively rugged construction and a wide temperature range. Disadvantages include higher cost, lower sensitivity, and non-linear output, which require a built-in reference. The infrared thermometer quickly registers surface temperatures, which facilitates general food safety system surveillance by allowing the scanning of numerous food temperatures over a short period of time. This type of thermometer is intended only for measuring surface temperatures of food products and should not be used to measure and verify critical internal temperatures such as cooking temperatures. Whatever devices are used, it shall be maintained and recorded.

Time/Temperature Indicators or Integrators (TTI) is a simple label-like device that continuously monitors cumulative time and temperature of food products. Some of these devices are threshold-sensitive or change in appearance when a certain threshold for temperature or time is reached. The appearance changes only if the threshold has been breached. Applications would include products such as sous vide or vacuum-packaged foods and some fresh products which are temperature-sensitive, such as milk and seafood.

Thermometers used for regulatory inspections should be calibrated initially, and then regularly thereafter, to ensure that accuracy of measurement is maintained. This calibration should be in the range of normal regulatory concern, 5°C (41°F) to 74°C (165°F). Calibrations should include both the instrument and any interchangeable probes used with that instrument. Each piece should be separately identified in the calibration records with serial numbers or agency equipment numbers. The National Institute of Standards and Technology (NIST) should calibrate the thermometer against a thermometer, which has been certified. Standard laboratory calibration protocol such as American Public Health Association (APHA) Standards for the Examination of Dairy Products should be followed. Proper calibration documentation is essential.

Calibration of pH Meters should be followed for both laboratory and portable pH meters. The calibration procedure must take into consideration the expected pH range of food. This factor is extremely important if a pH of 4.6 is used as a critical limit. A 2-point calibration using standard buffers of 4.0 and 7.0 is most common for working with potentially hazardous foods. Calibrations are usually performed immediately before the pH of the food samples is measured. Compensation for the temperature of the sample is required if the pH meter does not automatically address this variable.

Calibration of Water Activity Equipment should be followed for both laboratory and portable a_w instruments. The expected food moisture should be taken into consideration during the calibration procedure. The critical limit of 0.85 is the crucial point at which the instrument should be calibrated if the question is whether or not the food is potentially hazardous.

Sanitizing of Carton before the product goes inside and filled in to the cartons is a critical factor and requires continual monitoring and interval maintenance. This system introduces an atomizing spray of a Hydrogen Peroxide (H_2O_2) solution (or ozone water, or steam) into the carton, followed by a sterile hot air or ultraviolet light drying of the carton before filling. Spray Sanitizing of Machine Parts atomizing nozzles are placed in the machine to spray a sterilizing solution (typically iodine) onto the forming mandrel components and the filler nozzles. The system is activated whenever the machine enclosure is breached, and when the machine sanitizing sequence is activated. An operational log of the machine shall include this feature, be maintained, and referenced.

Preventive Maintenance Objectives:

- ❑ Reduce major repairs by correcting minor difficulties as soon as they are evident. This means listening to your operators who usually recognise before management that machinery is making a "funny noise" or other irregularity in performance of equipment. Do not punish employees who are trying to report a defect beyond their control.

- ❑ Maintain equipment in a more productive state. Keep it clean; repair or replace lost or worn parts immediately. Follow the machinery manual recommendations.

- ❑ Improve scheduling of repairs. Do not postpone needed repairs. Delaying repairs usually results in much more costly problems later on.

- ❑ Maintain safety. Some parts as they become worn become dangerous, as in worn chain or belt drives. Staffs are valuable and injuries are costly from the standpoint of lost time and training replacements, not to mention adverse impacts on employee moral.

- ❑ Improved customer service. A well-maintained mill looks good to the customer and helps assure the customer that the feed is made correctly the first time.

- ❑ Reduce overall operating costs. The miller of aquaculture feeds benefits from a well-maintained facility through reduced costs of operation and customer satisfaction.

- ❑ Provide trained maintenance personnel. Training of maintenance staff should be a high priority with high-level management oversight. Too often maintenance is seen as the bottom of the ladder, when in reality the quality and training of staff for this important responsibility should be paramount.

- ❑ The building grounds shall be adequately drained and maintained to be reasonably free from litter, waste, refuse, uncut weeds or grass, standing water and improperly stored equipment.

❑ The buildings shall be maintained in a reasonably clean and orderly manner.

❑ Adequate space, ventilation, and lighting shall be maintained for the proper performance of all manufacturing, storing, labelling, quality assurance and maintenance aspects of aquaculture feed manufacturing.

For implementation, the rule calls on the establishment to identify the employees, by positions rather than by the names of a specific employee, who will be responsible for the Plant and machinery maintenance team by monitoring the program and documenting adherence to the SOP and corrective actions taken. All the formats, SOPs, machine manuals, equipment manuals, instructions, maintenance log, Calibration procedures, and records, repair requests and job completion records must be maintained separately and referenced in HACCP manual.

14. Recall Procedure:

Since any system can fail, a recall Procedure might be in order, hopefully never to be used but available in the event it is needed. It is best that such a procedure be designed proactively, rather than put together in the event of an emergency.

A Recall Procedure for human food supplies defines the action to be taken by health regulatory authorities and food manufacturer whose product is in question when that food product for use in humans, for reasons relating to their quality, safety or efficacy, are to be removed from supply or use, or subject to corrective action.

A vital component of a food safety system is a recall program. The written recall program outlines plant's specific procedures that can be implemented at any time in the event of a recall. The overall objective of the establishment's written recall procedure is to ensure that an identified food is removed from the market as efficiently, rapidly, and completely as possible with out causing any health damage to consumers. Therefore, an understanding of the documentation requirements of a recall program and its reference in the HACCP manual is vital to food processing facility's food safety system.

Good Manufacturing Practices requires that an alert system be developed and maintained in expectation of a probable recall. The intention of the alert system is to promptly notify authorities of quality defects, recalls, counterfeiting and other problems concerning quality which could necessitate additional actions or suspension of the distribution of food, pharmaceutical/medicinal products. Potential product recalls should be quickly reported and investigated by a responsible decision-maker who has the authority to assign the recall classification to the situation. When warranted, a Recall Committee should be appointed.

The HACCP team members dealing with recall must realise, The importance and benefits of a recall program and how it fits into the HACCP system, The requirements of an effective recall program - recall team, code-dating, record keeping requirements etc., The requirements for effective communication strategy during a recall, How to document and ensure an effective Recall Program is in place for your food establishment and Learn what the CFIA's Food Safety Enhancement Program (FSEP) in Canada or FSIS in United States require in a documented Recall Program.

CFIA specifies Recall procedure in FSEP, which outlines the procedures the company would implement in the event of a recall. The objective of the establishment's written recall procedure is to ensure that an identified food is removed from the market as efficiently, rapidly, and completely as possible and can be put into operation at any time. The program is tested periodically to validate its effectiveness. Every manufacturer of a food product maintains a system of control that permits a complete and rapid recall of any lot of food product.

The written recall procedure includes the following:

1. Documentation pertaining to the product coding system. All products shall be identified with a production date or code identifying each lot. Sufficient coding of product is used and explained in the written recall program to permit positive identification and to facilitate an effective recall.

2. Finished product distribution records are maintained for a period of time that exceeds the shelf life of the product and is at least the length of time specified by respective commodity specific inspection manuals or by regulations. Records shall be adequately designed and maintained to facilitate the location of product in the event of a recall. Records are available on request.

3. Health and Safety complaint file must be maintained. Records documenting all Health and Safety related complaints and action taken must be filed.

4. Responsible individuals who will be part of the recall team along with their respective business and home telephone numbers are listed. For each individual, an alternate is designated to act on his or her behalf in case of absence. The roles and responsibilities of every member of the recall team are clearly defined.

5. The systematic procedures to follow in the event of a recall are described. These procedures will include the extent and the depth of the recall (i.e. consumer, retailer or wholesaler level) according to the recall classification.

6. Means of notifying the affected customers in a manner appropriate to the type of hazard are defined. The channels of communication (fax, telephone, radio, letter, or other mean) to be used for trace back and recovery of all affected product must be identified. Typical messages directed to retailers, wholesalers or customers, according to the severity of the hazards, must also be included.

7. Control measures for the returned recalled food is planned. This includes both returned product and product still in stock on the premises. The control measures and the disposal of the affected product are described according to the type of hazard involved.

8. Means of assessing the progress and efficacy of the recall are stated. A method of checking the effectiveness of the recall shall be defined.

Recall Initiation: Any manufacturer who initiates a recall of a food notifies the regulatory agency having jurisdiction immediately with information including:

1. The reason for the recall;

2. Recalled Product Identification: Name, code marks or lot numbers, Establishment number (Canadian or Foreign), date of production, date of importation or exportation if applicable, etc;

3. The amount of recalled product involved, broken down as follows:

    a. Total quantity of the recalled food originally in the company's possession,

    b. Total quantity distributed at the time of the recall,

    c. Total quantity remaining in the company's possession;

4. Areas of distribution of the recalled food: by areas, cities, provinces and, if exported, by country, along with retailers' and wholesalers' names and addresses;

5. Information on any other product, which could be affected by the same hazard

15.HACCP Audit: – See Chapter 12.

16.Standard Operating Procedures: –

Standard Operating Procedures (SOPs) provide guidance on policies and procedures associated with individual plants operational processes. In the professional world, they usually refer to the components of a procedures manual. It is possible to design a perfect practice, create a mission statement that defines it, and then develop SOPs that make that practice happen by adhering to the mission statement. That is, the desired outcome of each SOP is a reflection of the mission statement. It is possible to perform objective plant operation performance reviews by using the measurements of the SOPs as a key criterion as to an operational efficiency.

Standard Operating Procedures are intended to be flexible. Standard Operating Procedures are living documents and shall be reviewed and amended as deemed appropriate by the HACCP team. Wide format flexibility is extended in order to facilitate the needs of the content while still respecting the time constraints and situations at the time. Approved operating procedure documents shall include the date upon which the management approved the current document. Standard Operating Procedures shall be maintained by the HACCP coordinator and made available to the operators in each section, Auditors during an audit and members of HACCP management team as requested.

Standard operating procedures (SOPs) are a written set of work practices, which are most up to date and provide maximum safety and reliability of the desired results with out hindering the quality and safety of food. Sometimes many food managers may be needed to write their own SOPs for a particular operation. The complete details, authorization, and date of issuance or amendments shall be provided.

Sanitation Program: Sanitation standard operating procedures (SSOP's) are written methods that specify practices to address general hygiene and measures to prevent food from becoming contaminated due to various aspects of food environment at a food facility. Managers must train new crew members about SSOP's during the first days of employment. SSOP's must be a part of any food manufacturing culture. Good management system for food safety in a restaurant must include several prerequisite programs for an effective overall system. It is kind of like developing your own basic personal values and a moral code for food safety before you even start preparing and selling food.

The FDA Food Code has addressed the structural design of food establishments and equipment as well as acceptable operational practices. SSOP procedures ensure that Foods are purchased from approved suppliers / sources; Potable (safe) water is used in contact with food, food contact surfaces, and ice; Food contact surfaces are cleaned, sanitized, and in good condition; Un-cleaned or non-sanitized surfaces don't contact our foods; Raw animal foods don't contaminate ready-to-eat foods; Toilet facilities are accessible, properly equipped and maintained for crew.

Hand washing sinks are located in food preparation area, front service counters, and dishwashing areas. The sinks are all equipped with soap and paper towels (nailbrush, hand sanitizer, and gloves too); An effective pest control program is in place; Toxic materials are properly labelled, stored, and safely used; Food, food packaging materials, and food contact surfaces don't come in contact with physical hazards such as broken glass from light fixtures, jewellery, etc.

In a typical Dairy Food Farm, few of the SOPs may be required for the following operations. Additional SOPs could be developed for specific needs.

SOP-01: Animal Health Management
SOP-02: Animal Handling
SOP-03: Duodenal and Rumen Cannula Maintenance
SOP-04: Body Condition Score Determination
SOP-05: Body Weight Measurement - Cows and Calves
SOP-06: Management of Newborn Calves
SOP-07: Dehorning Heifer Cattle Feeding
SOP-08: Determination of Feed Refusal & Feed Issue
SOP-09: Diet Change Criteria
SOP-10: Equipment Maintenance and Lubrication
SOP-11: Cow Milking
SOP-12: Drying Off
SOP-13: Identification of Animals with Untellable Milk
SOP-14: Diagnosis and Treatment of Common Health Problems
SOP-15: Therapy Administration
SOP-16: Medicated Foot-Bath
SOP-17: Cattle Receiving and Shipping
SOP-18: Pest Control and Yard Maintenance
SOP-19: Biosecurity
SOP-20: Ingredients Procurement
SOP-21: Manufacturing Process
SOP-22: Processing Machine Maintenance
SOP-23: Packaging Machine Maintenance
Sop-24: Utility Maintenance Procedure

SOP-25: Cleaning In Place (CIP)
SOP-26: Cleaning On Place (COP)
SOP-27: Thermal treatment of Food Product
SOP-28: Laboratory Analytical Procedures
SOP-29: Food Staff Management
SOP-30: Clean-up and Sanitation
SOP-31: Employee Hygiene
SOP-32: Pest Control
SOP-33: For Inspection and Storage of Cleaning Agents, Sanitizers, and Lubricants
SOP-34: For Receipt and Storage of Packaging Materials and Ingredients
SOP-35: For Sanitation and Cleaning of Processing Facilities
SOP-36: For control of temperature of raw material being held and time of processing.
SOP-37: Manure and Runoff Collection
SOP-38: Standard Operating Procedures for Milking
SOP-39: Identify and Handle Mastitis Cows
SOP-40: Bacteriophage treatment in fermented dairy operations

Excellent quality will be produced on a continuous basis if all mentioned every person-involved works consistently according to his/her job description follows SOPs. Best Management Practices (BMPs) are the foundation of a quality assurance program and establishing standard operating procedures (SOPs) is the first step in applying BMPs in a consistent manner. Consistency with a repetitive task, such as milking, is necessary not only to produce quality milk, but also to produce it efficiently. Standard operating procedures help you and your staff to know which animals produce milk that cannot go into the bulk tank-- to prevent contamination of milk in the bulk tank, detect clinical mastitis-- to help with the treatment and prevention of mastitis; and apply the same milking routine with each milking-- essential to obtain good milking performance.

SOPs need to be accessible and regularly updated. Employees need to be trained and evaluated on a regular basis to ensure consistency. SOPs differ from farm to farm. However, the procedure to develop them often uses the following steps:

Name the SOP using a descriptive action word. For example: Identification of Animals with Unsellable Milk, Identify and Handle Mastitis Cows, Management of Newborn Calves.

If you're developing SOPs for several areas of your farm system, give each an identifying code and number. This will make it easier for an employee to find the specific list of procedures for a given task. Keep these in a manual. Include the date the SOP took effect, any revision dates, and the authors' names.

Write a scope for the SOP. To do this, answer these questions: What specific operations will be covered? What are not covered? Who is the SOP written for? For example: "This Milking SOP is for all regular and relief milker's. The SOP covers pre-milking sanitation, milking and post-milking sanitation of healthy cows. It does not cover safety around animals, bringing cows to the parlour, filling the parlour, milking sick or mastitis cows, or returning cows to the barn. For procedures covering these areas, see the appropriate SOP." (This is where code numbers come in handy.)

Identify the main tasks. Include the number of people required for the task; their skill levels; and equipment, supplies, and any personal protective equipment required. A Milking task list might include the following broad areas:
- Load the parlour.
- Pre-milk preparation.
- Milking.
- Post-milking sanitation.
- Release cows.

Describe each task in detail. In this section include the following:
- Specific order in which things are done.
- Timing sequences and times allowed.
- Materials or tools used and how they're used.
- Safety or health considerations.
- Expected outcomes or desired results.

Define terms and concepts when needed. Place health and safety warnings prominently in the SOP. People can't remember more than 10 or 12 steps, so they tend to ignore long SOPs. If your SOP goes beyond 10 steps, either break it into logical sub-job SOPs, or write a shortened SOP listing only the steps, not the detailed explanation of the steps. Use the long-form SOP for training and reference.

Get everyone on board. Successful SOP development demands that all people affected by a given SOP be involved in team-based problem solving. To achieve that: Have trained employees checked the written procedures against actual practices before implementation. Make revisions if necessary. Talk with employees to gain agreement that procedures and expectations are appropriate and achievable. Inform everyone about the written SOP. Train them on its contents and tell them where they can find it for future reference. Be aware that all your employees may not be able to read the SOP.

Set up a system to monitor the SOP regularly. The minute you write and implement SOPs, it's time to evaluate and update them. Employees should report needed changes to their supervisor. You and your veterinarian, or other consultants, should review each SOP annually. Take a team approach to modifying SOPs whenever needed. SOPs are worth the effort. Properly developed and implemented, they can result in consistent employee performance, improved milk quality and positive cow attitude.

Importance of SOPs: Standard operating procedures (SOPs) may seem like a lot of work. And once you invest the time, you might well wonder whether all those lists will ever get read. Fear not. Consider that SOPs provide:

- ❑ **A** guide for the new recruits who have less experience and new for the job
- ❑ **A** reference for employee training, cross-training and retraining
- ❑ **L**ess chaos and confusion when employees leave
- ❑ **C**onsistency a job is performed correctly every time
- ❑ **A**pproved procedures that reduce the risk of job failures and interruptions
- ❑ **A** basis for effective performance evaluation
- ❑ **I**mproved acceptance of practices because people support what they help create
- ❑ **A** means for everyone to think through the whole process of a task
- ❑ **A** statement of who does what, where, when, why and how
- ❑ **L**egal protection since a detailed process is documented in print
- ❑ **R**eference document in accident investigations
- ❑ **An** opportunity to build unity around attainable standards and
- ❑ **A** checklist for co-workers to observe performance and reinforce it if it's corrects
- ❑ **A**n aid in writing job descriptions and identifying skill requirements

17. Forms: Formats are designed to indicate a processing plant's compliance with the HACCP principles, Current Good Manufacturing Practices (CGMP's) and, Standard Hygiene Practices (SHPs), Regulatory requirements and to also provide a comparison with reference manufacturing plant. HACCP format is a tool in which hazards (things that can go wrong) are assessed based on collected data and control measures are established on that basis to prevent or minimise these hazards from occurring.

As a tool to collect data, it helps in reference, identification, a valuable record to plan and subsequently been used to address not only food safety but also quality. In a food-manufacturing situation, dozens of forms are used to record day-to-day activity, which reflects the degree of compliance as well as a monitoring tool.

The HACCP forms should include the following generic points.

- The title of the form reflecting the source of data and place of work
- The document should contain a reference number and revision
- Date of & Time of collecting data or writing an observation
- The collected information must be helpful in food safety
- Information recorded must identify the source of deviation
- It must reflect capability of the process
- The individual authority collecting data must sign the format
- A typical dairy plant may use construction checklist
- Equipment Inspection checklist
- Plant Sanitation Checklist
- Raw Material Receiving record
- Raw Material Laboratory Testing Record
- Testing of food and drink for nutritional information
- Final product labelling
- Final product surveillance
- Food testing for all major vitamins
- Testing for pesticide residues in food
- Testing for food additives
- Major Mineral and Trace Element Analysis
- Raw milk quality testing
- Technology upgrading
- Innovation practices
- Food Manufacturing Process Record
- Environment Monitoring Record
- Environmental Quality Standard
- Productivity Monitoring
- Personnel Efficiency Monitoring Record
- Processing Monitoring Record
- Quality Control Record
- Waste Minimization Record
- Water Quality Record,
- Dairy Effluent Monitoring Record
- Volatiles Monitoring record

18.Other Documents:

1. Copies of Standards to be used if not CFIA/FSIS Standard.
2. Copies of audit procedure to be followed when verifying controls applied at the farm.

Chapter: 12
HACCP AUDITS

Overview:

Auditing is held to account for the proper, efficient, and effective use of specified procedures to achieve complete safety in food manufacturing environment so that consumer health can be assured.

A HACCP auditing is a systematic and independent examination to determine whether food safety activities and related results comply with planned arrangements and whether these arrangements are implemented effectively and are suitable to achieve the objectives of food safety operations.

HACCP is a non-traditional, non-continuous and announced assessment technique that provides a more scientific, analytical, and economical approach than that provided by traditional inspection and quality control methods.

The subject knowledge required to perform a successful food safety audit is substantial. This requires significant experience, knowledge, and food industry background. For an effective and comprehensive audit in the food system, one should acquire following knowledge to contribute in a food safety audit system. Normally such knowledge should be imparted to HACCP Coordinators, Members of HACCP Teams, Quality Assurance and Personnel Manager, Operations Managers or anyone responsible for auditing prerequisite programs and HACCP plans. Such knowledge may require to: -

❑ Understand the Canadian Food Inspection Agency's (CFIA's) and US Food Safety Inspection Service (FSIS) standards and expectations.

❑ Consolidate others in the HACCP teamwork to boost overall understanding and participation.

❑ Auditing Fundamentals must form the basis of HACCP auditing.

❑ Develop Audit Program well ahead of schedule HACCP auditing.

❑ Audit Checklists may be generic but should include specifics of the plant.

❑ **M**aintain HACCP documentation consistent with ISO 9000 principles.

❑ **U**nderstand the knowledge role of auditing in food safety and HACCP system.

❑ **U**se auditing as a tool for preventive recurrence and corrective action.

❑ **U**nderstand the human food safety factors and human psychology while implementing food safety programs.

❑ **P**resent effective and open reports to the assessors to ensure objectivity and satisfactory results with in HACCP system operations.

In some countries, it is a condition of a dairy farmers licence that a certified HACCP system be in place on the farm to control both food safety and quality issues. In Australia, Safe Food certifies a dairy farm HACCP system through a certification audit. Following this system, Safe Food conducts a six monthly compliance audit. Once it is shown that the farm HACCP system is running effectively, Safe Food Safety Officers then audit the system on an annual basis. The HACCP manuals cover both quality and safety issues and both areas are audited. The quality areas are audited on behalf of the farmers' supplying to respective factories. Once a farm audit is completed, the Dairy Farm HACCP Audit Checklist and Dairy Building Inspection Reports are completed.

Prerequisite programs and HACCP plan development are only the initial steps in HACCP process implementation. The food manufacturing business organizations need to be ready for a government or customer audit of HACCP plan. HACCP team coordinator would appoint from members of his team one or more internal auditors who will assess the segments of system in places other than their work segments. They should be equipped to audit prerequisite programs and HACCP plan effectively.

Those who are concerned that some part of the HACCP system has been missed, or have questions, they may join for a hands-on workshop or refer the FSEP manual where they could review Prerequisite Programs and HACCP plans in relation to program requirements and CFIA expectations.

A continuous process of auditing HACCP system should be in place and to report on any deviations and non-conformance. It involves a thorough review of record keeping system and verification procedures by conducting independent audits to ensure the smooth running of the HACCP system. Audits should also be conducted prior to audit by authority as to prepare your plant and prepare/update your staff. Submit a complete audit report to your office for further action. That will contain useful advice on necessary changes to HACCP system based on the audit. Follow up audits on the necessary changes will be conducted on a regular basis depending on its necessity.

Classification of non-conformities in a dairy system may include the following points. The Critical Defects encountered in dairy husbandry are:

Critical Defects:
- Identification of treated cows
- Contagious human diseases
- Observe pesticides and identify paddocks sprayed with chemicals

Serious Defects
- Correct quantities of sanitizer, test dip/spray and detergents
- Teat dip/spray to manufacturer's recommendation
- Purchased feed declaration

Major Defects (Records)
- Vat cooling time
- Wash up procedure
- Sanitizer residue
- Recording treated cows
- Test milk of doubtful cows
- Tested milk of agisted / purchased cows
- Identify sold stock
- Record treated cows
- Record drug and medicine purchases
- Record chemical and spray purchases
- Record feed purchases
- Internal Audit

Major defects (Procedures)
- Drain sanitizer from plant
- Use accredited detergent, sanitizer and teat dip/spray
- Consult with vet on type, dose rate, administration method of drugs
- Do not feed antibiotic treated milk to claves for slaughter
- Milk treated cows last or into test bucket
- Dairy buildings to be maintained at A or B rating
- Use veterinary drugs and medicines purchased from approved outlets
- Store drugs and medicines in a secure area or to manufacturers recommendations
- Restricted dairy animals from effluent sprayed paddocks for at least 14 days

- ❑ **M**ix sprays according to label of Agronomist advice
- ❑ **S**tore and mix Agricultural sprays away from the dairy premises

Minor Defects

All other areas of non-conformance are minor

Types of HACCP Audit:

Most people appreciate that completing the HACCP study and implementing its requirements for a particular product or process is really just the starting point. It is necessary to verify the system to ensure that it continues to be complete, current, and fully effective, and this is where the many benefits of HACCP are seen. Auditing quality and safety systems is an often-underestimated function, which requires expert knowledge of industry standards and practical experience of operating quality and safety management systems. Auditors need to be technically up to date but also need to have the appropriate personal communication and negotiating skills and the ability to manage the audit process effectively. Audits in the food industry may include diversity in scope and that leads to many kinds of audits. HACCP audits are not different because it deals with the safety of food, which involves sanitation, food hygiene, regulatory, customary, and internal requirements.

We will discuss some of the audit types, which make part of the HACCP enforcement process that leads to confidence in the food safety system.

Regulatory System Audit: Under FSEP, a regulatory system audit is used to verify that prerequisite programs and HACCP plans are in fact being implemented as described and are effective on a continuous basis. The regulatory system audit under FSEP will consist of regulatory partial audits performed at frequencies according to the risk category of the processed involved, the level of inspection in the non-FSEP environment and the compliance record. The regulatory partial audits will consist of a partial review of the HACCP system.

For further details and study please refer to Canadian HACCP Audit requirements page in this chapter. As per the CFIA, an establishment may appeal the results of either a partial or full regulatory system audit. The appeal must be fully documented and forwarded in writing to the Area FSEP/HACCP coordinator (not implicated in the regulatory system audit). The Area FSEP/HACCP coordinator should consult with other regional/national experts for advice. The results of the appeal will be documented, forwarded to the establishment, and copied to HAQ. If the establishment is not satisfied with the decision it has the option of forwarding its request to the respective national association for further consultation prior to submission to CFIA for final decision.

The system audits are most extensive covering all aspects of the control system extending two to three working days. Regulatory system audits are conducted to verify, through objective evidence whether the HACCP system is implemented adequately and effectively, and meet the requirements set forth by CFIA/FSIS or any corresponding and applicable regulatory agency.

For a comprehensive auditing of a food plant, two or three auditors are often considered effective where a breakdown of the auditing team in to smaller system audit identified by a topic category. However, the number of auditors needed for any audit is dependent upon the purpose, scope, and depth of audit. The numbers of available auditors make a significant impact on positive side of the regulatory system audit. A full regulatory system audit includes and may exceed the scope of the process and product audit. The auditors would probe the interactive food product manufacturing of the organization as a whole and the effect of the system on the product safety, elimination of recurrence, corrective actions, and enhanced preventive measures. The time consumed in regulatory system audit is mainly cantered on process and its preventive controls.

The audited food plant as an extrinsic audit could also refer some times this type of audit. As a supplier and producer of any food item in Canada, the supplier is always liable for the regulatory system audit. The purpose of the audit is to safeguard the interest of customers and consumers who are never audited.

HACCP Accreditation Audits: HACCP is an internationally recognized means of assuring food safety from harvest to consumption. Recognized by "Codex Alimentarius" and other leading food safety agencies, HACCP has become the market standard for food safety worldwide. For the HACCP accreditation, an external auditor will scientifically review HACCP manual, Critical Control Points (CCPs), Critical Control Limits (CCLs), HACCP Plan, any discrepancies or non-conformities (major or minor) in any of these areas, on-site audit of plant based on the seven HACCP Principles and the six required Prerequisite Programs, actual implementation of the HACCP plan, employee training, data collection and record-keeping.

Following a successful on-site audit, the organization will receive a "Certificate of HACCP Accreditation," valid for up to three years, providing that follow-up audits verify that HACCP records are being properly maintained, Prerequisite Programs remain in place.

3rd Party Audit (Certification audit): Third party is an evaluation of a company by a certification body, and it lends its name to the concept that there are three parties involved: the company, the Certification body and the theoretical customer, which the certification body is auditing on behalf of. Both 2nd and 3rd party audits are classified as External audits.

A third party audit utilises an outside source to conduct the audit which is an independent source not affiliated or associated by any connection to the auditee's company business. The process of a third party audit could be a prelude to a regulator system audit. The company may contract with an outside professional to conduct an audit of its system. A third party audit could also be contracted to conduct audit on one or more suppliers.

In certain countries, a registered body conducts a third party audit where regulatory agencies of the country allow such a certification as recognition of a HACCP implementation system.

Sanitation Audit: Sanitation audits are part of the food hygiene audits, which are conducted to evaluate the ability of plant sanitation to adequately clean and sanitize food facilities before plant production begins. These audits are normally coordinated with food safety audits to provide a more complete set of observations, especially suited to high-risk ready-to eat products. Sanitation audits may also be considered as partial audit of a food safety system.

All the food safety conscious countries have special sanitation standards. Pre-Operational Sanitation Audits assess a plant's standard sanitation operating procedures for compliance to regulatory requirements as well as procedures established by the food organization. Actual plant performance is reviewed against planned and written sanitation procedures. It evaluates chemical handling and sign-off documents necessary to confirm that proper and regularly scheduled cleaning and sanitation have taken place.

The sanitation audits will be including observations made before production begins, sanitation process during the processing and packaging and after production is over. It analyses the critical factors and documents that confirm that the impact of proper sanitation continues throughout the manufacturing of the food products.

Food Hygiene Audit: A food hygiene audit is the first step towards identifying weaknesses in an operation. The first link is the cleaning process and HACCP must be applied to this process whether it is a clean or a deep clean. Auditing is the last link in the chain and is used to assess whether the cleaning procedures have been effective. Regulatory constraints and current management practices put the onus on food manufacturers to take all responsible precautions where hygiene is concerned. It was essential that managers acted on the audit results to drive improvements through the area or business audited, and that subsequent audits confirmed the actions had been implemented effectively.

Food hygiene audits have many facets. One is to ensure food is safe and that relevant legislation is being complied with. To meet these aims the auditors complete a prepared standard audit form when auditing premises. A food hygiene audit form will normally entail in the front a business name and address, registration no., auditors name, scope of audit and authority to audit. It may include any other necessary information required by the system. The regulatory food hygiene audit details could well include areas of concern since previous audit, a complaint to investigate, and overview of the business and staff of the premise.

The full food hygiene audit shall include Premises and Facilities, Maintaining standards, Personal Hygiene, Operational Controls and storage of food products.

Food Hygiene Audit could well be a third-party assessment of the establishment's hygiene standards based on routine food hygiene audit and food microbiological monitoring. It is relevant to organisations involved in the catering, processing, preparation, and retailing of food and beverage products. The hygiene audit report recognises the commitment to improving standards of food hygiene throughout the factory and the valuable role they play in protecting the public health.

The scope of a hygiene audit shall be with the agreement between auditor and the auditee. A regulatory audit is a compliance audit and auditee shall conform to the laid standards. An audit normally starts with a visual inspection of the key areas of the business, e.g. kitchens, storerooms, customer areas, and plant room. An assessment of the standard of the premises, in respect of the suitability and adequacy of the structure, ventilation, lighting, drainage, refuse facilities etc., general facilities and equipment. The audit can involve random food sampling and swabbing for analysis. A review of the practices, safety systems, services and staff personal hygiene standards to include: food handling (delivery / storage / date coding / temperature control etc.), food preparation, cleaning standards and procedures, pest control, dangerous machinery, accident reporting, chemical storage and handling, and protective clothing, staff appearance, and cleanliness and adequacy of staff facilities. Check of 'due diligence' records and procedures shall include training records and advice on legal compliance.

The benefits of food hygiene audits may include the report, which provides a checklist for auctioning non-compliances. It provides a measurable benchmark of compliance status and a target to achieve improved standards. It helps to keep key management up to date with current legislation and industry's best practices. It contributes to the business's 'due diligence' and consumer protection requirements. Improves relationships with local food regulatory authority and minimises the risk of prosecution and litigation. Raises both management and staff awareness and can act as a motivational tool.

Compliance audit: Compliance Audits are an integral part of HACCP audits. These food safety audits seek to confirm that specific food legislation; directions and regulations have been adhered to by food manufacturing and handling units. Compliance audits assess an enterprise's compliance with food legislation administered by the FDA, CFIA. The audits are unannounced and are conducted in accordance with the procedures and protocols set out in the government regulatory system. The findings of each audit and a follow-up action program based on the audit findings are reported in a Compliance Audit Report, which is sent to the concerned auditee.

In case of internal compliance audits, in such audits on a planned basis, the integrity of the process and product are maintained. In addition, organizational learning is fostered, in that a corporate memory is developed regarding usage of the defined process. Development of Internal Evaluation Programs will help to ensure that any apparent violations are promptly identified and corrected. HACCP managers and coordinators should encourage team members to make an Internal Compliance Audit an integral part of their everyday management process so that the full benefit of their voluntary disclosure can be realized. Programs that allow HACCP members to identify and correct their own instances of non-compliance and invest more resources in efforts to preclude their recurrence, rather than pay liabilities best serve food safety. The audit results are also one valuable input to the continuous improvement cycle.

Through the combined talents of trained experts and recognized investigative food safety specialists, allows a dedicated and qualitative evaluation of the significant factors involved in the creation and implementation of an Internal Evaluation and Compliance Audit. It is only through a well developed program that a company can be assured that it's policy and procedures are responsive to safety, change and that the procedures comply with appropriate safety requirements. A time-to-time Process and Product audits are healthy moves in fulfilment of overall quality and safety strategy.

Internal Audit: Internal audits are the part of compliance audit with a sense that its conformance to the laid standards are monitored and documented for continual improvements with consistency in the system. An internal audit is performed to measure and assess one's own performance, strengths, and weaknesses against its established and laid procedures for the HACCP system.

These audits are programmed with a timetable mentioning time intervals, which may range from once in a month to thrice in a year. It could vary according to one's own requirements. The system, process, and product audits are most frequently performed internally.

External Audit: This type of HACCP audits could be ordered by the customer company on an outside supplier of ingredients for its use in manufacturing food products. This could very well include packaging materials and containers coming in direct touch to food products. When auditors from the customer company audit a supplier, it is referred as an external audit. This is also very well understood as suppliers and 2nd party audit.

1st Party Audit: This is an internal evaluation of the food safety or quality management's systems in place within one's own organisation to ensure that the documented systems have been adequately implemented. The persons conducting this audit should be adequately trained.

All internal HACCP audits or QMS audits are considered to be 1st party audits. These are the audits authorized by the management to conduct an internal assessment on itself before inviting a third party audit, which is completely independent.

In internal audits, arrangements are made that the auditors who are affiliated with the same section do not perform section audits. Thus an engineering employee trained as an auditor could not perform audit in the engineering department. He could perform an audit in laboratory, process control, stores etc.

2nd Party Audit: 2nd Party Audit is an evaluation of a supplier by the customer to assess if planned arrangements by the supplier are implemented effectively and are suitable to achieve the objectives of food safety or quality issues. A 2nd party audit is also referred as external and supplier audit.

Supplier's Audit: Supplier audits are focused primarily on process control. They are the same as 2nd party audits and evolve the necessity to develop confidence in the process and supplies through a proper audit. Many organisations have a need to audit their suppliers. Sometimes, a buying company may request certain changes in order to make the auditee's product eligible for procurement. But purchaser assures that they intend to work together with the auditee to guarantee that the products they purchase are as per their expectation.

Purchasers recognise the importance of supplier assurance. This is essential to prevent poisoning or legal problems that could affect your business or reputation. Effective management of your supplier's chain with thorough HACCP audits will ensure that all products are covered. The food manufacturers should recognise these limitations and should develop a management system to help with due diligence systems.

Performance Audit: Performance Audits seek to determine whether a food business is carrying out activities efficiently, economically, and in compliance with the food control regulations applicable in host country. These audits may review all or part of a manufacturing operation. Qualitative survey based on qualitative data on critical points adds value to the food safety audits but partial audits are not seen as complimentary to the program. A complete componential evaluation with criticality serves the purpose of audit. Components responsible for food health risks to human are identified, isolated, eliminated, controlled and recurrence prohibited. That is where performance to conformance fits an acceptable outcome of HACCP process and system. Performance audits are normally initiated by internal HACCP management and prepares for an external audit. It could be considered a prelude to Accreditation Audits.

Process audit: They are the defined process, associated standards, and procedures actually being followed consistently and uniformly in a food manufacturing organization. The process audit is the most performed and the most convenient audit, often yielding swifter results. The food manufacturing auditor's team would like to perform process audits more frequently to comply with specific process upgrading, alteration, or modifications.

Process audits are actually compliance audits conducted to concentrate only one specific process element, product, or service. The process audits for the purpose of HACCP could be performed internally or externally. These audits are very useful in improving processing and could be performed in little duration of time.

Product audit: Do the various work products and deliverables conform to established standards as laid down in the product specifications by the manufacturing company. This is an evaluation of the product characteristics and typically does not form a part of a systems audit. This audit would usually be conducted against product specifications standards or in-house standards.

The product's audit is an assessment of the final food product or food supply service. Product audits are normally conducted on the request of customer, which may be conducted externally at the supplier site, the customer site or sometimes with the final consumer. The product audits are very rarely conducted at the consumer level and would not qualify as Quality Assurance Audit or HACCP audit unless mandated by the organization's HACCP manual.

Partial Audit: Partial audit is the process of auditing a food manufacturing plant in phases due to constraints in time. Due to time constraints, it is possible to be initially listed by CFIA as an establishment, which would only need to comply with the Basic Compliance Checklist (BCC) pending to the establishment FSEP recognition providing it did submit its request of recognition under FSEP. Following completion of the FSEP recognition process, establishments will be periodically subjected to FSEP regulatory partial audits. Each time such an audit is performed, a report is generated which takes the place of the Establishment Inspection Report.

Security Audit: Security Audits concerning food safety may be the audits of future as U.S. congressional auditors say the country's food supply is vulnerable to terrorist attacks partly because the government cannot ensure the security of processing plants. Without the ability to require food processing facilities to provide information on their security measures, these federal agencies cannot fully assess industry's efforts to prevent or reduce the vulnerability of the nation's food supply to deliberate contamination". Thus it may be required to share security plans with regulators otherwise lack of security would make them susceptible to terrorist attacks. However, security and safety plans could not be released to the public.

Audit Checklists Should Be Used:
When developing an audit checklist for the HACCP system, the following items should be considered:
- The scope of the audit
- List of CCPs

- ❑ **L**ist of CCLs
- ❑ **L**ist of reference standards
- ❑ **A** structured list of critical manufacturing process
- ❑ **L**ist of SOPs
- ❑ **D**ocumented procedures to gather objective evidence
- ❑ **A**n annual audit timetable
- ❑ **F**ollow up and corrective action
- ❑ **R**eporting procedures
- ❑ **R**ecord of HACCP review meeting/Management review meetings
- ❑ **H**ACCP Internal Audits Plan; Audit Frequency
- ❑ **H**ACCP Internal Auditors Record
- ❑ **A**udit Reporting

Scope of Food Safety Audits:

A food safety audit, which will be in fulfilment of HACCP process mainly, focuses on the elements of HACCP system, which includes the gathering of information about a food business to identify any area of potential risks from procurement to processing, packaging, and subsequent consumption of that food item.   With overall perception, we could safely say it is an improvement in the business's food safety process and system.

It definitely identifies areas of the food manufacturing, handling and trading in such a way that it identifies the irregulatories, eliminates it or reduce the risk up to safe levels, establishes the upper and lower levels scientifically and continually searches the means to improve the process and controls.

Through Food Product or Process Certification schemes, a registrar verifies the conformity of one's products or process to quality and safety criteria described in the laid company's standards that answer the needs of the consumers, the regulatory authorities, and stakeholders' requirements. Key aspects of any audit program include product Traceability, procured ingredients, manufacturing process, shelf life of the products, personnel, and hygiene systems of the food manufacturing or handling company.

In Canada, food businesses that produce different types of product for multicultural customers are increasingly expected to implement multiple food safety and quality systems. Multiple audits are often then needed to demonstrate compliance with the various regulatory, industry-driven, and customer-specific requirements. All these elements of audit impose additional costs on suppliers but develop confidence and trust of the consumers. To a minority of sceptically driven customers, it may create a lack of confidence in the integrity of auditing food safety and quality systems as inconsistencies are emerging with the implementation and auditing of these systems. Thus a confidence in the integrity of auditing food safety and quality systems is to be developed and emerging inconsistencies if any are to be eliminated in the implementation and auditing of these systems.

Under the food safety audit program, audition is designed to allow its auditors to cut to the chase, and focus on critical elements, on big-ticket items such as risks, which endangers human health. In food safety audit, what is material and what is important is to pin point critical stigma in food safety issues. The audit system has been developed for the purposes of auditing food safety programs. A food safety program is based on the Hazard Analysis and Critical Control Point (HACCP) principles and is a documented program that systematically identifies critical points in food handling operations that, if not controlled, may lead to preparation of unsafe food.

The audit system is integrated with elements of food safety. Elements of food safety are based on certain criteria laid down by CFIA and FSIS separately and respectively for Canada and the United States. Beside regulatory criteria, certain philosophical elements are also included which reflect the common human sense in safety matters. The elements of a HACCP audit are mentioned as follows:

- **A** Criterion of legality
- **A** Perception of food safety audit
- **A** Commitment of auditee
- **A** Jurisdictional basis
- **A** Regulatory audit requirement
- **A** Liability towards consumers
- **A** Demonstration of company's commitment
- **A** Commitment to code of practice in a profession
- **A** Recognition of value
- **A** Marketing tool
- **A** strategy of implementation

Benefits of HACCP Audit:
- Builds team knowledge of the food safety issues
- Critical Control Points are identified to prevent risks
- Reference point for the Master Batch Records
- Rational basis for process validation plans
- Reference point for quality assurance audits
- Excellent training tool for staff of the line
- Useful for self-control of quality by line teams
- Ensures that food safety continues to be fully effective
- Ensures that food safety continues to be complete and

current
- Imparts a good working knowledge of HACCP
- Paves the way for better Design of food plant
- Paves the way for better Construction of Food Premises
- Paves the way for improvements in Equipment
- Reduced consumer complaints
- Reduced potential for illness or injury
- Reduced potential for adverse publicity
- Overall cost savings
- Enhanced efficiencies among workability of plant
- Increased revenues if HACCP audits implemented
- More desirable co-packer or supplier
- The opportunity to mandate HACCP for a company's suppliers
- Enhanced product quality
- Reduced waste due to correct products
- Improved employee morale due to confidence
- Reduced product liability and other insurance
- Discount on their liability insurance.
- Operation's prerequisite programs systemised
- Sanitation standard operating procedures correctly implemented
- Good manufacturing practices followed
- Preventive maintenance implemented
- Workers education record checked to verify training
- HACCP audits could reduce insurance premiums
- Product Traceability maintained and documented
- Review of records to verify that things are being done
- Existing systems be upgraded
- HACCP Audits can protect business from liabilities

Who should do HACCP Audit?

It is very important in HACCP audits that integrity and non-biased auditing is not only ensured but also mandated. Who should be requested to perform internal, external, regulatory, third party audits and additional assistance in the selection and evaluation of certification bodies for the food manufacturing and handling companies evolves a situation of conflicting interest.

Neutrality in an auditing team is the most desired factor. The most important factor in deciding a right Auditor or a right Auditing team is to look into the neutrality of the auditing body or individual. Independent it goes without saying that an auditor should be completely independent from the area's being audited. This is a requirement of ISO 9001 for internal audits, and of the International Register of Certified Auditors (IRCA) * for certification and professional auditors. Probably one of the main reasons for this requirement is that an auditor should not have any links to the area being audited as this may severely impeach their judgement and impartiality to the areas being assessed.

Experience in the specific food industry is the deciding factor in the selection of auditors. When making evaluation of certification bodies, an enquiry to evaluate their back ground experience, and once more, for companies, which do not fit into the "normal" mould, it is extremely important to study carefully who will be performing your audit. In auditing individual auditors make more impact than the reputation of the auditing company. Thus the audit will only be as productive as the auditor's knowledge of the specific food industry and their experience as an auditor.

Respectability of an auditing organization may attract the importance of an auditee. Exposure of the Lead Auditor and the 2nd auditors to the concerned industry are paramount to a respectable audit. Accreditation bodies typically require a knowledgeable person of that industry to be present during the audits, however when auditing in a team, it would be physically impossible for that specialist to be present with each individual auditor as they go about their audits, and thus the 2nd auditors will still require a reasonable knowledge about the nature of the industry being audited.

Testimonials of an auditor or the background record in the form of resumes will help identify the educational and work experience background prior to becoming a certification auditor.

Credentials type an individual auditor may bring in the form of educational qualification and certificates may add value to auditor's credibility. One could draw similarities with the selection of a University and the degree provided. Here a standing reputation of a university or association may play a role in the selection of an auditor.

Regulatory agencies and professional in the industry may also advise in the selection of an auditing team as their certification and licenses would depend upon certain criteria and examination.

Language factor or communication factor is vital for any audit. As we all know, having knowledge of English and the French languages is an important part of a good audit, and persons not familiar with the above will find it more difficult to perform a good audit as they will waste a lot of time in translations, and may overlook important evidence due to the lack of understanding of the language.

Communication factor is by no means a least factor. Our food manufacturing systems are based on human factors. By default, we are fallible. If we decide to couple the riskful nature of food safety system along with the human factors, then supervisor to operators, and operator-to-worker communication is a natural next step in avoiding errors. A verbal friendly communication overcomes the cloud of fear among the members of auditee's manufacturing team. There are a lot of gaps in understanding, trust, and expectation.

HACCP Lead auditor and the auditors need to get everyone in the audit system involved, but until it's a kinder, gentler system, people involved will still immerse in the "shame and blame" environment. Auditing is the name of objectivity and fame to shame and then to blame does not have any place in quality or food safety audits. Communication is one of the important skills — it's critical and it must be learned to make change in the system. As an auditor make it relevant, practical, with solutions based on plenty of real-life examples. It's also about acknowledging that failures within the system are a primary reason for errors, which can make communication skills education an easier doze to digest.

Canadian HACCP Audit requirements:

The Canadian Food Inspection Agency (CFIA) has its HACCP Audit program for the food industry nationwide and continues to strengthen its program audit function to improve the effectiveness and efficiency of compliance actions. The Canadian Food Inspection Agency, in consultation with the Office of the Auditor General of Canada, engage in discussions with its provincial and territorial counterparts to identify and develop a satisfactory method to carry out a proper overall risk assessment of the non-federally registered sector. Please visit www.inspection.gc.ca for detailed and up-to-date information.

Quality Management Program (QMP): The QMP program was one of the first mandatory HACCP programs in the world, and has evolved to include prerequisite safety components, recall procedures and other regulatory action points (quality, packaging and labelling). The FSEP program is presently voluntary. The government is in the process of introducing mandatory HACCP requirements for the federally registered meat sector. Establishments, which have developed and implemented HACCP plans on a voluntary or mandatory basis are moved from a traditional inspection approach to a more audit-based government verification of the establishment's controls. Quality Management Program (QMP) is for the fish and seafood sector of the Canadian

Food Industry. Please visit www.inspection.gc.ca for detailed and up-to-date information.

Canadian Food Safety Adaptation Program: The Canadian Food Safety Adaptation Program (CFSAP) is an opportunity for national associations or groups who are involved directly or indirectly in the production, marketing, distribution and preparation of food to develop risk management strategies, tools and systems to enhance food safety throughout the total food chain. In order to be eligible, these activities must use the Hazard Analysis Critical Control Point (HACCP) definitions and principles as defined by the Codex Alimentarius Commission. Please visit www.inspection.gc.ca for detailed and up-to-date information.

On-Farm Food Safety Program: In support of the Agriculture Policy Framework (APF), the Agency is working with Agriculture and Agri-Food Canada, provincial governments, and industry associations to develop and implement a recognition process for industry-developed On-Farm Food Safety Program (OFFSP). For a further and detailed study, please refer Chapter: 11 HACCP: Its Implementation. Please visit www.inspection.gc.ca for detailed and up-to-date information.

Regulatory System Audits under FSEP: Under FSEP, a regulatory system audit is used to verify that prerequisite programs and HACCP plans are in fact being implemented as described and are effective on a continuous basis. This is consistent with the ISO 10011 approach to audit, which is defined as "A systematic and independent examination to determine whether quality activities and related results comply with planned arrangements and whether these arrangements are implemented effectively and are suitable to achieve objectives". The regulatory system audit should not be confused with "surveillance" or "inspection" activities performed for the sole purpose of process control or product acceptance. Please visit www.inspection.gc.ca for detailed and up-to-date information.

The Multi-Commodity Activities Program (MCAP) is a computerized program to be used in all registered and licensed establishments under the Meat Inspection Act and Canada Agricultural Products Act after FSEP/HACCP recognition and in all registered and licensed establishments under the Fish Inspection Act. The Multi-Commodity Activity Program details the activities related to a Regulatory (system) audit under FSEP and other non-food and safety activities. As an alternative to the computerized program for the regulatory system audit under FSEP, an appendix developed details the activities, worksheets for the auditing of

HACCP plans and prerequisite programs and reflects the logical sequence of the audit portion of the software program. Please visit www.inspection.gc.ca for detailed and up-to-date information.

Audit Report Form:

The benefits of any audit report are immeasurable. An audit conducted by third party identifies deficiencies and opportunities for further improvements in the system. By doing so it leaves an impact among the food-manufacturing employees, HACCP team, HACCP Coordinator, the management team and sometimes on stakeholders, which reinforces the importance of the food safety process to all employees. Among the customers and consumers it creates credibility to the process and make it easier to get accepted with improved confidence in the food products and the food service. Auditing of HACCP system ought to improve the whole safety system.

The HACCP Verification Audit is a comprehensive review of how one's HACCP plans are being implemented. A continuous process of auditing HACCP system shall be currently in place to report on any deviations and non-conformance. It involves a thorough review of record keeping system and verification procedures. An audit of the work highlights much good work and some areas for further improvement.

Audit Report Contents:

The audit report will be completed by the lead auditor and includes the following:

Introduction: The identification of the lead auditor and audit team members if applicable. The Lead auditor, together with Audit team and specialists in areas constitute a formidable team that need to succeed in the auditing. The identification and introduction of the team, right people behind each single aspect of a full audit provide a better understanding and a better communication.

The identification of company representative(s) is also arranged in the same way to facilitate the presence of right people at right place. Thus identification of those concerned with auditing including auditor and auditee should be mentioned in the audit report.

Reference Standards:
Food safety regulation in Canada
Food safety regulations in the United States of America
Food safety regulations in a host country i.e. China, India, Japan, Mexico, Pakistan, UAE etc

Scope of Audit: The scope of the HACCP audit shall include the elements of prerequisite program, CCLs, CCPs, SOPs, GMPs, outstanding CARs, company's log book and sanitation. The adoption and implementation of HACCP with a documented and effective quality management system, control of factory environment standards, product, process, and personnel eventually may expand the scope of a comprehensive HACCP audit. The scope of audit is mentioned objectively to avoid confusion between Auditor and Auditee.

Scope of any quality or safety audit is designed to increase the efficacy of a newly introduced food quality and safety systems. Studies have demonstrated very significant increases in performance over the two-year period for each of the attributes, namely - condition of raw material (20% increase), process (32%), product quality (15%), hygiene (10%), equipment (10%) and quality (15%)-111.

Audit Objectives: The Objective of any audit is the verification of a system or products by meeting planned standards of activities. It produces instigation to plan implementation, discuss status, and implement any changes found necessary. The objective is not one stick aim but multiple achievements, which agglomerates the safety and quality of products for human consumption.

Thus in a HACCP process, the objective becomes to review and verify all elements; HACCP Plan Verification, Validation Checklist, verification of Flow Charts, Hazard Analysis for each process step, CCP Records for the current day production, SSOP and CCP Records, Review all Non-Compliance Records, Review of written SSOP and HACCP Plan to assure accuracy, completeness, and proper validation, validation techniques and literature to support HACCP Plan CCP's and critical limits, status of working relationship with CFIA, USDA etc., In Depth Verification Audit Report and to continue food safety process growth. The bottom line of all these objectives is identifying deficiencies and opportunities for improvement. Objectives of a HACCP audit are clearly stated in the audit report to put a convincing impact on the concerned employees and the management.

Audit Observations: Audit observations and their relative impact on the integrity of the system is an idealistic approach. This is to include any immediate corrective/compliance action taken at the time of the audit to address food safety concerns. The auditor should complete an Observation Form (AO) whenever the auditor identifies a possible opportunity for operational improvement, discrepancy, error, irregularity, weakness or deviation from internal control standards, regulations, or policies. Prior audit reports and linked audit observations should be reviewed and used to the extent possible to avoid re-creating an observation already developed.

Employee development in the field of safety and quality are critical to an effective HACCP program. HACCP coordinators, team members, and production supervisors must learn and develop observation techniques to manage and continuously improve overall HACCP system. Critical HACCP principles and observing what their roles could bring to overall safety of the manufactured food products is a motivating step. Many times during the auditing process or in the beginning the auditor realizes they have an audit concern, they should begin to complete the Observation Form and discuss the observation with the auditee.

The discussion between the auditing officer and the auditee's representative should be documented in the applicable fields of the Observation Form. The Observation Form should stand-alone and should document the auditor's analysis (criteria, condition, cause, consequence, and corrective action) related to the finding. That information should not be elsewhere in the work papers. Documenting the analysis assists the auditor in preparing to discuss the observation with the auditee. The Observation Form should document the results of the problem analysis/resolution process. In order to get best out of the documented observations the auditor should analyze such findings and generate corrective action requests with advice if applicable.

The identification and chronology of the problem that exists, its effects, risk associated with it, control measures, self analysis to verify observations, finding critical solutions and also if auditee's management agrees with recommended corrective action or they may formulate their own corrective actions. Such observations do become part of an audit report.

Sometimes an observation may not result in CAR. The observation may not pose a direct threat to the safety of products but it could indirectly affect the operation and the HACCP system. This observation should still be brought to the notice of Auditee and advice could be given to pre-empt future risks. Based on additional information provided by the auditee or further consideration of available solutions, the auditor may be convinced that their initial concern is not worth pursuing. This should be explained on the Audit Observation form and the applicable disposition should be selected. Dispositions for such observations may include that controls are in place which reduce the risk below the cost of the control or not a significant observation as immaterial errors have been identified or it may not be a concern at all as determined issue was unsubstantiated. Such observations are not included in the audit report but mentioned verbally to the auditee.

Key Findings: The auditor should verify the key facts with applicable auditee personnel before loosing the momentum considering the importance of key finding. Document the date and discussion with the auditee as outlined on the observation form. The auditor should document the analysis of the problem in this section. References to applicable standards and/or good business practice should be included. If possible, the auditor should identify probable causes (as opposed to the symptoms) for the audit observation. This section should not contain information that is redundant to that found on the work paper.

The Key Findings provides critical information about food safety loopholes and presents insights. The audit report will include the key findings and CAR referenced accordingly.

Corrective Actions Requested: The Corrective Action Request (CAR) forms are used to notify auditee where the auditee takes the charge to implement corrective actions and subsequent verification from the auditor. A time based CAR may also be issued to expedite the process. The CAR could also be presented to stakeholder meeting by the Auditee management in case of financial approvals and extended advice. HACCP team coordinator may advise to the management that a continuance of pre-approval as an option rather than mandatory which may seek stakeholders advice. From this suggestion, management may form a focus group to work out details of the change in the process required by the HACCP audit and develop a proposal for the stakeholders or Steering Committee. Several meetings may be held, to finalize the corrective actions proposal. It gives an opportunity to all to get complimented and everyone involved in the focus group for the work that has been done and may recommend that the committee hear from consultants as well as owners/operators with respect to food safety risk prioritization. In such cases, a special time may be asked from regulatory agencies/second party/third party auditors to compliment CAR. All the CARs form the part of an audit report and should be properly referenced and listed.

Any detected nonconformity in the food safety and Quality System, i.e. areas which did not meet the requirements of the applicable HACCP Standard, need to be corrected before approval of the system can be issued. In cases minor observations and auditing team may require that auditee sends confirmation of corrective actions to the auditing team leader to confirm that the agreed actions have been performed.

In the case of key findings which are considered serious errors lead auditor may have to revisit or send one of his team auditor to auditee manufacturing or service location to confirm that all the requested corrective actions have been carried out.

Audit Findings and Overall conclusions: As a result of the audit, the status of the HACCP implementation system can be confirmed (traditional inspection when applicable, normal or reduced audit frequency). HACCP audit focuses on the food inspection programs. An audit may find good progress on a number of CFIA's initiatives. It could also find that progress on other initiatives has varied. It is possible that lead auditor may like to discuss some of these in more detail. Findings may include observations on the implementation of the hazard analysis and critical control points (HACCP) approach in general. It may conclude that further enhancements to the HACCP-based system in the factory are badly needed. A review of a number of high-risk products manufactured in the factory may require more CCPs and CCLs.

The findings may identify weaknesses in the company's options for dealing with non-compliance and some problems with previous compliance actions. The CFIA may identify a number of initiatives that it believes are important to fulfilling its mandate. In doing so, it has created expectations for improvement by the food manufacturing company. All findings with bottom line conclusions are included in the audit report.

Recommendations: The auditor should include a statement of risk which is sufficient to answer the "so what?" question so that the reason for reporting the observation is clear. This section should also include the corrective action to be presented to the auditee.

For reporting purposes, audit observations are often combined for the purposes of clarity or conciseness. When such a combination is appropriate, this should be documented in this field. The auditor should indicate on both the individual observations and the summary/combined observation that concerns were combined for reporting purposes (i.e., different concerns with the same risk). For those documents combined, only the observation used in the report will have a disposition of audit report. Supporting observations that were combined should have a disposition of "combined for report". Only the recommendation section of the combined form will be updated to reflect the final report language. Doclink's should be created on both the individual observations and the combined observation for easier review and subsequent follow-up. A Combined Audit Observation Form may include: Finding, Discussion and background, Recommendation, Disposition, Discusses with, Date, Comments, Management Response, Person(s) Responsible, Auditor Responsible, Planned Follow-up Date, Follow-up Comments, Recovered Follow-up Work papers, Report Item, and Actual Completion Date.

Review Requests:
- Developing and reviewing standards
- Management of food recalls
- Progress towards an Integrated Food Safety Strategy
- Coordination of food surveillance
- Surveillance and Monitoring Strategy
- Information on food safety issues
- Local Regulatory Agency's enforcement
- Internal Reporting

The final written report, including any CARs issued (if applicable) will be given to establishment management and copied to the responsible inspector, for follow-up action. The report is also copied to the Area HACCP coordinator and HQ program chief. The characteristics of Audit report are normally maintained as per the following criteria.

- **Be** concise and clearly written;
- **Include** only information that is needed for a proper understanding of the findings, conclusions and recommendations when provided;
- **Provide** appropriate context by describing the objectives and timing of the assessment, the activities assessed, their importance and how they fit into the overall operations of the Agency;
- **Clearly** expose the limits of the assessment in terms of scope, methods and conclusions;
- **Provide** an accurate presentation of the findings; and
- **Present** the conclusions and recommendations, when provided, so that they flow logically from the findings.

Manufacturing HACCP Plan Development
- Documented project plan with time line
- Current program evaluation - GMP's, SOP's and SSOP's
- Creation of necessary GMP's or SOP's
- HACCP team training
- Facilitation of HACCP team meetings
- Documentation of HACCP team meeting minutes
- Employee training programs and assistance
- Completion of Process Descriptions

- ❑ Completion of Flow of Food Diagrams
- ❑ Completion of Potentially Hazardous Food List
- ❑ Hazard Analysis process
- ❑ Complete HACCP Plan development
- ❑ HACCP Plan documentation
- ❑ HACCP Ready Recipe Manual documentation
- ❑ HACCP Plan implementation assistance
- ❑ Initial plan verification
- ❑ Recall Program

Food Manufacturers Employees:

All manufacturers that supply the United States or Canada will have to develop a HACCP plan and train employees in HACCP procedures.

Re-assessment of food handlers may form an important aspect in food safety issues. If an establishment performed a reassessment and concluded that the employee needs extra training or isolation for food safety reasons then it should be done as per the schedule.

Sometime during the production time frame and the audit plan, HACCP plan may need modification and inspection program employees may be required to verify the modification to the HACCP plan through performance HACCP internal audit or inspection procedures. Signed and dated modifications to the HACCP plan must be done. That is where an audit expertise is important in the HACCP team.

Manufacturing in today's environment has needs that totally differ from other industries. A quality and HACCP coordinator have many concerns that require attention on a daily basis. Food manufacturing should understand that employees need a safe, happy, and productive workplace, balanced with the need to reduce costs and enhance safety.

Food Managers need to be aware of hidden costs of safety and quality failures associated with using the wrong or inferior product for the application. A food technologist expertise is needed for the purpose.

An exporting food manufacturer in Canada may need expertise in the fields of exporting, market identification, and technical requirements for food exporting and importing. Either someone who has more than specified years experience in the food and Agriculture industry with extensive international activity in the marketing of foods and Agricultural products would fill the gap or one may like to impart the special training to cover quality and safety matters involved.

Traditionally, stakeholders in the food industry have practiced and depended on spot-checks of manufacturing conditions and random sampling of final products to ensure food safety and quality. This approach, however, tends to be reactive, rather than preventative and can be less efficient than the HACCP and ISO-9001 systems. It is vital that the management and the stakeholders obtain critical information necessary to develop a workable efficient HACCP team to program a geared HACCP process specifically to the concerned food manufacturing and handling facility.

Adding a food line to a traditionally non-food plant raises special challenges to the food safety. Earlier, Mohawk Canada, a Western Canadian retailer and manufacturer of environmentally-friendly fuels and lubricants enlisted GFTC's help in making a major change, adding a food division to their non-food repertoire. Mohawk Canada Ltd. is marketing a high-fibre food ingredient, derived from a by-product of its ethanol production, that it hopes will appeal to health-conscious consumers. With the establishment of a new Fibrotein Cereal Products division they are able to invert the process and produce a food-grade wheat flake that is clinically proven and recognized by Health Canada as a source of dietary fibre. GFTC assisted in designing, implementing Good Manufacturing Practices (GMPs), implementing HACCP program and to train employees in these systems. So diversity is possible through a proper implementation plan and employee's education-62.

A day doesn't go by in this world without hearing about food borne illnesses, food recalls, or the implementation of new technology to make foods healthier, safer and more convenient. Nowhere else is this more prevalent than at the retail level where all the production and processing of food come together in foods offered to consumers. Faced with more complex and sophisticated food safety challenges, food manufacturers should understand the need to change for a comprehensive food manufacturing system, which guarantees profit and assures quality and safety. All involved in the system should understand the theme.

All the food scientists agree and regard HACCP (Hazard Analysis and Critical Control Points) systems as the most effective way to prevent physical, chemical, and microbiological hazards in foodservice operations. To determine where safety might be compromised, operators must:
- ❑ Understanding the basics of HACCP
- ❑ Basic training in food safety handling

In the plainest terms, outbreaks of food borne illness stem from human errors and human infection. Estimates indicate that as much as 85 percent to 95 percent of cases may be caused by improper food handling, despite HACCP and other controls.

A management system directs employees to control errors because structure and accountability for verifying food safety are part of the process. A large part of the industry doesn't have a staff in place with HACCP expertise. Now it is not a time to mom and pop to run a business. Complain of "simply don't have a lot of time to sit down and write detailed plans" is not valid any more. It is a regulation, which is meant to assist food manufacturers to be safe and earn in the business. In addition, if we're expecting ordinary food employees to go in and get a quantity that sells, we're kidding ourselves that is where enforcement and training comes from the management.

In many observations, the author himself focussed the operators and workers on addressing risk factors—those items directly attributed to food borne disease outbreaks—items such as time and temperature management for food products, personal hygiene, preventing cross contamination, proper storage, proper transportation and getting products from reputable suppliers. These areas are the foundation to an effective food safety management system within any retail food operation and in manufacturing establishments. The missing piece in any operation should be analysed and system for monitoring and evaluating food safety procedures and practices within their establishments should be followed as principled in HACCP.

One of the most common food safety mistakes operators make is not properly training their employees. To make matters worse, sometimes it's difficult to retrain people and get them to understand that what they've always done is not necessarily correct. It all comes down to employee training, it may sound expensive exercise to traditional businessmen, but training and supervision are necessary steps and shall be considered as an investment for a healthier food manufacturing and handling business.

<u>REFERENCES</u>

A

1. Abdussalam, M. & D. Grossklaus (1991) Food-borne illness: a growing problem. *World Health*. 18: 9

2. A Federal-Provincial-Territorial Initiative Food Safety and Food Quality (2003). Putting Canada First - An Architecture for Agricultural Policy in the 21st Century. Web Site: http://www.agr.gc.ca/puttingcanadafirst/index_e.ph p?section=fd_al&group=docu&page=fd_pres0203

3. Ahmed, Farid E., Editor. 1991. Seafood safety. Washington, DC, National Academy Press. 3031 WEYMOUTH ST., #204 DURHAM NC 27707 USA

4. Anna M. Lammerding and Greg M. Paoli (1999); Quantitative Risk Assessment: An Emerging Tool for Emerging Food borne Pathogens; Health Canada, Guelph, Ontario, Canada; and †Decisionalysis Risk Consultants, Ottawa, Ontario, Canada Gisèle Albrough, Access to Information and Privacy Coordinator, Health Canada, 12th floor, Jeanne Mance Building, Tunney's Pasture, Ottawa, Ontario, K1A 0K9 E-Mail: copyright.droitdauteur@communication.gc.ca

5. An International Outbreak of Salmonella Infections Caused by Alfalfa Sprouts Grown from Contaminated Seeds," Journal of Infectious Diseases, Vol. 175 (1997), pp. 876-882;

6. Annual Report (2001 - 2002) Canadian Food Inspection Agency Executive Summary Of Our Results Commercial Affairs, Canadian Food Inspection Agency (CFIA); 59 Camelot Drive, Nepean, Ontario, Canada, K1A 0Y9. Web Site: http://www.inspection.gc.ca

7. Approach to Valuing Food Safety Risks (1998); Victoria Salin

   Assistant Professor, Department of Agricultural Economics, Texas A&M Universities- E-mail: v salin@tamu.edu Tel: (409) 845-8103 Web Site: http://www.umass.edu/ne165/haccp1998/salin.html

8. Australia's Integrated Quality Assurance and Food Safety Programs Web Site: http://www.ausmeat.com.au/cs/training/foodsafety/ E-mail ausmeat@ausmeat.com.au

9. A.W. Randell, K. Miyagishima and J. Maskeliunas (2002); Protecting food today and in the future; Alan Randell is Senior Officer and Jeronimas Maskeliunas is Food Standards Officer, Codex Alimentarius Commission: Joint FAO/WHO Food Standards Programme. Kazuaki Miyagishima is Associate Professor, Department of Public Health, Faculty of Medicine, and Kyoto University.

10. A. Zugarramurdi, M.A. Parin, L. Gadaleta and H.M. Lupin (1998); Utilisation of the PAF Model to Evaluate the Economics of HACCP Application: Summary- Poster Session Decision Makers' Summaries of Papers; The Economics of HACCP: New Studies of Costs and Benefits June 15-16, 1998 A Conference Organized by the NE-165 Regional Research Project and Sponsored by the Farm Foundation, Food Marketing Policy Center, University of Illinois, and University of Massachusetts Washington DC Web Site: http://www.umass.edu/ne165/haccp1998/zugarr.html

B

11. BACKGROUND ON Genetically Engineered Food Issues prepared by Center for Food Safety Web Site: http://www.icta.org/projects/cfs/backgrd.htm

12. Bakery Merchandising and Marketing Specialists (2003); the largest non-profit resource site for professional pastry chefs and bakers Web Site: http://caima.net/research_reports.htm;   E-mail: info@caima.net Telephone: 905-528-8371, Fax: 905-528-3589

13. Barbara King, Robin Foroutan Aronow & Pollock Communications, Inc. New Study Provides Evidence That Tea Consumption Reduces Low Density Lipoprotein ("Bad" Cholesterol) Levels 212-941-1414. E-mail: bking@aronowandpollock.com E-mail: rforoutan@aronowandpollock.com   Web   Site: http://www.tea.ca/press-trends-sep24.asp?section=media

14. Blast Chilling: A Critical Control in the Preparation Of Food; North Blast Chillers. 61 Broadway, Suite 1900, New York, NY 10006, (212) 898-9699 Web Site:http://www.bmil.com/bally/nwnotwi.htm

15. Belzer, Richard B. & Richard P. Theroux (1995) Criteria for evaluating results obtained from contingent valuation methods. *In* Julie A. Caswell, ed. *Valuing food safety and nutrition,* pp. 341-362 Boulder, Colorado, Westview Press.

C

16. Canada and Alberta Agri-food exports to Saudi Arabia: Canada and Alberta-MENA Trade Relations. Alberta Agriculture, Food and Rural Development, J. G. O'Donoghue Building, 7000 - 113 St. Edmonton AB T6H 5T6 Canada Duke at duke@gov.ab.ca Web Site:
http://www.Agric.gov.ab.ca/marketnews/middle_eas t/trade_relations.html#arabia

17. Canadian Code of Recommended Handling Practices for Frozen Foods", Food Institute of Canada; 350 Sparks St., Suite 605, Ottawa, Ontario K1R 7S1 Webmaster: joy@foodprocessors.ca Web Site: http://foodnet.fic.ca/

18. Canadian Food Safety Adaptation Program (CFSAP-2003); Canadian Food Inspection Agency (CFIA) 59 Camelot Drive, Ottawa, Ontario, K1A 0Y9. E-mail: cfiamaster@inspection.gc.ca Web Site: http://www.agr.gc.ca Tel: (613) 225-2342, Fax: (613) 228-6125 Web Site: http://www.agr.gc.ca/policy/adapt/national_initiativ es/cfsap.phtml

19. Canadian Government Publishing Directorate (2003), Constitution Square Building, 4th Floor, 350 Albert Street, Ottawa, Ontario, and Canada.K1A 1M4 E-mail: copyright.droitdauteur@communication.gc.ca

20. Canadian Research Institute for Food Safety; Officially Opens September 18, 2002. Mansel Griffiths; Director, Canadian Institute for Food Safety Research; Professor, Department of Food Science. Canadian Research Institute for Food Safety University of Guelph, 43 McGilvray St., Guelph, Ontario, Canada N1G 2W1. Telephone: 519-824-

4120 ext. 8010. Fax: 519-763-0952 Email: crifs@uoguelph.ca Web Site: http://www.oac.uoguelph.ca/CRIFS/

21. Caroline Smith DeWaal (1997); "Delivering on HACCP's Promise to Improve Food Safety: A Comparison of Three HACCP Regulations," (1997), Food and Drug Law Journal, Vol. 52, No. 3 (1997), pp. 331-335

22. Caroline Smith DeWaal (1998) Director of Food Safety: A Blueprint For the Future - Institute of Food Technologists Annual Meeting. Center for Science in Public Interest (CSPI), 1875 Connecticut Ave. N.W., Suite 300, Washington, D.C. 20009, Main switchboard: (202) 332-9110 Fax: (202) 265-4954, General e-mail address: cspi@cspinet.org Web Site: http://www.cspinet.org/reports/blueprint.html

23. C. Colatore and J.A. Caswell (1998) The Cost of HACCP Implementation in the Seafood Industry: A Case Study of Breaded Fish; University of Massachusetts Department of Resource Economics Amherst Campus, College of Natural Resources and the Environment, Department of Resource Economics, E-Mail: caswell@resecon.umass.edu. Web Site: http://www.umass.edu/ne165/haccp1998/caswell.html

24. Centers for Epidemiology and Animal Health, USDA: APHIS: VS, attn. NAHMS, 2150 Center Ave., Bldg., B, MS 2E7,Fort Collins, CO 80526-8117, World Wide Web: http://www.aphis.gov/vs/ceah/cahm

25. Charles E. Morris (2000); HACCP Under the Microscope, Joyce Fassl Editor in Chief Food Engineering, 901 S. Bolmar Street, Suite P, West Chester, PA 19382, Tel: 610 436-4220 ext. 19, Fax: 610 436-6277 E-Mail: fasslj@bnp.com Website:http://www.foodengineeringmag.com/articles/2000/1000/0010haccp.htm

26. Chris Gallagher (1996) Odwalla expresses condolences to Denver Family. Odwalla press release, Odwalla Inc., Chris Gallagher, Odwalla, Inc. Odwalla 120 Stone Pine Road, Half Moon Bay, CA 94019, Phone: 650-726-1888, Email: eprice@odwalla.com Tel: (650) 712-5512

27. Cigarette Butt in Loaf; F2 Network, The Sydney Morning Herald, 201 Sussex St Sydney 2000 GPO Box 506 Sydney NSW 2001E-Mail: readerlink@smh.com.au Website: http://newsstore.f2.com.au/apps/browseArchive.ac?sy=smh&cls=3469

28. Citizens Against Lawsuit Abuse (CALA) Web Site: http://www.cala.com/caesar.shtml

29. Clearer Standards Needed For Food Safety Protection; GROWMARK, Inc, 1701 Towanda Avenue Bloomington, Illinois, 61701 Tel: (309) 557-6000 Fax: (309) 829-8532, Web Site: http://www.growmark.com/Room/News/food_safety.htm

30. Code of Practice for the Production and Distribution of Unpasteurized Apple and Other Fruit Juice/Cider in Canada (2000); Recommendations for the Production and Distribution of Juice in Canada Approved June 20, 2001: Mr. Robert Forrest Manager - HORTICULTURE Ontario Ministry of Agriculture, Food and Rural Affairs, 1 Stone Road West 5th Floor NW, Guelph, Ontario N1G 4Y2 Web Site: http://www.cfis.agr.ca

31. Codex Alimentarius, FAO/World Health Organization (WHO). 1997a. Suppl. to Vol. 1B, General requirements (food hygiene) Rome 2nd Ed. (187)

32. Codex Alimentarius in Canada (2003) Web Site: http://www.hc-sc.gc.ca/food-aliment/friia-raaii/ip-pi/codex/e_index.html

33. Codex Committee Report "Report of the 30th session of the Codex Committee on Food Hygiene" Appendix IV FAO/WHO 1997b ALINORM 99/13 Rome

34. Competencies for Bakery Personnel; CDC Web Site: http://cdc.aibonline.org/education/trainingguide/bakcomps.html

35. Consumer Groups to USDA: Don't Feed Irradiated Food to School Children Web Site: http://www.citizen.org/pressroom/release.cfm?ID=1286

36. Consumer Safety behaviours and Safety Concern; Economic Research Service, (2002) Katherine Ralston; USDA Web Site: http://www.ers.usda.gov/Briefing/ConsumerFoodSafety/consumerconcerns/

37. Contributing to the Quality of Canadian Life (2002) P0175E-02 July 2002. Commercial Affairs, Canadian Food Inspection Agency (CFIA); 59 Camelot Drive, Nepean, Ontario, Canada, K1A 0Y9 Web Site: http://www.inspection.gc.ca

38. Covello, V., Sandman, P. and Slovic P. (1988) Risk Communication, Risk Statistics and Risk Comparisons: A Manual for Plant Managers - Chemical Manufacturers Association, Washington, D.C. Peter M. Sandman 59 Ridgeview Rd. Princeton NJ 08540-7601 Phone: 1-609-683-4073 Fax: 1-609-683-0566 Email: peter@psandman.com

39. Covello, V.T. and Merkhofer, M.W. 1994. Risk Assessment Methods; Approaches for Assessing Health and Environmental Risks", Plenum Press, New York. 319 pp. NY 1993

40. Critical Controls for Juice Safety; Carol Lewis (1999) Publication No. (FDA) 99-2324- U. S. Food and Drug Administration-Web Site: http://www.cfsan.fda.gov/~dms/fdjuice.html

41. Critical Steps Toward Safer Seafood; Paula Kurtzweil (1999) - Publication No. (FDA) 99-2317; U. S. Food and Drug Administration FDA Consumer. Web Site: http://www.cfsan.fda.gov/~dms/fdsafe3.html

42. Cost of Johne's disease; Dairy '96 Study, National Animal Health Monitoring System (NAHMS) US Department of Agriculture-Animal (USDA) and Plant Health Inspection Service-Veterinary Services, Centers for Epidemiology and Animal Health, Ft. Collins, Colorado and Robbinsville, NJ, USA. E-Mail: NAHMSweb@aphis.usda.gov.

43. Council for Agricultural Science and Technology (CAST), Food borne Pathogens: Risks and Consequences (Ames, IA: CAST, 1994), p. 1.

44. Cross Contamination (2000); Tel: 1-800-444-4094 E-Mail: Nicole@allergicchild.com Subject Web Site: http://www.allergicchild.com/cross_contamination.ht m

D

45. Dairy Food Safety; UC Davis School of Veterinary Medicine (UCDAVIS), School of Veterinary Medicine, Office of the Dean, University of California One Shields Avenue, Davis, CA 95616E-Mail:webmaster@vmtrc.ucdavis.edu Web Site: http://www.vmtrc.ucdavis.edu/dfs/dfs.html

46. Dairy Program (2000); P0179E-00 July 2000. Food Inspection Agency (CFIA); 59 Camelot Drive, Nepean, Ontario, Canada, K1A 0Y9 Web Site: http://www.inspection.gc.ca

47. Dairy Quality & Safety From Farm to Refrigerator; Dairy Food Safety Controls; National Dairy Council, 10255 W. Higgins Rd., Suite 900, Rosemont, IL 60018 Web Site: http://www.nationaldairycouncil.org/about_us.htm

48. Dave Martin (2002): Government Proposes to Expand Food Irradiation; Nuclear Campaign - Sierra Club of Canada. E-mail: nucaware@web.ca Web site: www.sierraclub.ca/national

49. Dealing With HACCP Criticism: University of Washington Box 357234, Seattle, Washington USA 98195-7234, Phone (206) 543-3199 Fax (206) 543-9616 E-mail ehadmin@u.washington.edu Web Site: http://depts.washington.edu/foodrisk/problem.html

50. Department of Health and Human Services, Office of the Inspector General, FDA Food Safety Inspection, August 1991.

51. Description Of The U.S. Food Safety System; FSIS U.S. Codex Office, Room 4861, South Building, Washington, DC 20250-3700, Web Site: http://www.fsis.usda.gov/OA/codex/system.htm

51A. Dr. Douglas Powell (1998) Risk-Based Regulatory Responses in Global Food Trade: Guatemalan Raspberry Imports Into the U.S. and Canada, 1996-1998. Dept. Plant Agriculture, University of Guelph, Ont. N1G 2W1 Tel: 519-824-4120 x2506 E-Mail:

dpowell@uoguelph.ca   Subject   Website: http://www.foodsafetynetwork.ca/food/cyclospora-ppr.htm

51B. Dr. Douglas Powell (1998) Setting the stage: understanding communication issues with Food borne pathogens Dept. Food Science, University of Guelph, Guelph, Ont. N1G 2W1, Tel: 519-824-4120, ext. 2506, Fax: 519-763-8933. Website: http://www.foodsafetynetwork.ca/risk/oca-talk/oca-talk.htm

51C. Dr. Douglas Powell (1998) Impacts of Biotechnology, Environment, Food Safety: Communications. A Presentation Prepared for the Agriculture Risk Management Conference, October 28-29, 1998, Holiday Inn, Plaza la Chaudière, Hull, QC Dept. Plant Agriculture, University of Guelph, Ont. N1G 2W1 Tel: 519-824-4120 x2506

52. Dr. Douglas Powell (1999); On-Farm Food Safety Program Ontario Vegetable Growers' Marketing Board-Assistant Professor Dept. Plant Agriculture, University of Guelph, Guelph, ON N1G 2W1 Tel: 519-821-1799, fax: 519-824-6631, e-mail: dpowell@uoguelph.ca.

53. Dr. Douglas Powell (1999); Food Safety Guidelines For Greenhouse Vegetables; Ontario Greenhouse Vegetable Growers Association assistant professor, Dept. Plant Agriculture, Mauricio Bobadilla Ruiz and Amanda Whitfield, graduate students, Dept. Food Science, University of Guelph, Ont., N1G 2W1 Tel: 519-821-1799, fax: 519-763-8933, e-mail: dpowell@uoguelph.ca; Web Site: http://www.foodsafetynetwork.ca/food/ogvga/report.htm

E

54. *E. coli* O157:H7 Outbreak Associated with Odwalla Brand Apple Juice Products," HHS News, P96-17, Oct. 31, 1996;

54A. Economics of food borne disease (2001); Economic Research Service; United States Department of Agriculture: Web Site: http://www.ers.usda.gov/briefing/Food-borne Disease/

55. Egg Usages in the Irish Hotel, Restaurant and Commercial Catering Industry (1999); Food Safety Authority of Ireland. Web Site: http://www.fsai.ie/industry/egg_usage/egg_survey.htm

56. Elizabeth Dahl and Caroline Smith DeWaal (1997), Scrambled Eggs: How A Broken Food Safety System Let Contaminated Eggs Become a National Food Poisoning Epidemic; Elizabeth Dahl Staff Attorney, Food Safety Program, Caroline Smith DeWaal Director, Food Safety Program, Center for Science in the Public Interest, 1875 Connecticut Avenue, NW, Suite 300 Washington, D.C. 20009-5728, Tel: (202) 332-9110, p. 11. General e-mail address: cspi@cspinet.org

57. Ensuring Safe Food — A HACCP-Based Plan for Ensuring Food Safety in Retail Establishments; Bulletin 901, Chapter 6 The Seven HACCP Principles; The Ohio State University, Food Science and Technology 2015 Fyffe Road, Columbus, OH 43210-1007 Web Site: http://ohioline.osu.edu/b901/chapter_6.html

58. Ensuring a Safe Food Supply for Manitobans (1999); Manitoba Agriculture and Food, Home Economics Section, 915 - 401 York Avenue, Winnipeg MB, R3C 0P8. Web Site: http://www.gov.mb.ca/Agriculture/homeec/cbe01s01.html

59. Ensuring Safe Food — A HACCP-Based Plan for Ensuring Food Safety in Retail Establishments; Bulletin 901; Chapter 2 — HACCP and Retail Food Operations, Ohio State University; Food Science and Technology 2015 Fyffe Road, Columbus, OH 43210-1007. Web Site: http://ohioline.osu.edu/

60. Epidemiologic Notes and Reports Lead Poisoning Following Ingestion of Homemade Beverage Stored in a Ceramic Jug -- New York. CDC Web Site: http://www.cdc.gov/mmwr/preview/mmwrhtml/00001401.htm

61. Establishing Preventive Measures With Critical Limits For Each Control Point; Auditing Tip of the Month July (1999). GMP Institute, A Division of ISPE3109 West Dr, Martin Luther King, Jr Blvd Suite,

250 Tampa, FL 33607. Web Site: http://www.gmp1st.com/autp/autp0799.htm

62. Nancy Boomer (1997) Ethanol Co-product Utilization-Food, Mohawk Debuts High-Fibre Food Ingredients, Internet Information Services for Canadian Agriculture and Bioenergy Technology. Web Site: http://members.shaw.ca/bethcandlish/etoh1.htm

63. EU Sets Up New Food Safety Body (2002); News Center, International Dairy Foods Association (IDFA) 1250-H street, NW Suite 900, Washington DC 20005, P: 202.737.4332 – F: 202.331.7820. Web Site: www.idfa.orghttp://www.idfa.org/news/stories/intlhap/02-02.cfm

F

64. Facility Compliance Requirements (2002) Fish Inspection Regulations, Schedules I and II. Canadian Food Inspection Agency (CFIA); 174 Stone Road West, Guelph, Ontario, N1G 4S9 Web Site: http://www.inspection.gc.ca

65. Facilitate record keeping with recordHACCP^{TM} Jean Allen; CIBUS Consulting, PO Box 501 1095 O'Connor Drive, Toronto, ON M4B 3M9. Web Site: http://www.norbackley.com/record_keeping_frame.htm

66. Facilities Inspection Manual; QMP Reference Standard and Compliance Guidelines. Canadian Food Inspection Agency Animal Products Directorate, Fish, Seafood and Production. Web Site: http://www.inspection.gc.ca

67. Facts about Juice Safety (2003); The National Food Processors Association Web Site: http://www.nfpa-food.org/pubpolicy/juice_facts.htm

68. Fact Sheet (2001) PO174E-01 - May 2001 The Canadian Food Safety System; Canadian Food Inspection Agency (CFIA), 59 Camelot Drive, Nepean, Ontario, Canada, K1A 0Y9. Web Site: http://www.inspection.gc.ca Tel: (613) 225-2342, CFIA Media Relations: Tel: (613) 228-6682

69. FAO/WHO/General Agreement on Tariffs and Trade (GATT) 1991 FAO/WHO Conference on Food

Standards, Chemicals in Food and Food Trade, Vol. 1, Report. Rome, 18-27 March 1991. Rome.

70. Fast food firms responsible for obesity. Bell Globe Media Inc. Updated Sat. Mar. 30 2002 11:56 AM ET Web Site: http://www.ctv.ca/servlet/ArticleNews/story/CTVNew s/20020330/ctvnews854709/

71. FDA Announces Pilot Food Safety Program For Retail Settings (1998); Press Office Food and Drug Administration, U.S. Department of Health and Human Services. Web Site: http://vm.cfsan.fda.gov/~lrd/hhsfsret.html

72. FDA Proposal on Safety of Juices; HHS press release, 4/21/98
US Apple document, 5/26/98.Christina Stark, M.S., R.D.
Nutrition Specialist, Cornell Cooperative Extension. E-mail:cms11@cornell.edu Web Site: http://www.cce.cornell.edu/food/fsarchives/050698/f dajuices.html

73. FDA still studying raw milk cheese (2003); Web Site: http://www.foodengineeringmag.com/articles/2001/ 0901/0901mfgnews.htm

74. Fischoff, B. and Downs, J.S. (1997) Communicating food borne disease risk. Emerging Infectious Diseases, Volume: 3, No: 4 Carnegie Mellon University, Pittsburgh, Pennsylvania, USA. Emerging Infectious Diseases, National Center for Infectious Diseases, Centers for Disease Control and Prevention Atlanta, GA

75. Fish Inspection Regulations Amended to Update Quality Management Program (1999); Cameron Prince Canadian Food Inspection Agency, 59 Camelot Drive, Nepean, Ontario, K1A 0Y9 Canada

76. Food and Beverage Industry Distribution Channels Study: Opportunities for Canadian Companies in the Southwest U.S.; Prepared for the Canadian Consulate General in Dallas by Economic Development Services Irving, Texas March 1997 update to the October 1995 study. Web Site: http://atn-riae.agr.ca/info/us/e0078.htm

77. Food borne Illness: Implications for the Future. Emerging Infectious Diseases, Richard L. Hall (1999) National Center for Infectious Diseases. Centers for Disease Control and Prevention, Atlanta, GA.

78. Food Distribution System in Gulf Cooperation Council (GCC) Countries, Wissem Ben-Marzouk, Research Assistant, European and Emerging Market Team, Alberta Economic Development, Phone: (780) 422-7887 E-mail: Wissem.Ben-Marzouk@gov.ab.ca

79. Food Poisoning Outbreaks in Secondary School; Web Site:http://www.soceh.org.sg/publication_food.html

80. Food Safety and Quality: Salmonella Control Efforts Show Need for More Coordination U.S. General Accounting Office (GAO), (Washington, D.C.: GAO, April 1992) [hereinafter cited as Salmonella Control Efforts]; Food Safety and Inspection Service (FSIS), USDA

81. Food Safeties and Inspection Service (FSIS), United States Department of Agriculture, Washington, D.C. 20250-3700. Web Site:http://www.fsis.usda.gov

82. Food safety and product liability; Jean C. Buzby and Paul Frenzen (1999); In Food Policy Volume 24, Issue 6 December 1999 Pages 637-651 Oxford, U.K.: Elsevier Science Ltd. Web Site: http://www.ers.usda.gov/briefing/IndustryFoodSafet y/pdfs/liability.htm

83. Food Safety, HACCP, And Future Regulation (2000) Office of the Under Secretary for Food Safety, U.S. Department of Agriculture Food Safety and Inspection Service, United States Department of Agriculture, Washington, D.C. 20250-3700. Web Site:http://www.fsis.usda.gov/oa/speeches/2000/c w_rfa.htm

84. Food Safety (2003), Agri Food Trade Service Web Site:http://atn-riae.agr.ca/safety/food-e.htm

85. Food Safety From Farm To Table: A National Food Safety Initiative. A Report to the President, May 1997, Appendix B

86. Food Safety Enhancement Program (FSEP-2000) Canadian Food Inspection Agency (CFIA), Commercial Affairs, Canadian Food Inspection

Agency, 59 Camelot Drive, Nepean, Ontario, Canada, K1A 0Y9. Web Site: http://www.inspection.gc.ca FSEP homepage: http://www.cfiaacia.agr.ca Toll-Free: 1-800-442-2342, Tel: (613) 225-2342, Fax: (613) 228-6634

87. Food Safety From Farm to Table, pp. 3, 39; National Marine Fisheries Service, National Oceanic and Atmospheric Administration, Department of Commerce

88. Food Safety From Farm to Table, p. 37; FSIS, USDA, "Pathogen Reduction; Hazard Analysis and Critical Control Point (HACCP) Systems; Proposed Rule," *Federal Register*, Vol. 60, No. 23 (1995), p. 6780.

89. Food safety related actions, Web Site: http://www.bigclassaction.com/class_action/complaint_form_capers.html

90. Food Science & Technology; Research Strengths of the Food Science and Technology Group, Department of Agricultural, Food and Nutritional Science, 1-18 Agriculture/Forestry Centre, University of Alberta, Edmonton, Alberta, Canada T6G-2P5. Web Site: http://www.afns.ualberta.ca/Teaching_Research/food_science.asp

91. Food technologies and public health: food safety issues. WHO. (1995), Geneva, Switzerland

92. FS_ANNOUNCE CHINESE BAKERY SOURCE OF SALMONELLA POISONING; Sun, 10 Dec 2000 20:29:33 −0500 Web Site: http://www.freedomsite.org/pipermail/fs_announce/2000/000290.html

94. FSNET October 26, 1998 − II, Dr. Douglas Powell, dept. of plant Agriculture University of Guelph, Guelph, Ont., N1G 2W1, Tel: 519-824-4120 x2506, fax: 519-763-8933 E-Mail: dpowell@uoguelph.ca Web Site: http://131.104.232.9/fsnet/1998/10-1998/fs-10-26-98-02.txt

94. Frank F. Busta (2000); Evolution and Current Trends in HACCP and Risk Assessment; ABSTRACT Dr. Richard S. Johnston IIFET 2000 Conference Organizer, 213 Ballard Extension Hall, Dept. of Agricultural and Resource Economics Oregon State University, Corvallis OR 97331-

3601USA. Phone: 1 541 737 1427 Fax: 1 541 737 2563 Website: richard.s.johnston@oregonstate.edu Subject Web Site:http://oregonstate.edu/dept/IIFET/2000/abstracts/busta.html

95. Fred W. Leak (1996) HACCP: Hazard Analysis Critical Control Points; Animal Science Department; University of Florida; Gainesville, Florida.

96. FSIS Eliminates Requirements for Partial Quality Control Programs; Organic Consumers Association. Web Site: http://www.organicconsumers.org/irrad/pqc.cfm

97. Future Direction for HACCP Web Site: www.cdc.gov/od/oc/media/pressrel/r990917.htm

G

98. General Food Safety Daily News, This site is designed for fast and simple food safety communications. Web Site http://www.foodhaccp.com/0503.htmlE-Mail: (Online)

99. G. M. Jones (199); Proper Dry Cow Management Critical for Mastitis Control; Professor Of Dairy Science, Extension Dairy Scientist, Milk Quality and Milking Management, Virginia Tech Publication Number 404-212, posted May 1999 Web Site: http://www.ext.vt.edu/pubs/dairy/404-212/404-212.html

100. GMP / HACCP Good Manufacturing Practices (GMP) And Hazard Analysis Critical Control Points (HACCP); WebSite:http://www.panalimentos.org/Panalimentos_ing/haccp2/GUIA9.htm

101. Good Transportation Practices Code (2001) Web Site:http://www.cfis.agr.ca/english/cnsltdoc/gtp2001jan-e.htm

102. Government Response to the Fourteenth Report of the Standing Committee on Public Accounts (2002); Canadian Food Inspection Agency (CFIA), 59 Camelot Drive, Ottawa, Ontario K1A 0Y9 Web Site: http://www.inspection.gc.ca

103. Guide to Food Labelling and Advertising; Canadian Food Inspection Agency; Section I: Introduction

Sections 1.1 to 1.4 Web Site: http://www.inspection.gc.ca/english/bureau/labeti/guide/1-0-0e.shtml

H

104. HACCP and Meat Safety Quality Assurance (MSQA) 2001Meat & Livestock Australia, 1401 K Street NW, Suite 602,Washington, D.C   20005. Web Site: http://www.australianmeatsafety.com/haccp-msqa.html

105. HACCP: A State-of-the-Art Approach to Food Safety; BG   01-4;   USFDA   Website: http://www.fda.gov/opacom/backgrounders/haccp.html

106. HACCP Based Inspection Models Project United States Department of Agriculture, Food Safety and Inspection Service, Office of Policy, Program Development and Evaluation, Web Site: http://www.fsis.usda.gov

107. HACCP Curriculum Guidelines; Food Safety Enhancement Program, The Canadian Food Inspection Agency (CFIA). Commercial Affairs, Canadian Food Inspection Agency, 59 Camelot Drive, Nepean, Ontario, Canada, K1A 0Y9. Web Site: http://www.cfia-acia.agr.ca

108. HACCP Plan Requirements and Meat and Poultry Product Processing Categories; Policy Clarification; Food Safety and Inspection Service. Web Site: http://www.fsis.usda.gov/OPPDE/rdad/FRPubs/98-006N.htm

109. HACCP Overview: Hazard Analysis & Critical Control Point (1996); Guelph Food Technology Centre: 88 McGilvray Street, Guelph, Ontario, N1G 2W1, Canada

110. HACCP Software; Web Site: http://www.arrowscientific.com.au/dohaccp_sw.html

111. HAZARD ANALYSIS CRITICAL CONTROL POINT (HACCP): FROM THE FARM TO THE FORK; Web Site: http://www.camib.com/camib/publications/haccp.htm

112. Hance, B.J., Chess, C. and Sandman, P.M. 1988. Improving dialogue with communities: A Risk Communication Manual for Government.

Environmental Communication Research Program, Rutgers University, New Brunswick, NJ 83 pp.

113. Health Advisories/Press Releases (2001): CFIA safety alert on mini cup jelly products - choking hazard Michael Hiscock (English) Canadian Food Inspection Agency, Office of Food Safety and Recall. CFIA web site at: http://www.inspection.gc.ca. Tel: 613) 755-3324

114. Health Guidelines: Peace Country Health, Corporate Office, Health Region 8, Provincial Building, 2101 10320 - 99th Street, Grande Prairie, Alberta T8V 6J4, Phone: 1-800-732-8981 or (780) 538-5387, Fax: (780) 538-5455 COMMUNICATIONS, Vicki Swan, Communications Director Phone: (780) 538-6181 E-Mail: vswan@mhr.ab.ca Web Site: www.mhr.ab.ca/Inspect/Water

115. Helen H. Jensen (1998); HACCP in Pork Processing; Costs and Benefits: (Iowa State University) and Laurian J. Unnevehr (University of Illinois): Web Site:http://www.umass.edu/ne165/haccp1998/jensen.html

116. Hepatitis A Outbreak In Michigan Schools, USDA Release No. 0100.97, April 2, 1997; Barbara Mahon et al.,

117. High-efficient dough cooling system during mixing; Contact: loesche@ttz-bremerhaven.de

118. Hofmann, J., Liu, Z., Genese, C., Wolf, G., Manley, W., Pilot, K., Dalley, E., Finelli, and L. 1996 Update: Outbreaks of Cyclospora cayetanensis infection — United States and Canada, 1996. CDC MMWR 611 Vol. 45 / No. 28

I

119. IAMFES, Procedures to Implement the HACCP System, 1991, Ames, Iowa 50010-6666, U.S.A.

120. Irradiation in the Production, Processing, and Handling of Food; FDA Final Rules, *Federal* Register, Vol. 62, No. 232 (1997), pp. 64102-64121; (60)

J

121. Jack Guzewich & Marianne P. Ross (1999); Evaluation of Risks Related to Microbiological

Contamination of Ready-to-eat Food-by-Food Preparation Workers and the Effectiveness of Interventions to Minimize Those Risks; Food and Drug Administration, Center for Food Safety and Applied Nutrition. Web Site: http://vm.cfsan.fda.gov/~ear/rterisk.html

122. James C. Cato (1998); Visiting Scientist (Economics) Estimates of HACCP Implementation Costs FAO Fisheries Technical Paper – 381; Food and Agricultural Organization of The United Nations; Fish Utilization and Marketing Service Fishery Industries, Division FAO Fisheries Department, Rome, 1998. Web Site; http://www.fao.org/DOCREP/003/X0465E/X0465E00.HTM#Contents

123. James C. Cato (1998) Practical Approaches to Valuing Seafood Safety. Seafood Safety - Economics of Hazard Analysis and Critical Control Point (HACCP) programmes; FAO FISHERIES TECHNICAL PAPER – 381 FOOD AND AGRICULTURE ORGANIZATION OF THE UNITED NATIONS; Fish Utilization and Marketing Service Fishery Industries Division FAO Fisheries Department Rome, 1998 Web Site: http://www.fao.org/DOCREP/003/X0465E/X0465E06.htm

124. Jeff Chilton (1998); HACCP Principles 2-6, Reality of Record Keeping; Chilton Consulting Group, P. O. Box 129, Rocky Face, Georgia 30740, Office Phone (706) 694-8325, Cell Phone (706) 264-1054, Fax:(706) 694-8316; Web Site: http://www.chiltonconsulting.com/mpfeb98.htm

125. J. E. Hobbs, A. Fearne and J. Spriggs, (2002); Incentive Structures for Food Safety and Quality Assurance: An International Comparison," Food Control 13, 77-81, University of Saskatchewan, Canada; A. Fearne, Wye College, University of London, UK; and J. Spriggs, Charles Sturt University, Australia

126. Jensen, Helen H., Tanya Roberts, Laurian Unnevehr, & Shannon Hamm 1995 Setting priorities in food-borne pathogen data: public and private response. *In* Julie A Caswell, Ed *The economics of reducing health risk from food, proceedings of NE-165 conference,*

pp. 47-53. Storrs, University of Connecticut, Food Marketing Policy Center

127. J. M. Juran and F. M. Gryna (1993); Quality Planning and Analysis, 3rd ed. p12 McGraw Hill: New York.

128. John M. Antle (2002) The Cost of Quality in the Meat Industry: Implications for HACCP Regulation; Professor of Agricultural Economics and Economics, Montana State University. Web Site: http://www.umass.edu/ne165/haccp1998/antle.html

129. J. R. Skees, A. Botts, and K. Zeuli () "The Potential for Recall Insurance to Improve Food Safety," Department of Agricultural Economics, 310 CEB Building, University of Kentucky, Lexington, Kentucky 40546-0215 USA E-Mail: jskees@uky.edu Web Site: www.globalAgrisk.com Subject Web Site: http://www.uky.edu/Ag/AgEcon/skeesvita.pdf

130. Juice Safety Debate; Journal of American Medical Association Reports Unpasteurized Juices Caused Illnesses at Disney World: Article Endorsed by the Center for Disease Control and Prevention. National Food Processors Association, The Food Safety People, 1350 I Street, NW Suite 300, Washington, DC 20005, Phone 202.639.5900E-Mail: nfpa@nfpa-food.org Web Site: http://www.nfpafood.org/pubpolicy/juice_jama.htm

131. Julien Destorel (2001); Quarterly Agri-Food Trade Highlights; Fourth Quarter 2001, Agriculture and Agri-Food Canada Web Site: http://www.agr.gc.ca/policy/epad/english/pubs/qrthigh/2001/4quart01.htm

K

132. Kevin T. Higgins (2001) How Emmpak Manages HACCP: Kevin T. Higgins is Senior Editor of Food Engineering Magazine Contact RSi-Copyright Customer Support: support@rsicopyright.com 800-217-7874 web Site; http://www.foodengineeringmag.com/CDA/ArticleInformation/coverstory/BNPCoverStoryItem/0,6326,95003,00.html

133. Kevin T. Higgins (2002), The Culture of clean (2002), there is no shortage of sanitation tools to keep food plants safe. Web Site:

http://www.dairyfoods.com/articles/2002/1102/PO_Culture_of_Clean.htm

134. Key Facts: Economic Impact Analysis (1996) Food Safety and Inspection Service United States Department of Agriculture Washington, D.C. 20250-3700

135. Kimberlee J. Burrington (1998); Prolonging Bakery Product Life; 3400 Dundee Rd. Suite #100, Northbrook, IL 60062 Website: www.foodproductdesign.com

136. Kim, Dong-Kyoon and Wen S. Chern. 1995. Health Risk Concern of Households vs. Food Processors: Estimation of Hedonic Prices in Fats and Oils. In Valuing Food Safety and Nutrition, ed. NE-165 PROJECT PROPOSAL Julie A. Caswell, 155-172 Boulder, CO: Westview Press, Inc. Kinnucan, Henry W., Stanley Thompson, and Hui-Shung Chang. 1992. Commodity Advertising and Promotion. Ames, IA: Iowa State University. University of Massachusetts Amherst, Massachusetts, 01003 Tel: (413) 545-0111 E-Mail: caswell@resecon.umass.edu

L

137. Lawsuit filed in pasta poisoning case (2002) http://cbc.ca/stories/2002/05/30/Consumers/Shigellasuit_020530

138. Layoff, G. and Johnson, M. 1980 Metaphors We Live By. University of Chicago Press Chicago

139. Location of Food Mishandling (1994) Centers For Disease Control Centers For Disease Control, U.S. Department of Health and Human Services, Atlanta GA.

140. Louis Carson and Philip Spiller; (1998) Remarks & comments-Food Regulatory Update; Food and Drug Administration, at Food Regulatory Update '98, Food and Drug Law Institute, Washington, D.C.

141. Lynn Knipe (1999) Listeria Control and Your HACCP Plan. Web Site:http://www.ag.ohio-state.edu/~meatsci/listeriahaccp.htm

M

142. Marriott, N.G., Principles of Food Plant Sanitation, 1989, Van Nostrand Rheinhold, New York, N.Y., U.S.A.

143. Masters, B.A. 1997. Tainted basil shows the challenges of tracking a microbe. Washington Post July 28, B1

144. Making the most of HACCP; Learning from others' experience; Woodhead Publishing Limited, Woodhead Publishing Ltd, Abington Hall Abington Cambridge, CB1 6AH, UK.

145. M.C. van der Haven, B.A. Slaghuis (2003); Hygiene protocols for pathogens in farmhouse dairy products Practical Scientific Report 22, P.O. Box 2176, NL-8203 AD Lelystad, Netherlands, E-mail: info@pv.agro.nl Web Site; www.pv.wur.nl
Subject Web Site: http://www.pv.wageningen-ur.nl/index.asp?english/products/books/praktijkrapp ort/rsp/22.asp

146. Mel Coleman (1999); An interview; A Cowboy in the Meat Business; Mel Coleman, Sr. Colorado In Motion Magazine, Rural America. Sr. and Photo Series by Nic Paget-Clarke Denver and Saguache, Colorado Web Site:http://www.inmotionmagazine.com/coleman.ht ml

147. Michael F. Jacobson, Ph.D.; executive director (2001); Does the Fragmented Structure Really Make Sense?" Federal Food Safety Oversight Center for Science in the Public Interest (CSPI), Washington, D.C. Web Site: http://www.cspinet.org/foodsafety/food_contaminati on.html

148. Michael Taylor, (1995); Privatization of In-plant Seafood Inspections and Related Services; Notice of Inquiry, *Federal Register*, Vol. 60, No. 184 (1995), pp. 49242-49245.

149. Mickey Parish (1998); *Escherichia coli* and *Salmonella Serovars* Associated with a Citrus-Processing Facility Implicated in a Salmonellosis Outbreak, Coliforms, Journal of Food Protection, Vol. 61, No. 3 (1998), pp. 280-284.

150. Milk Protein Concentrate; c/o Canadian Dairy Commission, MILKINGREDIENTS.CA, Building 55,

NCC Driveway, Central Experimental Farm, 960 Carling Avenue, Ottawa ON K1A 0Z2 Web Site: http://www.milkingredients.ca

151. Modernized Poultry Inspection Project: A Science-Based Evolution (1997) Canadian Food Inspection Agency (CFIA). Web Site: http://www.inspection.qc.ca

152. Modern Meat; Web Site: http://www.pbs.org/wgbh/pages/frontline/shows/me at/evaluating/haccp.html

153. Multispectral Imaging in Food and Agriculture; Contents of this website   Is Copyright © 2000-1990 Duncan Technologies, Inc. Duncan Tech, 11824 Kemper Rd., Auburn, CA 95603,Phone: (530)-888-6565,Fax: (530)-888-6579,   Email: info@duncantech.com,   Web   Site: http://www.duncantech.com/AG_applications.htm

N

154. Nationwide Broiler Chicken Microbiological Baseline Data Collection Program, July 1994-June 1995 (Washington, D.C.: USDA, April 1996).

155. Nelkin, D. (1987) Selling Science: How the Press Covers Science and Technology. W.H. Freeman and Company. New York. 224 pp.

156. New Federal Initiative Will Enhance Canada's Food Safety System (2003); Contact: Frank Massong, Canadian Food Inspection Agency, Ottawa Web Site: http://www.agr.gc.ca/cb/news/2000/n00925ae.html

O

157. Outbreaks of Escherichia _coli_ O157:H7 Infection Associated with Eating Alfalfa Sprouts -- Michigan and Virginia, June-July 1997," Morbidity and Mortality Weekly Report, Vol. 46, No. 32 (1997), pp. 741-744.

158. On Farm Food Safety Program (2003); The Canadian Turkey Marketing Agency 969 Derry Road East, Unit 102 Mississauga, Ontario, L5T 2J7 Web Site: http://www.albertaturkey.com

P

159. Pam Belluck and Christopher Drew (19980; Tracing

Bout of Illness to Small Lettuce Farm, New York Times, Jan. 5, 1998, p. A1; HHS

160. Pam Erickson (1992); A HACCP Primer; Weeks Publishing Company, 3400 Dundee Rd. Suite #100, Northbrook, IL 60062, Phone: 847-559-0385, Fax: 847-559-0389, E-Mail: info@foodproductdesign.com, Website: www.foodproductdesign.com Web Site: http://www.foodproductdesign.com/archive/1992/10 92PE.html

161. Plant Inspectors Hit the Field on FDA Juice HACCP, Biosecurity (2002) Web Site: http://www.idfa.org/news/stories/2002/11/juicehacc p.cfm

162. Possible future Codex regulations (1999); Codex Alimentarius & HACCP E-Mail: Sqeditor@aol.com Web Site: http://www.supplementquality.com/stdregs/futureco dex.html

163. Powell, D.A. and Leiss, W. (1997) Mad Cows and Mother's Milk: The perils of Poor Risk Communication. McGill-Queen's University Press Montreal 308 pp

164. Preparing for the Twenty-First Century, p. 18; Food Safety From Farm to Table, p. 37. Cebter for Science in the Public Interest (CSPI), Center for Science in the Public Interest, 1875 Connecticut Ave. N.W., Suite 300, Washington, D.C. 20009, Main switchboard: (202) 332-9110, Fax: (202) 265-4954, General e-mail address: cspi@cspinet.org, Web Site: http://www.cspinet.org/reports/24

165. President's Council on Food Safety (1999) August 1998 under E.O. 13100, An Introduction; Food Safety from Farm to Table: A National Food-Safety Initiative. Steve Teasley; United States Department of Agriculture (USDA) and Health and Human Services (HHS) E-Mail: steasley@usda.gov. Web Site: http://www.foodsafety.gov/~fsg/cwelcome.html

166. Prevention of Vibrio vulnificus Infections," Eric Mouzin, et al., Journal of the American Medical Association, Vol. 278, No. 7 (1997), pp. 576-578; CDC.

167. Preparing America's Food Safety System for the Twenty-First Century -- Who is Responsible for What When it comes to Meeting the Food Safety Challenges of the Consumer-Driven Global Economy? *"Food and Drug Law Journal,* Vol. 52, No. 1 (1997), p. 18.

168. Procedures for the Safe and Sanitary Processing and Importing of Fish and Fishery Products; Final Rule, Food and Drug Administration (FDA), HHS," Federal Register, Vol. 60, No. 242 (1995), pp. 65096-65202; FSIS, USDA, "Pathogen Reduction; Hazard Analysis and Critical Control Point (HACCP) Systems; Final Rule," *Federal Register,* Vol. 61, No. 144 (1996), pp. 38806-38989.

169. Progress Report on Salmonella Testing of Raw Meat and Poultry Products, Code "A" sample 1998-2001; Food Safety and Inspection Services, U.S. Department of Agriculture, Washington, DC 20250-3700 Web Site: http://www.fsis.usda.gov/OPHS/haccp/salm4year.htm

170. Purpose of On-Farm Food Safety Programs (2002) Ministry of Agriculture and Food Government of Ontario-Canada Web Site: http://www.gov.on.ca/OMAFRA/english/crops/radio/food/radio_foodpro_0102.htm

Q

171. Quality Eggs for Volume Buyers (1996)- Brochure No AMS-6277 C.F.R. § 59.28; Poultry Division, AMS, USDA, August 1996

172. Quality Management Program (2003); Animal Products Directorate, Fish, Seafood and Production Canadian Food Inspection Agency

(CFIA); 174 Stone Road West, Guelph, Ontario, N1G 4S9 Web Site: http://www.inspection.gc.ca

R

173. Randell, A. (1995); 1995 Codex Alimentarius how it all began. Food Nutr. Agric., 13/14: 35-40.

174. Recall background and definition; U.S. Food and Drug Administration Food Safety and Inspection Service, Regulations and Directives Development

Staff, Telephone: 202-720-5627,Fax: 202-690-0486, E-Mail: FSIS.Regulations@fsis.usda.gov Web Site: http://www.fda.gov/oc/po/firmrecalls/recall_defin.html

175. Recommendations for the Production and Distribution of Juice in Canada; (2001) CFIS; Web Site: http://www.cfis.agr.ca/english/regcode/hrt/juc_e.htm

176. Red Meat Industry major Accomplishment (2001) Web Site: http://www.cmccvc.com/docs/about/majoracc2001.htm

177. Regulation 593/99 (1999), To Amend Ontario Regulations 403/97 Made Under The Building Code Act, 1992 Ministry of Municipal Affairs and Housing Ontario. Web Site: http://obc.mah.gov.on.ca/New/Oreg593-1999.html

178. Report of the WHO Commission on Health and Environment WHO (1992) our planet, our health Geneva, Switzerland

179. Richard B. Belzer, Ph.D. (2000) Senior Economist Office of Information and Regulatory Affairs, Office of Management and Budget, NEOB Room 10202 Washington, DC 20503

180. Richard Durbin; (1999); Senator – United States Congress, Statement on the Introduction of the Safe Food Act. Web Site: http://www.senate.gov/~durbin/Legislation/s1281.htm

181. Richard Zurbrigg; Director-Fish, Seafood and Production Division Facilities Inspection Manual (2002); Web Site: http://www.inspection.gc.ca/english/anima/fispoi/manman/fimmii/bull24e.shtml

182. Risk Communication and Government; Theory and Application for the Canadian Food Inspection Agency; Website: http://www.inspection.gc.ca/english/corpaffr/publications/riscomm/riscomme.shtml

183. Roberts, Tanya & Suzanne Marks. 1995. Valuation by the cost of illness method: the social costs of *Escherichia coli* O157:H7 food-borne disease. *In.* Julie A. Caswell, ed. *Valuing food safety and nutrition*, pp. 173-206. Boulder, Colorado, Westview Press. NE-165 PROJECT PROPOSAL; Iowa State University. University of Massachusetts Amherst, Massachusetts, 01003. Tel: (413) 545-0111 E-Mail: caswell@resecon.umass.edu

184. Role of food safety in health and development WHO (1984), Report of a Joint FAO/WHO Expert Committee on Food Safety WHO Technical Report Series No. 705 Geneva, Switzerland

185. Role Of Ministry Of Agriculture, Forestry And Fisheries-Japan Web Site: http://www.maff.go.jp/ROLE.html

186. Ronald Pilchik Mocon (2001); HACCP and Its Implications For Sterile Medical Device Packaging, Minneapolis, Minnesota, USA; © Copyright 2001 Advanstar Communications Inc. Corporate Office Advanstar, Inc. 545 Boylston Street Boston, MA 02116 Tel: 617-267-6500, 617-267-6900 E-Mail: info@advanstar.com Web Site: http://www.advanstar.com/ Subject Web Site:

http://www.medicaldevicesonline.com/features/story .epml?features.REF=45

187. Rosanna Mentzer Morrison, Jean Buzby, and C. T. Jordan Lin (1997); Irradiating Ground Beef to Enhance Food Safety, Food Review, Vol. 20, No. 1 (1997), p. 34; FDA, HHS.

S

188. Sandman, P.M. 1987. Risk communication: facing public outrage. EPA Journal 13: 21 Peter M. Sandman, 59 Ridgeview Rd., Princeton NJ 08540-7601, Phone: 1-609-683-4073, Fax: 1-609-683-0566, E-Mail: peter@psandman.com

189. Seafood HACCP Regulation; PART 123--Fish and Fishery Products; U.S. Food & Drug Administration, enter for Food Safety & Applied Nutrition, Fish and Fisheries Products, Hazards and Controls Guide, Second Edition, January 1998, Web Site: http://vm.cfsan.fda.gov/~dms/haccp-2z.html

190. Sheila A. Martin and Donald W. Anderson (1998) Components of HACCP Costs to Industry; Research Triangle Institute 306 GOODELL BLDG, University of Massachusetts, Amherst, MA   01003 -9272 Tel: (413)   545-0111,   E-Mail webcomments@oit.umass.edu   Web   Site: http://www.umass.edu/ne165/haccp1998/martin.ht ml

191. Simpson, A.C.D. 1994. Integrating Public and Scientific Judgments into a Tool Kit for Managing Food-Related Risks, Stage II: Development of the Software. A report to the U.K. Ministry of Agriculture, Fisheries and Food ERAU Research Report No. 19, University of East, Anglia, Norwich, Norfolk, NR4 7TJ, Tel: 01603 593280, Fax: 01603 458596 E-Mail: intl.office@uea.ac.uk

192. Slovic, P. 1987. Perception of risk Science 236: 280-285 (258)

193. Smith, Gary C. (1999) Red Meat Safety; Center For Red   Meat   Safety,   The   Department   of   Animal Sciences, Colorado State University, Fort Collins, CO 80523-1171   E-Mail: gcsmith@ceres.agsci.colostate.edu

    Web   Site: gcmiller@ceres.agsci.colostate.edu http://www.colostate.edu/Depts/AnimSci/ran/meat/r edmeatsafety.html

194. Smith, G.C., J.N. Sofos, J.B. Morgan, J.O. Reagan, G.R. Acuff, D.R. Buege, J.S. Dickson, C.L. Kastner and R. Nickelson, II. (1995). Fecal-Material Removal and Bacterial-Count Reduction by Trimming and/or Spray-Washing   of   Beef   External-Fat   Surfaces; Proceedings of the Conference On New Technology to Improve Food Safety (April 12, 1995; Chicago IL) Food   Safety   and   Inspection   Service,   U.S. Department of Agriculture, Washington DC.

195. Soby, B.A., Simpson, A.C.D. and Ives, D.P. 1993. Integrating Public and Scientific Judgments into a Tool Kit for Managing Food-Related Risks, Stage 1: Literature Review and Feasibility Study. A report to the U.K. Ministry of Agriculture, Fisheries and Food ERAU Research Report No. 16, International Office, University of East, Anglia, Norwich, Norfolk, NR4 7TJ,

Tel: 01603 593280, Fax: 01603 458596 E-Mail: intl.office@uea.ac.uk

196. Sofos, J.N. and G.C. Smith (1993); New headache of the U.S. meat industry: E. coli O157:H7. Meat Focus International 2(7): 317-325. (178)

197. Starr, C. 1969 Social benefit versus technical risk Science 165: 1232-1238

198. Steahr, Thomas & Tanya Roberts's 1993 Microbial food-borne disease: hospitalizations, medical costs and potential demand for safer food. NE-165 Working Paper Series-32 Storrs, Connecticut, Department of Agricultural Economics

199. Steve Ingham, (2000); BASICS OF MICROBIOLOGY FOR APPLE PROCESSORS; Food Safety Extension Specialist, UW-Madison, Dept. of Food Science, 1605 Linden Drive, Madison, WI 53706. E-Mail: scingham@facstaffwisc.edu

Web   Site: http://www.wisc.edu/foodsci/cider/inspect_mb.html

200. Summary of Current Lawsuits on the Frankenfoods Front Summary of Lawsuits & Litigation on GE Food Issues in the US and Canada. Issue #6 G E An Update Dec. 20, 2000. Published by Genetic Engineering Action Network, USA Editor: Andy Zimmerman, E-Mail: turtle@westnet.com Organic Consumers Association. Web Site: http://www.organicconsumers.org/ge/gelawsuits.cfm

201. Systematic risk identification analysis (2003) Granimex NV. Granimex N.V - I.Z. E17/2, Wolfsakker 4, B-9160 Lokeren Belgium E-mail: info@granimex.be Web Site: http://www.granimex.be

T

202. Tasks Force on Good Farming Practices (2000), Canadian Dairy Information Center; Agriculture and Agri-Food Canada, CANADIAN DAIRY INFORMATION CENTRE, 1341 Baseline Road, Tower 7, 7th floor, Ottawa, Ontario, K1A 0C5, Facsimile: (613) 759-6313, E-mail: dairyinfo@agr.gc.ca Web Site: http://www.dairyinfo.agr.ca/cdicidftask.htm#Canada

203. Tea has less caffeine than coffee (2002), Tea Council of Canada-Tea Association of Canada, Web Site: http://www.tea.ca/press-trends-caffeine.asp?section=media

204. Transportation and Storage Requirements for Potentially Hazardous Foods; Docket Clerk (1997) FSIS DOCKET #95-049ARoom 3806, South Agriculture Building Food Safety and Inspection Service, U.S. Department of Agriculture, Washington, DC 20250 Web Site: http://www.asmusa.org/pasrc/fsistra.htm

205. Thomas Grein, Darina O'Flanaga, Tom McCarthy, Tom Prendergast (1996); An outbreak of *Salmonella enteritidis* food poisoning in a psychiatric hospital (1997), Dublin, Ireland; Eastern Health Board, Dublin European Programme for Intervention Epidemiology Training. E-Mail: carole.desmoulins@smi.ki.se Epiet Website - www.epiet.org Subject Web Site: http://www.epiet.org/seminar/1997/grein.html

206. T. Riggs, E. Elbasha, and M. Messonnier, The Effects of Information on Producer and Consumer Incentives to Undertake Food Safety Efforts: A Theoretical Model and Policy Implications," Centers for Disease Control and Prevention, USA.

U

207. United States Food Safety System (2000); Precaution in U.S. Food Safety Decision Making: Annex II to the United States' National Food Safety System Paper; Food and Drug Administration U.S. Department of Agriculture. Web Site: http://www.foodsafety.gov/~fsg/fssyst4.html

208. United States Food Safety System (2000); U.S. Food Safety System. U.S. Food and Drug Administration U.S. Department of Agriculture Web Site: http://www.foodsafety.gov/~fsg/fssyst2.html

209. U.S. National Research Council 1989 Improving Risk Communication Committee on Risk Perception and Communication National Academy Press, Washington, D.C. 332 pp.

210. Impacts of Biotechnology, Environment, and Food Safety: Communications. *A* Presentation Prepared

for the Agriculture Risk Management Conference, October 28-29, 1998, Holiday Inn, Plaza la Chaudière, Hull, QC Background Information, Ag-West Biotech annual meeting, Oct. 29, 1998, Saskatoon, SK. by: Dr. Douglas Powell, Dept. Plant Agriculture, University of Guelph, Guelph, Ont. N1G 2W1 E-mail: dpowell@uoguelph.ca. Web Site: http://www.foodsafetynetwork.ca/risk/CFBMCppr/CF BMC.html

211. United States Department of Agriculture, Animal and Plant Health Inspection Service, USDA/APHIS/DMB, 4700 River Road Suite, Unit 33, Riverdale, MD. Web Site: http://marketingoutreach.usda.gov/info/99Manual/h ealth.htm

212. Update: Outbreaks of Cyclosporiasis -- United States and Canada, 1997, Morbidity and Mortality Weekly Report, Vol. 46, No. 23 (1997), pp. 521-523; United States Department of Agriculture (USDA) and U.S. Department of Health and Human Services (HHS),

213. USDA, "USDA Researchers Create New Product That Reduces *Salmonella* in Chickens," USDA Release No. 0121.98, March 19, 1998.

V

214. Valerie Strand; The British Consulate-General Office, The British Trade & Investment Office 777 Bay Street, Suite 2800, Toronto, Ontario, M5G 2G2 Canada Tel. (416) 593-1290, Ext.2229, Fax. (416) 593-1229 Email: Valerie.Strand@fco.gov.uk Web Site: http://www.uk-canadatrade.org/sectors/beverage.htm

215. Value-Added Food Processing; Manitoba Trade & Investment Corporation 410 - 155 Carlton Street, Winnipeg, MB R3C 3H8Telephone: (204) 945-2466; Fax: (204) 957-1793; Toll Free in Canada & U.S.: 1-800-529-9981 Web Site: http://www.gov.mb.ca/itm/trade/invest/busfacts/bu siness/valfood.html

216. Viral Gastroenteritis Associated with Eating Oysters - - Louisiana, December 1996-January 1997," Morbidity and Mortality Weekly Report, Vol. 46, No.

47 (1997), pp. 1109-1112; USDA, HHS, and the U.S. Environmental Protection Agency.

W

217. Water Quality Report (2003) South Peel Mississauga, Brampton, Bolton. Region of Peel, 10 Peel Centre Drive, and Brampton ON L6T 4B9 Web Site: http://www.region.peel.on.ca/rop-survey.htm

218. What is the Government of Canada's role in food safety (2002)? Canadian Food Inspection Agency (CFIA); 59 Camelot Drive, Nepean, Ontario, Canada, K1A 0Y9 Web Site: http://www.inspection.gc.ca

219. William L Bennet and Leonard L Steed (1999); History of HACCP; Quality Progress/February 1999 - An Integrated Approach to Food Safety, Merrion Hall, Strand Road, Sandymount, Dublin 4, Ireland

220. W. Michael McCabe; Deputy Administrator and EPA Employees (2001 Risk characterization; Science Policy Council Handbook; Science Policy Council, U.S. Environmental Protection Agency; USEPA Office of Science Policy, 1300 Pennsylvania Ave. NW MC 8104R, Washington, DC 20460 Web Site: http://www.epa.gov/osp/spc/2riskchr.htm

GLOSSARY OF TERMS

A

ADI
Allowed Daily Intake of certain food ingredient which will not cause any illness for a non-allergic person to that ingredient

ADIC
Australian Dairy Industry Council (ADIC) is Australia's peak policy body for the national dairy industry, representing all aspects of this highly successful rural sector.

AFPP
Agri-Food Processed Product means any meat, fruit, vegetable, egg, dairy, honey or maple product, which is canned, cooked, pasteurized, sterilized, ultra heat-treated, dehydrated, refrigerated or otherwise preserved.

AIB
American Institute of Baking

Albumin
A type of protein widely distributed in the tissues and fluids of plants and animals. It is the single most abundant protein in blood. Albumin acts as a carrier for numerous substances in the blood.

Animal and Plant Health Inspection Service (APHIS)
The Animal and Plant Health Inspection Service (APHIS) is responsible for protecting and promoting U.S. Agricultural health, administering the Animal Welfare Act, and carrying out wildlife damage management activities. The APHIS mission is an integral part of U.S. Department of Agriculture's (USDA) efforts to provide the Nation with safe and affordable food.

APEDA
Agriculture Processing and Export Development Authority (APEDA) is an autonomous organization attached to the Ministry of Commerce of the Government of India. The main function of APEDA is to build links between Indian producers and the global markets. APEDA undertakes the briefing of potential sources on government policy and producers. It is along with providing referred services and suggesting suitable partners for joint ventures.

Appeal
Appeal means that it shall be the process by which a consultancy and certification agency can request reconsideration of decision

taken by APEDA / CFIA / FSIS or any other regulatory or certifying agency.

Approved source
Means acceptable to the regulatory authority based on a determination of conformity with principles, practices, and generally recognized standards that protect public health.

Applicant
Means it shall be the consultancy and certification agency that has applied for recognition by APEDA.

AQIS
The Australian Quarantine and Inspection Service (AQIS) is responsible for ensuring that products imported into Australia do not lead to the introduction, establishment and spread of pests and diseases which may endanger plants, animals and human life or health. Products regulated by AQIS include animals and animal products, plants and plant products and biological products containing or derived from microorganisms, animal, human or plant material. Genetically manipulated products imported into Australia that may pose a pest and disease risk fall, amongst other Commonwealth Acts, under the Quarantine Act 1908 administered by AQIS.

AQIS
Edmund Barton Building
Kings Avenue
BARTON ACT 2600
Website: www.affa.gov.au
Tel: 1 - 800 020 50

ARMCANZ
Agriculture and Resource Management Council of Australia and New Zealand (ARMCANZ) consists of the Australian Federal, State/ Territory and New Zealand Ministers responsible for Agriculture, soil, water (both rural and urban) and rural adjustment policy. The objective of the Council is to develop integrated and sustainable Agricultural and land and water management policies, strategies, and practices for the benefit of the Australian community.

ARMCANZ Secretariat   Tel: (02) 6272 5216
Department of Agriculture,   Fax: (02) 6272 4772
Fisheries and Forestry
GPO Box 858
CANBERRA ACT 2601 AUSTRALIA
E-mail: armcanz.contact@affa.gov.au

Artiodactyls
A taxonomic order, within super order Laurasiatheria - the even-toed ungulates. Artiodactyls include such familiar animals as sheep, goats, camels, pigs, cows, deer, giraffes, and antelopes — most of the world's species of large land mammals are artiodactyls.

Audit
It means that an appraisal shall include an independent assessment on-site to verify that the performance of an operation/ a product / a quality system / a safety system is in accordance with the laid procedure or standards.

Audit Checklist
It means that a tool, which is prepared by the auditor(s), (lead auditor or team), which lists what must be checked during the audit to assess if the written program is implemented as described and it is effective. This checklist is also used to record information found during the audit.

Audit Finding
A statement of fact made during an audit and substantiated by objective evidence.

Audit Frequency
It means the rate at which partial audits are to be conducted.

Audit Observation
Audit Observation means a statement of fact made during an audit and substantiated by objective evidence.

Auditor
Auditor means that it shall be the person who is identified by CFIA or FSIS or certified by a recognised institution in a host country and has the qualifications to perform regulatory recognition / system audit / third party audit / second party audit / product audit / process audit / audits of food manufacturing and management systems.

Audit team
Audit team means a group of auditors including at least the lead auditor / responsible regulatory inspector / one regional reviewer.

B

Bacteria
Bacteria are living single-cell organisms measuring less than a micron to five micron and in some cases beyond that limit. Water, wind, insects, plants, animals can carry bacteria, and so the people where bacteria survive well on skin, clothes and in human hair. Bacteria also thrive in scabs, scars, the mouth, nose, throat,

intestines, and room-temperature foods.

BMP
Butter Milk Powder

BMPs
Best Management Practices (BMPs)

Bovine Spongiform Encephalopathy (BSE)
BSE is a fatal brain disease of cattle with unusually long incubation periods measured in years and caused by an unconventional transmissible agent. Bioassays have identified the presence of the BSE agent in the brain, spinal cord, retina, dorsal root ganglia (nervous tissue located near the backbone), distal ileum, and the bone marrow of cattle experimentally infected with this agent by the oral route. Milk and milk products from cows are not believed to pose any risk for transmitting the BSE agent.

Bovine Somatotropin (BST)
Bovine Somatotropin (BST) is a natural protein hormone that stimulates the production of milk.

British Columbia Centre for Disease Control (BCCDC)
British Colombia Centre for Disease Control (BCCDC) is British Columbia's Centre of Excellence for the prevention, detection and control of communicable disease, and a provider of specialty health support and resource services. BCCDC provide the coordinated services essential to efficiently and effectively prevent and control communicable disease in the province which are Hepatitis Services, Epidemiology Services, Laboratory Services, STD/AIDS Control , Tuberculosis Control , Drug and Poison Information Centre , Food Protection Services and Radiation Protection Services. BCCDC works in close partnership with the province's health authorities, Medical Health Officers and the Provincial Health Officer. BCCDC collaborates with the University of British Colombia Centre for Disease Control in the advancement of academia, research and teaching.

C

Canada Beef Export Federation (CANADA-BEEF)
CANADA-BEEF is an independent non-profit organization committed to improving export results for the Canadian cattle and beef industry. The Federation's Mandate is to identify and develop markets to increase the sale of Canadian beef and beef products with the cooperation of all companies, organizations and institutions, which will benefit from this success. The federation was established in 1989.

CANADA-BEEF   Tel: (403) 274-0005

235, 6715-8th Street NE   Fax: (403) 274-7275
Calgary, AB T2E 7H7
E-Mail: canada@cbef.com

Canada Pork International (CPI)

Canada Pork International (CPI) is the association of Canadian pork exporters. Its membership is comprised of provincial hog producer organizations and Canadian pork packing and trading companies. CPI's mandate includes seeking and maintaining access to foreign markets as well as coordinating the generic promotion of Canadian pork products.

CANADA PORC INTERNATIONAL Tel: (613) 236-9886
75 Albert, Suite 1101   Fax: (613) 236-665
Ottawa, Ontario
K1P 5E7

Canadian Cattlemen's Association (CCA)

CCA is the association of more than 100,000 beef producers, which was established in 1932. Wide range of issues affecting Canadian beef are tackled by CCA and some of the important issues are beef trade, animal health, environment and animal care, fiscal and monetary policy, and grading/inspection. CCA works closely with other sectors of the Agriculture and food industries on matters of mutual concern.

Canadian Cattlemen's Association Tel: (613) 233-9375
#1403, 150 Metcalfe St.   Fax: (613) 233-2860
Ottawa, ON K2P 1P1

Canadian Dairy Information Center (CDIC)

The Canadian Dairy Information Centre (CDIC) is an organized centre of Canadian partnership between Agriculture and Agri-Food Canada (AAFC), the Canadian Dairy Commission (CDC), & the Dairy Farmers of Canada (DFC), these three organizations have worked in partnership to create a comprehensive site on the Canadian Dairy Industry.

CANADIAN DAIRY INFORMATION CENTRE Fax: (613) 759-6313
1341 Baseline Road
Tower 7, 7th floor
Ottawa, Ontario
K1A 0C5
E-mail: dairyinfo@agr.gc.ca
Web: http://www.dairyinfo.gc.ca/cdicmain.htm

CEPA

Canadian Environmental Protection Act (CEPA) is an Act respecting pollution prevention and the protection of the environment and human health in order to contribute to sustainable development.

Canadian Food and Drugs Act (CFDA)

Canada's Food and drug Act is a regulatory document respecting foods, drugs, cosmetics and therapeutic devices. Food and Drug Regulations with in CFDA outline the standards and requirements with respect to food that have been established by Health Canada. Requirements pertaining to the advertising, labelling and packaging of food, drugs, medical devices and cosmetics are set out in the Food and Drugs Act ("FDA") and the Regulations thereto.

Health Canada   Tel (613) 957-1316
Bureau of Food Regulatory, Fax (613) 941-3537
International & Interagency Affairs
Canadian Food and Drugs Act (CFDA),
Food Directorate
Building #7, Tunney's Pasture (PL 0702C1)
Ottawa, ON K1A 0L2

Canadian Food Inspection Agency (CFIA)

Canadian Food Inspection Agency (CFIA) created in April 1997 incorporates the activities of four federal government departments – Agriculture and Agri-Food Canada, Fisheries and Oceans Canada, Health Canada and Industry Canada. The establishment of the CFIA consolidated the delivery of all federal food, animal and plant's health inspection programs. The CFIA delivers 14 inspection programs related to foods, plants and animals in 18 regions across Canada. Activities range from the inspection of federally-registered meat processing facilities to border inspections for foreign pests and diseases, to the enforcement of practices related to fraudulent labelling, verify the humane transportation of animals, conduct food investigations and recalls, perform laboratory testing and environmental assessments of seeds, plants, feeds and fertilizers. CFIA is Canada's federal food safety, animal health and plants protection enforcement agency.

Canadian Food Inspection Agency
Headquarters
59 Camelot Drive
Ottawa, Ontario
K1A 0Y9
Tel: (613) 225-2342 / 1-800-442-2342
Fax: (613) 228-6601

Canadian Food Safety Adaptation Program (CFSAP)

The Canadian Food Safety Adaptation Program has been evolved to enhance food safety throughout the total food chain in the manufacturing, marketing, distribution and catering of food by using Hazard Analysis Critical Control Point (HACCP) definitions and principles as defined by the Codex Alimentarius Commission. It is an innovative national program to assist the Agri-food industry in designing comprehensive, collaborative food safety strategies and management systems. CFIA designed CFSAP.

Canadian Meat Council (CMC)

CMC is the organization of Canadian meat packing/processing industry. It procures the views of Canadian meat processing industry through membership to the organization. CMC promotes high standards, safety of Canadian meat, wholesomeness, nutritious meat products, free and expanding markets for products of Council's packers and processors, and suppliers of goods and services. It also maintains effective communications with various levels of government, and all elements of food production, processing, distribution and retailing, with consumer organizations, the research and academic community and the news media with respect to all matters that affects the meat processing industry in Canada.

Canadian Meat Science Association (CMSA)

Created in 1985, CMSA associates the professionals of Canadian meat industry, Canadian meat academics and government of Canada. The CMSA facilitates understanding of the meat science and constituents of meat animals to address the needs of the industry in Canada. The CMSA helps its members in professional development by providing a forum for the exchange and dissemination of new developments in meat science research, teaching and application of new technology in the meat industry.

Canadian Pork Council (CPC)

Created in 1966, CPC provide a leadership role in a concerted effort involving all levels of industry and government toward a common understanding and action plan for achieving a dynamic and prosperous pork industry in Canada. The CPC operates from a single office located in Ottawa, Canada's capital city. CPC works in the areas of opening new markets for pork, quality improvement, communicating research priorities, advising on animal health programs, addressing biotechnology, environment, food safety and animal care issues in Canada.

Canadian Pork Council Tel: (613) 236-9239 (phone)
1101-75 Albert Street   Fax: (613) 236-6658 (fax)
Ottawa, Ontario
Canada K1P 5E7

Canadian Registration Board of Occupational Hygiene (CRBOH)
The CRBOH is a not-for-profit organization, which sets standards of professional competence for occupational hygienists and occupational hygiene technologists in Canada. Registration with the CRBOH confers the right to use the title Registered Occupational Hygienist (ROH) or Registered Occupational Hygiene Technologist (ROHT), and indicates the attainment and maintenance of a high standard of professionalism, recognizable in all Canadian jurisdictions.

Canadian Registration Board of
Occupational Hygienists
Business Office
224, Park side Court,
Port Moody, British Columbia,
Canada V3H 4Z8

CCP Decision Tree (CCP-DT)
CCP-DT is a sequence of questions to determine whether a control point is a Critical Control Point (CCP).

Centers for Disease Control (CDC)
The Centers for Disease Control and Prevention (CDC) is the United States federal agency for protecting the health and safety of people - at home and abroad, providing credible information to enhance health decisions, and promoting health through strong partnerships. CDC serves as the national focus for developing and applying disease prevention and control, environmental health, and health promotion and education activities designed to improve the health of the people of the United States. The CDC is one of the major operating components of the Department of Health and Human Services. CDC's major organizational components respond individually in their areas of expertise and pool their resources and expertise on crosscutting issues and specific health threats.

Centers for Disease Control and Prevention
1600 Clifton Rd.,
Atlanta, GA 30333
U.S.A
Web Site: http://www.cdc.gov
Tel: (404) 639-3311
TTY: (404) 639-3312

Center for Food Safety and Applied Nutrition (CFSAN)
Center for Food Safety and Applied Nutrition carry out the mission of the United States Food and Drug Administration (US-FDA). CFSAN, in conjunction with the Agency's field staff, is responsible

for promoting and protecting the public's health by ensuring that the nation's food supply is safe, sanitary, wholesome, and honestly labelled, and that cosmetic products are safe and properly labelled.

CFSAN
Food and Drug Administration
5600 Fishers Lane
Rockville, Maryland 20857
Web Site: http://vm.cfsan.fda.gov

Center for Science in the Public Interest (CSPI)

Center for Science in the Public Interest has been a strong advocate for nutrition and health, food safety, alcohol policy, and sound science. CSPI carved out a niche as the organized voice of the American public on nutrition, food safety, health and other issues during a boom of consumer and environmental protection awareness in the early 1970s.

Center for Technology Assessment (CTA)

Center for Technology Assessment (CTA) is a non-profit, bi-partisan organization committed to providing the public with full assessments and analyses of technological impacts on society. CTA was formed to assist the public and policymakers had better understand how technology affects society.
Website: http://www.icta.org

Certification

Means it shall be the procedure by which a written assurance is given by APEDA recognised certification agency that a clearly identified production or processing system has been methodically assessed and conforms to the specified requirements

Chronic Disease

Chronic diseases are of long duration, denoting a disease of slow progress and long continuance

Chronic Fatigue and Immune Dysfunction Syndrome (CFIDS)

A synonym used for chronic fatigue syndrome used by some patients and physicians. It should be stressed, however, that no immune dysfunction or aberration has been persuasively linked to chronic fatigue syndrome.

Closed CAR

CAR means with an action plan to correct non-conformity, which is found to be completed and effective within the set period.

Code of Ethics

Means it shall be followed by all HACCP auditors, lead auditors, internal quality auditors as well as consultancy and certification agencies.

Codex Alimentarius Commission (CAC)

FAO and WHO created The Codex Alimentarius Commission in 1963 to develop food standards, guidelines and related texts such as codes of practice under the Joint FAO/WHO Food Standards Programme. The main purposes of this Programme are protecting health of the consumers and ensuring fair trade practices in the food trade, and promoting coordination of all food standards work undertaken by international governmental and non-governmental organizations.

Comprehensive Nutrient Management Plans (CNMP's)

Comprehensive Nutrient Management Plans (CNMP's) are conservation plans unique to livestock operations. These plans document practices and strategies adopted by livestock operations to address natural resource concerns related to soil erosion, livestock manure and disposal of organic by-products.

Consumer Packaging and Labelling Act (CPLA)

The Consumer Packaging and Labelling Act is a regulatory statute of Canada governing product packaging and labelling at both levels, federal and provincial governance. The Consumer Packaging and Labelling Act contain packaging and labelling requirements for 'pre-packaged products'.

Contingent valuation (CV)

Contingent valuation (CV) deals with subjective valuation of food attributes such as food safety

Control Point (CP)

CP means any step in a process whereby biological, chemical, or physical factors may be controlled.

Corrective Actions (CA)

CA means Procedures followed when a serious or critical deficiency is assessed or when a critical limit is reached or exceeded.

Contamination

It means the unintended presence in food of potentially harmful substances, including microorganisms, chemicals, and physical objects.

Continuous Monitoring

Uninterrupted collection and recording of data such as temperature on a strip chart

Control

To manage the conditions of an operation to maintain compliance with established criteria, and (b) the state wherein correct procedures are being followed and criteria are being met.

Corrective Action (CA)
Means an activity that is taken by a person whenever a critical limit is not met.

Corrective Action Request (CAR)
Means Formal request to the plant management for actions to be taken to correct non-conformity identified during an audit.

Criterion
A requirement on which a judgment or a decision can be based.

Critical Control Point (CCP)
The last point, step, or procedure at which control can be applied and a food-safety hazard can be prevented, eliminated, or reduced to acceptable levels. CCP means any step in a process, which, if not properly controlled, may result in an unacceptable safety, wholesomeness, or economic fraud risk

Critical Defect
A deviation at a CCP that may result in a hazard.

Critical Deficiency
Means a hazardous deviation from plan requirements such that maintenance of the safety, wholesomeness, and economic integrity is absent; will result in unsafe, unwholesome, or misbranded product

Critical Limit
The maximum or minimum value to which a physical, biological, or chemical hazard must be controlled at a Critical Control Point (CCP) to prevent, eliminate, or reduce to an acceptable level the occurrence of the identified food safety hazard. A criterion that must be met for each preventive measure associated with a Critical Control Point.

Cross Contamination (CC)
Means the transfer of harmful substances or disease-causing microorganisms to food by hands, food-contact surfaces, sponges, cloth towels and utensils that touch raw food, are not cleaned, and then touch ready-to-eat foods. Cross contamination can also occur when raw food touches or drips onto cooked or ready-to-eat foods.

Critical Control Point (CCP)
Means an operational step or procedure in a process, production method, or recipe, at which control can be applied to prevent, reduce, or eliminate a food safety hazard.

Committee
It shall mean panel constituted by APEDA for the purpose of

evaluation and assessment of consultancy and certification agencies.

Consultancy
Means it shall mean the advisory service extended by APEDA recognised consultancy agency to the operators.

Consumers Association of Canada (CAC)
Founded in 1947, CAC mission is to represent and articulate the best interests of Canadian consumers to all levels of government and to all sectors of society by continually earning recognition as the trusted voice of the consumer on a national basis.

Consumers Association of Canada
Po Box 18112
Delta, British Columbia
V4M 2M3
Tel: 604 454 7827

Creutzfeldt-Jakob Disease (CJD)
Creutzfeldt-Jakob disease (CJD) is a rare, degenerative, invariably fatal brain disorder. Typically, onset of symptoms occurs at about age 60.

Cycle
Means the length of time necessary to complete a moving or working object/function from a point of start to a point of completion in routine

Cytomegalovirus (CMV):
One of the eight known types of human herpes viruses, which are also known as human herpes virus 5 (HHV-5) belongs to the beta subfamily of herpes viruses. CMV can cause severe disease in patients with immune deficiency and in newborns when the virus is transmitted in utero.

D

Dairy Farmers of Canada (DFC)
Founded in 1934 as the Canadian Federation of Milk Producers, DFC is the Canadian organization representing Canada's 17,747 dairy producers. DFC runs for producers and by producers.

Dairy Farmers of Canada
1801 McGill College Avenue, Suite 1000
Montreal, PQ, H3A 2N4
E-mail: cdaragon@dfc-plc.ca
Tel: (514) 284-1092

Dairy Industry Association Ltd (DIAL)
Created in 2002, DIAL was formed because of The Dairy Industry

Federation (DIF) and The National Dairymen's Association (NDA) to represent the entire milk processing and distribution, and dairy manufacturing sector in England and Wales. This sector processes around 14 billion litres of milk a year and is worth £6 billion in retail sales. DIAL offers its members Political representation at all levels in the UK, Europe and beyond, provision of information targeted specifically at the needs and interests of members, Representation of members interests on and through organisations such as the European Dairy association, Dairy Council, National Dairy Farm Assured Scheme and farmers' organisations and policy formulation and issues management.

The Dairy Industry Association Limited
93-Baker Street
London W1U 6RI
E-Mail: sbates@dia-ltd.org.uk
Web: http://www.dia-ltd.org.uk
Tel: 020 7456 7244

Dairy Management Inc. (DMI)
DMI helps demand for American dairy products on behalf of dairy producers and it is dedicated to the success of the dairy industry.

Dairy Management Inc.
#900-10255 West Higgins Road
Rosemont, IL60018-5616
Tel: 1-800-853-2479

Danish Dairy Board (DDB)
DDB promotes the common commercial interests of the Danish dairy industry in Denmark and abroad and its common interests in relation to export of dairy products, and to safeguard the interests of Danish milk producers in relation to national and international policies, including EU policies.

Danish Dairy Board   Tel: +45 87312000
Fredericks Alle 22   Fax: +45 87312001
Dk-8000 Arhus C
E-Mail: ddb@mejeri.dk
Web: http://www.mejeri.dk

Deviation
Failure to meet a required critical limit for a critical control point.

Deviation Procedure
Means Pre-determined and documented set of corrective actions, which are implemented when a deviation occurs

E

Ecolab

Ecolab is the world's leading provider of cleaning, food safety and health protection products and services for the hospitality, foodservice, healthcare and industrial markets.

CORPORATE HEADQUARTERS
Ecolab Center
370 N. Wabasha Street
St. Paul, Minnesota 55102-2233
Telephone: 1 (651)293-2233

Electrolytes

Substances that dissociate in water to form a cation (positively charged ion) and anion (negatively charged ion) - Charged ions are central to a variety of important processes in the body, including muscle contraction and nerve impulse conduction.

Enterocolitis (EC)

"Entero" refers to the small intestine; "Colo" refers to large intestine, which is inflammation. Enterocolitis is an inflammation causing injury to the bowel. EC may involve only the innermost lining or the entire thickness of the bowel and variable amounts of the bowel.

Enterovirus

It is a genus of RNA viruses with over 70 types identified in humans. They reproduce in the intestinal tract, and various members can cause a variety of human diseases, including poliomyelitis, aseptic meningitis, hepatitis, inflammatory heart disease, and rhinitis.

Environment Canada

Environment Canada's mandate is to preserve and enhance the quality of the natural environment; conserve Canada's renewable resources; conserve and protect Canada's water resources; forecast weather and environmental change; enforce rules relating to boundary waters; and coordinate environmental policies and programs for the federal government.

Environmental Protection Agency (EPA)

The mission of the Environmental Protection Agency is to protect human health and the environment. Since 1970, EPA has been working for a cleaner, healthier environment for the American people.

U.S. Environmental Protection Agency
U.S. EPA, Region 10

1200 Sixth Avenue Suite 900
Seattle, WA 98101
Tel: 1 (206) 553-1200

Enzyme

Enzymes are specialized proteins that act as catalysts for virtually all-necessary chemical reactions that take place within the body. Like all catalysts, enzymes unchanged by the reactions they promote, and will initiate many reactions until they are degraded (usually by another enzyme).

Evaluation:

Means shall be the process of systematic examination of the performance of the consultancy and certification agency by APEDA to the extent it fulfills specific requirements of HACCP applications in all levels of food chain for exports.

F

FIL-IDF

Established in 1903, the International Dairy Federation (FIL-IDF) is an independent, non-profit association, which aims to promote scientific, technical and economic progress in the international dairy field through international cooperation and consultation. FIL-IDF and developing dairying countries to exchange views and to bring there combined expertise to bear on common problems. Currently, 32 countries are representatives of FIL-IDF.

International Dairy Federation
Diamante Building,
Boulevard Augusta Reyers 80, 1030 Brussels, Belgium
E-mail: info@fil-idf.org
Tel: +322 733 9888

FIL-IDF Canada

The Canadian National Committee of the International Dairy Federation (FIL-IDF Canada) groups the different partners of the Canadian dairy sector. FIL-IDF Canada brings together producers, processors, provincial governments, federal departments and agencies, universities, colleges, research institutes and private companies involved in the dairy business in Canada. FIL-IDF Canada is the only national forum where all partners of the Canadian dairy industry discuss issues relevant to the sector in a non-political way (e.g. the National Dairy Code).

FIL-IDF Canada
Agriculture and Agri-Food Canada
Dairy Section,
2200 Walkley Road,

Ottawa, Ontario
K1A 0C5
E-Mail: doylep@agr.gc.ca
Web: www.dairyinfo.gc.ca
Tel: (613) 759-6264

Fish
It means fresh or saltwater finfish, crustaceans and other forms of aquatic life (including alligator, frog, aquatic turtle, jellyfish, sea cucumber, and sea urchin and the roe of such animals) other than birds or mammals, and all molluscs, if such life is intended for human consumption. Includes an edible human food product derived in whole or in part from fish, including fish that have been processed in any manner.

Food
It means raw, cooked, or processed edible substance, ice, beverage, chewing gum, or ingredient used or intended for use or for sale in whole or in part for human consumption.

Food Animal Residue Avoidance Databank (FARAD)
FARAD is a food safety and human health support system designed to provide livestock producers, extension specialists, and veterinarians with practical information on how to avoid drug, pesticide and environmental contaminant residue problems. It is a National Food Safety Project of U.S. Department of Agriculture Cooperative State Research, Education, and Extension Service. The drugs and pesticides used in modern animal Agriculture improve animal health and thereby promote more efficient and humane production. The development of effective residue avoidance and quality assurance programs requires access to a vast array of information. The Food Animal Residue Avoidance Databank (FARAD) offers the means to provide this information. FARAD is authorized by the Agricultural Research, Extension, and Education Reform Act of 1998 (Public Law 105-185, Title 6, Subtitle A, Section 604)

Food establishment
Means an operation at the retail level, i.e., that serves or offers food directly to the consumer and that, in some cases, includes a production, storage, or distributing operation that supplies the direct-to-consumer operation.

Food Safety Enhancement Program (FSEP)
The Food Safety Enhancement Program (FSEP) is the CFIA's tool to encourage the development, implementation and maintenance of Hazard Analysis Critical Control Points (HACCP). The system is based and applicable in all federally registered Canadian processing

establishments and shell egg grading stations for which CFIA monitoring and verification programs have been established. The objective of FSEP is to ensure food safety through rigorous and scientific management of food processing activities. Thus all federally registered establishments of meat, dairy, honey, maple syrup, processed fruit and vegetable, shell egg, processed egg and poultry hatchery are eligible under FSEP.

Canadian Food Inspection Agency (CFIA), Commercial Affairs, Canadian Food Inspection Agency, 59 Camelot Drive, Nepean, Ontario, Canada, K1A 0Y9.

Web Site: http://www.inspection.gc.ca
FSEP homepage: http://www.cfiaacia.agr.ca
Toll-Free: 1-800-442-2342,
Tel: (613) 225-2342,
Fax: (613) 228-6634

Food Safety and Inspection Service (FSIS)
The Food Safety and Inspection Service (FSIS), is a public health regulatory agency of the U.S. Department of Agriculture, protects consumers by ensuring that meat, poultry, and egg products are safe, wholesome, and accurately labelled. Food Safety and Inspection Service is the food agency of United States of America to improve the management and effectiveness of regulatory programs, ensure that policy decisions are based on science, Improve coordination of food safety activities with other public health agencies, Enhance public education efforts and to Protect meat, poultry, and egg products against intentional contamination.

Food Safety and Inspection Service
Congressional and Public Affairs Staff
United States Department of Agriculture
Washington, D.C. 20250-3700
Phone: (202) 720-3897

Food borne Illness
It means sickness resulting from acquisition of a disease that is carried or transmitted to humans by food containing harmful substances.

Food borne outbreak
It means the occurrence of two or more people experiencing the same illness after eating the same food.

Foot and Mouth Disease (FMD)
Foot and Mouth Disease (FMD) is an acute, highly contagious *picornavirus* infection of cloven-hoofed animals. The virus (FMDV) is sensitive to environmental influences, such as pH less than 5,

sunlight and desiccation; however it can survive for long period of time at freezing temperatures.

G

Genetically Modified Foods (GMF)

Genetically modified (GM) foods are the edibles that have had their DNA altered through genetic engineering. The process is known by many different names such as gene, or DNA manipulation, gene splicing, transgenic and many others. In 2006, a total of 252 million acres of transgenic crops were planted in 22 countries by 10.3 million farmers. The majority of these crops were herbicide- and insect-resistant soybeans, corn, cotton, canola, and alfalfa. Other crops grown commercially or field-tested are a sweet potato resistant to a virus that could decimate most of the African harvest, rice with increased iron and vitamins that may alleviate chronic malnutrition in Asian countries, and a variety of plants able to survive weather extremes.

Technologies for genetically modifying (GM) foods offer dramatic promise for meeting some areas of greatest challenge for the 21st century. Like all new technologies, they also pose some risks, both known and unknown. Controversies surrounding GM foods and crops commonly focus on human and environmental safety, labelling and consumer choice, intellectual property rights, ethics, food security, poverty reduction, and environmental conservation.

Globulin

A family of proteins found with abundance in plasma. They include the gamma globulins, which in turn include the various antibody molecules produced by the immune system.

Glucose

A simple sugar, which is actively transferred into the blood following the digestive breakdown of starch and other carbohydrates in the gut.

Good Manufacturing Practices (GMP)

An extensive list of practices that, if not met, could cause an adulterated food product

Good Cleaning Practices (GCPs)

GLPs are the procedures applied to attain standard hygiene and sanitation in plant, machinery, and food processing area, which will safeguard the production activities and eliminate contaminants to food.

H

HACCP
Hazard Analysis and Critical Control Points

HACCP Generic Models
Means Generalized HACCP plans designed for a specific product or product category that can be used as an example or guideline for developing a plant specific HACCP plan.

HACCP Plan
It means a document that describes the firm's HACCP-based inspection system. It is the written document based upon the principles of HACCP and that delineates the procedures to assure the control of a specific process or procedure.

HACCP Plan Re-evaluation
One aspect of verification in which the HACCP team with the purpose of modifying the HACCP plan as necessary does a documented periodic review of the HACCP plan.

HACCP Plan Validation
The initial review by the HACCP team to ensure that all elements of the HACCP plan are accurate

HACCP system
HACCP system means the result of implementing the HACCP principles in an operation that has a foundational, comprehensive, prerequisite program in place. A HACCP system includes the HACCP plan and all SOPs.

HACCP Team
Means Group of people with different backgrounds (i.e. Team production, sanitation, quality control, food microbiology) who are responsible to assist the HACCP coordinator in the development, implementation and modification/updating of HACCP plans.

Haemolytic Uremic Syndrome (HUS)
Haemolytic uremic syndrome (HUS) is characterized by acute renal failure, micro-angiopathic haemolytic anaemia, fever, and thrombocytopenia. Diarrhoea and upper respiratory infection are the most common precipitating factors. HUS is one of the most common causes of acute renal failure in children. Haemolytic uremic syndrome (HUS) is characterized by renal failure due to the production of toxin, which damages endothelial cells, which triggers the clotting mechanism.

Haemorrhagic Colitis (HC)
Haemorrhagic Colitis (HC) is characterized by abdominal cramps and watery diarrhoea followed by hemorrhagic bleeding from the

large intestine, distinguishing it from other *E. coli* infections; onset of 4-8 days.

Hazard
Means a chance for or the risk of, a biological, chemical, physical, or economic property in a food product that could violate established program criteria or cause the consumer distress or illness.

Health Canada
Health Canada is the federal department responsible for helping the people of Canada maintain and improve their health. In partnership with provincial and territorial governments, Health Canada provides national leadership to develop health policy, enforce health regulations, promote disease prevention and enhance healthy living for all Canadians.

Health Canada
A.L. 0900C2
Ottawa, Canada
K1A 0K9
Tel: (613) 957-2991
TTY: 1-800-267-1245

Healthy Futures for Ontario Agriculture (HFOA)
Ontario government designed this program in 1999 to promote safe water, safe food, and develop new markets.

Hedonic Pricing (HP)
This technique is normally used to estimate the value that consumers place on various attributes of a food commodity.

Hepatitis B virus
A small DNA virus capable of causing both acute and chronic liver disease, possibly by eliciting tissue damage by the immune system - The virus may also be a risk factor for hepatic carcinoma. It is often transmitted through sexual activity or through exposure to contaminated blood.

Hepatitis C virus
An RNA virus related to the pest viruses and flaviviruses. It is capable of causing both acute and chronic liver disease. As with hepatitis B, the liver damage resulting from this infection may be the result of immune reactivity against virus-infected liver cells.

Herpesvirus
A family of large DNA viruses that infect a wide range of animal species - Eight distinct types have been associated with a variety of human diseases.

I

International Dairy Food Association (IDFA)
IDFA is the dairy foods industry's collective voice in Washington, D.C., throughout the country and in the international arena. IDFA has become a leading player in the formation of positive domestic and international dairy policies. Today, IDFA represents more than 500 dairy food manufacturers, marketers, distributors and industry suppliers across the United States and Canada, and in 20 other countries.

International Dairy Food Association's (IDFA)
Tel: (202) 737-4332 Fax: (202) 331-7820
1250 H Street, NW, Suite 900
Washington, DC 20005
Website: www.idfa.org

International Food Safety Council (IFSC)
The International Food Safety Council's mission is to heighten the awareness of the importance of food safety education throughout the restaurant and foodservice industry. The Council envisions a future where food borne illness no longer exists. Through its educational programs, publications and awareness campaigns the Council fulfills this mission.

International Occupational Hygiene Association (IOHA)
The IOHA provides an international voice of the occupational hygiene profession through its recognition as a non-governmental organization (NGO) by the ILO (International Labour Organisation) and WHO (World Health Organisation).

IOHA Secretariat
Suite 2, Georgian House,
Great Northern Road,
Derby DE1 1LT
United Kingdom
Email: admin@ioha.com
Tel: +44 1332 298101

Internal temperature
Means the temperature of the internal portion of a food product

Irish Dairy Board
Created in 1961, Irish Dairy Board is a co-operative exporting Irish dairy product. Kerrygold is a famous worldwide consumer brand. The Irish Dairy Board is the major international exporter of Irish dairy products, servicing the needs and quality demands of customers worldwide. It is now one of Ireland's biggest exporters

and a major food distribution company in overseas markets, with annual sales of €1.9 billion.

IRISH DAIRY BOARD
Grattan House
Mount Street Lower
Dublin 2
Email: idb@idb.ie
Web: http://www.idb.ie
Tel: +353 1 661 9599

J

Johne's disease (JD)
Johne's disease (JD) is a chronic, progressive, wasting disease of ruminants caused by *Mycobacterium avium paratuberculosis*. The disease is characterised by a long incubation period, with clinical disease usually only occurring in older animals. Clinical signs are rarely seen in cattle younger than 2 years and are usually observed between 2 and 6 years of age.

K

L

Low risk products
Means Seafood that poses no significant risk to the health of the public when prepared for consumption by conventional or traditional means

Lead Auditor (LA)
Means the auditor identified to lead the audit and responsible for making any final decisions.

Lean Meat
Lean meat is a portion of meat, which is low in animal fat, low in cholesterol, high in protein, high in iron and good for heart improvement programs. In calculated terms, less than 10 g fat, 4.5 g or less saturated fat, and less than 95 mg cholesterol per serving and per 100 g is termed as lean meet. A meat portion, which is less than 5 g fat, less than 2 g saturated fat and less than 95 mg cholesterol per serving and per 100 g, is extra lean meat.

Long Term Action Plan (LTAP)
Long Term Action Plan (LTAP) means an action plan to permanently correct the cause of the problem when the set period to correct non-conformity must be exceeded.

M

Major Deficiency

Means a significant deviation from HACCP plan requirements, such that maintenance of safety, wholesomeness, or economic integrity is inhibited.

Meat Safety Quality Assurance (MSQA)

The Australian beef and sheep meat industries have ADOPTED AN integrated HACCP system into a total quality management system that incorporates Standards Organisation 9002:1994 standards, Good Manufacturing Practices (GMP), Codex Alimentarius Commission Hazard Analysis Critical Control Points (HACCP) methodology and Standard Operating Procedures to provide process control. The program is called Meat Safety Quality Assurance (MSQA). Meat Safety Quality Assurance (MSQA) is a system developed by the Australian Quarantine and Inspection Service (AQIS).

Mega Regs

Mega-Regs are the United States Department of Agriculture's (USDA) meat regulations, which took effect on January 26, 1998, set new standards for control of Salmonella sp. and E. coli in food production, and require food manufacturing companies to improve monitoring and documentation of critical control points in their operations.

Milk Protein Concentrates (MPC)

A Milk Protein Concentrate (MPC) is a dairy protein product with protein content greater than 55% preferably greater than 75% on a dry matter basis. The casein: whey protein ratio is similar to that of the initial skim milk; lactose content of MPC varies according to protein concentration. As such, MPC-42 indicates a protein content of 42% and a lactose content of 46%, while MPC-82 signifies 82% protein and only 4% lactose.

Milk Protein Isolate (MPI)

A Milk Protein Isolate (MPI) is a dairy protein product with protein content greater than 85%, on a dry matter basis. The casein: whey protein ratio is similar to that of the initial skim milk. Isolates differ from the concentrates in that they possess high protein content with almost no lactose content.

Milk Protein Fractions (MPF)

Milk protein fractions are the milk proteins, which are separated individually from non-protein milk components with specific functional properties. By separating milk proteins into different fractions, specific functional and nutritional qualities are obtained and used for a particular food system or product. One primary application example is the use of the milk protein fraction beta casein in infant formula and whey protein chains that act as a hydrocolloid in foods such as yoghurt, ice cream, gravy and even gummy candy. Cow's milk contains more than 20 protein fractions. In the curd, 4 caseins (i.e., S1, S2, S3, S4) can be identified that account for about 80% of the milk proteins. The remaining 20% of the proteins, essentially globular proteins (e.g., lactalbumin, lactoglobulin, bovine serum albumin), are contained in the whey.

Minor Deficiency
Means a failure of the part of the HACCP-based system relative to facility's sanitation, which is not likely to reduce materially the facility's ability to meet acceptable sanitation requirements.

Meat
Means the flesh of animals used as food including the dressed flesh of cattle, swine, sheep, or goats and other edible animals, except fish, poultry, and wild game animals.

Microorganism
Microorganism means a form of living being that it is invisible to the naked eye and that can be seen only with a microscope; including bacteria, viruses, yeast, extremophiles and single-celled animals. Microorganisms can be helpful as in Agriculture, food science, and medicine, some are harmful as pathogens when, as parasites, cause infections and disease.

Ministry of the Environment (MOE)
It refers to the Japanese Ministry of Environment, which directs Waste Management, Environmental Policy, Environmental Health Department, Water Environment Bureau, Nature Conservation Bureau, National Institute for Minimata Disease and National Institute for Environmental Studies.

Minor non-conformity
Means An isolated non-conformity within the sub-element of the prerequisite program or CCP of the HACCP plan being audited.

Molluscan shellfish
Means any edible species of raw fresh or frozen oysters, clams, mussels, and scallops or edible portions thereof, except when the scallop product consists only of the shucked adductor muscle.

Monitor
To conduct a planned sequence of observations or measurements to assess whether a CCP is under control and to produce an accurate record for future use in verification.

Monitoring
It means the act of conducting a planned sequence of observations or measurements of control parameters to assess whether a CCP is under control and to produce an accurate record.

Monitoring Procedures
Means Scheduled testing and/or observations recorded by the firm to report the findings at each CCP.

Moving window
Means the number of consecutive planned partial audits to be conducted in order to determine if the audit level should be changed (e.g. normal to reduced or reduced to normal). It includes the most recent audit and the previous "x" audits required to complete the moving window size.

Multi-commodity activities program (MCAP)
Means Tool used by CFIA to perform regulatory system audits (partial and full audits).

N

National Animal Health Monitoring System (NAHMS)
The USDA initiated the National Animal Health Monitoring System (NAHMS) in 1983 to collect, analyze, and disseminate data on animal health, management, and productivity across the United States. NAHMS' first national study of the United States' dairy industry, 1991's National Dairy Heifer Evaluation Project (NDHEP), provided the snapshot of animal health and management that would serve as a baseline from which to measure industry changes in animal health and management. Before designing a study, NAHMS conducts a needs assessment of critical information gaps involving the industry and related groups. NAHMS performs evaluations of biologic samples in cooperation with the USDA: National Veterinary Services Laboratories and recruited university laboratories.

National Animal Health Monitoring
System (NAHMS)
2150 Center Ave., Bldg. B, MS 2E7
Fort Collins, CO 80526
E-mail: NAHMSweb@aphis.usda.gov
Tel: (970) 494-7000

National Animal Health Program (NAHP)
National Animal Health Program (NAHP) controls animal diseases, including those that would have a significant economic impact, and protects Canadians from diseases that can be transmitted by

animals. The NAHP is administered by the Canadian Food Inspection Agency under the authority of the Health of Animals Act.

National Dairy Code (NDC)
National Dairy Code is a Canadian federal/provincial/industry document, which standardizes dairy product standards and requirements.

National Dairy Development Board (NDDB)
Created in 1965, NDDB was founded to replace exploitation with empowerment, tradition with modernity, stagnation with growth, transforming dairying into an instrument for the development of India's rural people. NDDB began its operations with the mission of making dairying a vehicle to a better future for millions of grassroots milk producers. Since its inception, the Dairy Board has planned and spearheaded India's dairy programmes by placing dairy development in the hands of milk producers commonly known as Gwalas and the professionals they employ to manage their cooperatives. NDDB also promotes other commodity-based cooperatives, allied industries and veterinary biological on an intensive and nation-wide basis.

National Dairy Development Board
P.B. No. 40 Anand - 388 001
Gujarat INDIA
E-mail: anand@nddb.coop
Tel: 91-2692-260148, 260149, 260159,

National Food Safety Education Month (NFSEM)
The National Restaurant Association Educational Foundation (NRAEF)'s International Food Safety Council (IFSC) created this annual campaign of National Food Safety Education Month (NFSEM) in 1994 to heighten the awareness about the importance of food safety education. Each year a new theme and training activities are created for the industry to reinforce proper food safety practices and procedures.

National Restaurant Association
National Restaurant Association is the leading business association for the United States restaurant industry. Since its foundation in 1919, the Association has represented, educated and promoted a rapidly growing industry that is today comprised of 870,000 restaurants.

National Restaurant Association Educational Foundation (NRAEF)
National Restaurant Association Educational Foundation (NRAEF) is a United States not-for-profit organization dedicated to fulfilling the educational mission of the National Restaurant Association.

Focusing on three key strategies of risk management, recruitment, and retention, the NRAEF is the premier provider of educational resources, materials, and programs, which address attracting, developing and retaining the industry's workforce.

National Restaurant Association
Educational Foundation,
175 West Jackson Boulevard
Suite 1500, Chicago, IL 60604-2814
Tel: 1-312-715-1010

National Shellfish Sanitation Program (NSSP)

Means the voluntary system by which regulatory authorities for shellfish harvesting waters and shellfish processing and transportation and the shellfish industry implement specified controls to ensure that raw and frozen shellfish are safe for human consumption.

Netherlands Controlling Authority for Milk and Milk Products (COKZ)

The Netherlands Controlling Authority for Milk and Milk Products (Centraal Orgaan voor Kwaliteitsaangelegenheden in de Zuivel, COKZ) is a Netherlands's regulatory authority on milk and milk products dealing with Product Control, Inspection, Certification, Laboratory Research, Export Guarantee Certificate, Advice on Legislation and Regulations. COKZ has been testing milk and milk products for the presence of undesirable substances, and keep close scrutiny on other quality aspects of milk and milk products.
COKZ   Tel. +31 (0) 33 496 56 96
Netherlands Controlling Authority for Milk and Milk Products
Postbus 250
3830 AG Leusden
Kastanjelaan 7
Princenhof Business Park
3833 AN Leusden
The Netherlands
E-Mail: pr@cokz.nl
Web: http://www.cokz.nl

New Zealand Milk (NZM)

Created in 2001 as a separate company under the ownership of Fonterra Cooperative Group, New Zealand Milk has been providing nutritious dairy products for more than 50 years as part of the New Zealand Dairy Board. The company is responsible for 95 percent of milk produced in New Zealand.

Non-fat dry milk (NFDM)

Non-fat dry milk (NFDM) is dry milk powder, produced by

extracting fat and water from pasteurized, fresh cow's milk.

Non-conformity (N/C)
It means a failure to meet specified requirements of the HACCP system.

NSSP
Means National Shellfish Sanitation Program.

O

Objective evidence
It means Factual and verifiable information describing an audit observation. This may include photocopies of documents, notes made as a result of observations and interviews, etc.

Occupational Health and Safety Agency (OHSA)
It was created in 1971; its mission is to ensure safe and healthful workplaces in the United States of America. OSHA plays a vital role in preventing on-the-job injuries and illnesses through outreach, education, and compliance assistance OSHA offers an extensive educational site.

Occupational Safety & Health Administration Tel: 1-800-321-OSHA (6742)
200 Constitution Avenue, NW   TTY 1-877-889-5627
Washington, DC 20210
Web: www.osha.gov

Operational Step
It means an activity in a food establishment, such as receiving, storage, preparation, cooking, etc.

Operator
Means shall mean an individual or a business enterprise practicing food handling, food processing or allied activities.

P

Parasite
It means an organism that grows, feeds, and is sheltered on or in a different organism and contributes to its host.

Pasteurization
It is a process of heating a beverage or other food, such as milk or beer, to a specific temperature for a specific period of time in order to kill all disease causing Microrganisms without allowing recontamination of that milk or milk product or other food product during the heat treatment process. In the dairy industry, milk is heated to a temperature of 63° C for not less than 30 min. or 72° C for not less than 16 sec., or equivalent destruction of pathogens

and the enzyme phosphatase. Milk is deemed pasteurized if it tests negative for alkaline phosphatase.

Pasteurized Milk Ordinance (PMO)
Pasteurized Milk Ordinance (PMO) is An ordinance in the United States of America defining "milk" and certain "milk products", "milk producer", "pasteurization", etc.; prohibiting the sale of adulterated and misbranded milk and milk products; requiring permits for the sale of milk and milk products; regulating the inspection of dairy farms and milk plants, the examination, labelling, pasteurization, aseptic processing and packaging and distribution and sale of milk and milk products; providing for the construction of future dairy farms and milk plants; and the enforcement of this *Ordinance* and the fixing of penalties. Now titled the Grade "A" Pasteurized Milk Ordinance (PMO), 2001 Revision, represents the 24th revision since 1924 and incorporates new knowledge into public health practice. This ordinance establishes nationwide quality standards for milk.

Pathogen
It Means microorganisms (bacteria, parasites, viruses, or fungi) that is infectious and causes disease.

Perishable Agricultural Commodities Act (PACA)
The Perishable Agricultural Commodities Act (PACA) is the act in the United States of America, which fosters trading practices in the marketing of fresh fruits, frozen fruits and vegetables in interstate and foreign commerce. It prohibits unfair and fraudulent practices and provides a means of enforcing contracts. Under the PACA, anyone buying or selling commercial quantities of fruit and vegetables must be licensed by the U.S. Department of Agriculture. PACA was enacted in 1930 to promote fair trading practices in the fruit and vegetable industry.

Personal hygiene
It means individual cleanliness and habits.

Plant HACCP Coordinator
It means Plant employee responsible to liaise between senior plant management and the HACCP team. It is his / her role to lead the development, implementation and maintenance of HACCP plans.

Plant Specific HACCP Plan
It means a customized HACCP plan designed in accordance with the 12 logical sequence steps outlined in Volume II utilizing appropriate generic models as example, if applicable.

Potentially Hazardous Food
Means a food that is natural or synthetic and that requires

temperature control because it is capable of supporting:

a. The rapid and progressive growth of infectious or toxigenic microorganisms,

b. The growth and toxin production of _Clostridium botulinum_, or

c. In raw shell eggs, the growth of _Salmonella_ enteritidis.

Potentially hazardous food includes foods of animal origin that are raw or heat-treated; foods of plant origin that are heat-treated or consists of raw seed sprouts; cut melons; and garlic and oil mixtures that are not acidified or otherwise modified at a processing plant in a way that results in mixtures that do not support growth of pathogenic microorganisms as described above.

Preventive Measure
Physical, chemical, or other factors that can be used to control an identified health hazard

Procedural step
It means an individual activity in applying this Guide to a food establishment's operations.

Process approach
Means a method of categorizing food operations into one of three modes:

a. Process number one: Food preparation with no cook step wherein ready-to-eat food is stored, prepared, and served;

b. Process number two: Food preparation for same day service wherein food is stored, prepared, cooked, and served; or

c. Process number three: Complex food preparation wherein food is stored, prepared, cooked, cooled, reheated, hot held, and served.

Process
Means one or more actions or operations to harvest, produce, store, handle, distribute, or sell a product or group of similar products.

Prerequisite Programs
It means Universal steps or procedures that control the operational conditions within a food establishment allowing for environmental conditions that are favourable to the production of safe food. The six (6) programs cover premises, transportation and storage, equipment, personnel, sanitation and pest control, and health and safety recall procedures

Q

QCP (Quality Control Point)

QCP (Quality Control Point) is a living document during the manufacturing of food where quality assurance system is in effect and guarantees a quality product outcome as identified in documented procedure. Properly followed and completed by all the relevant parties QCP would mean to give assurance that everything is under control and the quality activities are being performed in accordance with the agreed requirements.

Qualitative Risk Assessment (QRA)

A Qualitative Risk Assessment (QRA) presents a logical and structured argument for defining particular risk levels. Typically, a qualitative risk assessment assigns frequency and consequence into broad bands and compares this to established risk acceptance criteria.

R

Random Checks

Random checks are the Observations or measurements that are performed to supplement the scheduled evaluations required by the HACCP plan.

Raw Farm Milk (RFM)

Raw Farm Milk (RFM) may be referred to a quality of milk, which is freshly drawn from milk animals from a dairy farm herd, and it has been not subjected to any heat treatment, which will alter its raw status. Raw Farm Milk could be chilled to store for a limited period until despatched for further processing.

Ready-to-Eat Food

It means a food that is in a form that is edible without washing, cooking, or additional preparation by the food establishment or consumer that is reasonably expected to be consumed in that form. Ready-to-eat food includes potentially hazardous food that has been cooked; raw, washed, cut fruits and vegetables; whole, raw, fruits and vegetables that are presented for consumption without the need for further washing, such as at a buffet; and other food presented for consumption for which further washing or cooking is not required and from which rinds, peels, husks, or shells have been removed.

Recognition:

It means Recognition means approval, by APEDA through a recognition mechanism, to consultancy and certification agencies for HACCP applications at all levels of the food chain for exports.

Regulatory requirements
It means all appropriate acts, regulations, manual of procedures and directives.

Regulatory Audit
A systematic assessment by CFIA of the establishment's conformance to and effectiveness of its written HACCP system (Note: During the audit of the HACCP system, CFIA will maintain its regulatory role and may take appropriate compliance action if required)

Regulatory authority
It means a federal, state, local, or tribal enforcement body or authorized representative having jurisdiction over the food establishment.

Regulatory system audit
The audit performed to assess the plant's ongoing conformance to and effectiveness of its recognized HACCP system.

Regulatory recognition audit
Means the audit performed as part of the review process leading to recognition of an establishment operating within a HACCP based environment.

Record
It means a documentation of monitoring observation and verification activities.

Regulatory requirements
It means all appropriate acts, regulations, manual of procedures and directives.

Retrovirus
It means a family of RNA viruses that have the unique characteristic of producing an enzyme that makes a DNA copy of its genetic information from an RNA template (the opposite of what normally takes place). The most widely recognized of these viruses is HIV, the causative agent in AIDS. Another virus from this family (HTLV-1) has been associated with T cell leukemia. Initial reports of an association of an HTLV-II-like retrovirus with CFS could not be confirmed in subsequent studies.

Risk
It means an estimate of the likely occurrence of a hazard.

Rubella
Also known as German measles, an acute disease marked by skin rash and swollen lymph nodes, but generally without fever. An RNA virus of the toga virus family is the cause of it.

Ruminant Animals

The ruminant animals , from a physiological point-of-view, are any artiodactyl mammal that digest its food in two steps, first by eating the raw material and regurgitating a semi-digested form known as cud from within their first stomach, known as the rumen. The process of again chewing the cud to break down the plant matter and stimulate digestion is called ruminating. Ruminating Mammals include cattle, goats, sheep, giraffes, American Bison, European bison, yaks, water buffalo, deer, camels, alpacas, llamas, wildebeest, antelope, and pronghorn.

Ruminantia

The biological suborder Ruminantia includes many of the well-known large grazing or browsing mammals: among them cattle, goats, sheep, deer, and antelope.

S

Sanitation Standard Operating Procedures (SSOP)

Developed by the Food Safety and Inspection Service (FSIS), USDA, as a Reference Guide to provide written directions in assuring good quality control and sanitation programs.

Sensitive Ingredient

This is an ingredient known to have been associated with a hazard and for which there is a reason for concern.

Severity

The seriousness of a hazard

Serious Deficiency

Means a severe deviation from plan requirements such that maintenance of safety, wholesomeness, and economic integrity is prevented; and, if the situation is allowed to continue, may result in unsafe, unwholesome, or misbranded product.

Severe Acute Respiratory Syndrome (SARS)

Severe acute respiratory syndrome (SARS) is an emerging, sometimes fatal, respiratory illness. The first identified cases occurred in China in late 2002, and the disease has now spread throughout the world. Although SARS is believed to be caused by a virus, the specific agent has not been identified, and there is not yet any laboratory or other test that can definitively identify cases.

Shellfish

Means bi-valve Molluscan shellfish.

SRIA

Systematic Risk Identification Analysis

SSOP
Sanitation Standard Operating Procedures

Stabilizers
These are food additives added to food to preserve flavour or improve its taste and appearance.

Standard Operating Procedure (SOP)
It means a written method of controlling a practice in accordance with predetermined specifications to obtain a desired outcome.

Substantial risk products
Means Seafood that may pose a significant danger to the health of the public when prepared for consumption by conventional or traditional means. For example, ready-to-eat; heat and/or brown and serve products; products which may contain a microbial pathogen, booting, or physical or chemical contaminant which may pose an unacceptable health risk at the time of consumption.

Systems Audit
Means On-site NMFS evaluation or any regulatory evaluation of the firm's effectiveness in following the quality/safety plan after validation.

T

Target Levels
Criteria that is more stringent than an operator uses critical limits and that

Temperature Measuring Device (TMD)
It means a thermometer, thermocouple, thermistor, or other device for measuring the temperature of food, air, or water.

Toxin
It means a poisonous substance that may be found in food.

TQM
Total Quality Management

U

UHT
Ultra Heat Treatment

Unit
It means Corresponds to one prerequisite program audit task to be performed during a partial audit. One unit could include one or two sub-elements according to the time required to audit them.

USDA
United States Department of Agriculture

US-FDA
United States Food and Drug Administration

USNRC
United States National Research Council

V

Validation
It means obtaining initial confirmation that the elements of the HACCP system are complete and effective in controlling biological, chemical, and physical hazards. This may include ingredient product sampling, end product sampling.

Verification
It means the use of methods, procedures, or tests by supervisors, designated personnel, or regulators to determine if the food safety system based on the HACCP principles is working to control identified hazards or if modifications need to be made.

Verification Audit
Unannounced on-site regulatory review of the effectiveness of regulatory field inspection personnel in complying with established quality/safety procedures.

Virus
It means a protein-wrapped genetic material, which is the smallest and simplest life-form known, such as hepatitis A Virus.

Vitamin
A group of organic micronutrients often referred as vital amines, present in minute quantities in natural foodstuffs that are essential to normal metabolism.

W

Water
Water is a common chemical substance that is essential for the survival of all known forms of life. In typical usage, water refers only to its liquid form or state, but the substance also has a solid state, ice, and a gaseous state, water vapour.

Water Activity
Water activity or a_w is a measurement of the energy status of the water in a system. It is defined as the vapour pressure of water divided by that of pure water at the same temperature; therefore, pure distilled water has a water activity of exactly one.

West Nile Virus (WNV)
West Nile virus is a cause of potentially serious illness. Experts believe WNV is established as a seasonal epidemic in North

America that flares up in the summer and continues into the fall.

World Health Organization (WHO)
World Health Organization is the directing and coordinating authority for health within the United Nations system? It is responsible for providing leadership on global health matters, shaping the health research agenda, setting norms and standards, articulating evidence-based policy options, providing technical support to countries and monitoring and assessing health trends.

World Trade Organization (WTO)
The World Trade Organization is the only global international organization dealing with the rules of trade between nations.

X

Y

Z

Zoonosis
A Zoonosis is any infectious disease that can be transmitted (by a vector) from other animals, both wild and domestic, to humans or from humans to animals. The word is derived from the Greek words *zoon* (animal) and *nosos* (disease). Many serious diseases fall under this category.

Lightning Source UK Ltd.
Milton Keynes UK
UKOW03n1128180514

231815UK00002B/28/P